Contents

Foreword

An invitation to write a second edition is always welcomed by authors – even if it does need nearly as much work as the first – because it suggests that the book has met the needs of those who bought it. Writing a foreword needs much less work, but the task has prompted me to look back over the years and reflect how much paediatrics has changed in the 35 years since I first invested in a (second-hand) textbook of paediatrics. For instance, thanks to preventive medicine, in this book measles now merits just two paragraphs, the devastating complications of intrauterine rubella infection get one line and rhesus disease (which kept my generation out of bed on many a night) is now stated to 'have almost disappeared'. These are wonderful achievements and it is a privilege to have lived through an era of such dramatic progress. Yet the need for enthusiastic dedicated paediatricians is greater than ever. As old diseases disappear, new challenges come on the scene. The neonatologists have made great strides, through the application of basic sciences and randomised trials – who would ever have thought that babies of less than 26 weeks' gestation could survive at all, let alone survive intact to lead useful lives? Cardiac surgery, oncology, genetics – every specialty has seen astonishing progress. There have been advances in less glamorous areas as well, like pain control and the support of families with disabled children.

And yet… there is also a little sadness in reading through the chapter headings in this book. Complex long-term illness and disability are actually more prevalent as we become more expert at sustaining life. With little malnutrition and fewer life-threatening infectious illnesses to pre-occupy us, our discipline has turned its attention to other problems – psychosomatic disease resulting from stress, family break-up or bullying, abuse and neglect in an almost infinite variety of forms, and mental health problems. Taken together, in the developed world these will in the future probably account for more wasted and blighted lives than all childhood physical illness put together. These socially induced 'diseases' have always been with us, both here in the UK and around the world, but it is only as children's physical health improves, and the economy supports more health professionals, that they are beginning to receive the attention they deserve.

If this is your first paediatric textbook, you will find that it offers an admirable balance between these many different perspectives of the problems and the healthcare needs of children and young people. It shows how each illness has physical, psychological and social dimensions – good paediatrics requires that all three be addressed and none be neglected. To provide the best possible care for children there must be no artificial boundaries between care in hospital and care at home or at school and no territorial disputes between disciplines. If you are already experienced in paediatrics, this book will give an excellent refresher course on topics in which you may have become just a little out of date (it does happen occasionally), and will be a valuable aide to planning a balanced curriculum for students.

Sir David Hall
Professor of Community Paediatrics
University of Sheffield
September 2005

Foreword

It is a pleasure to join Professor David Hall in writing a foreword to the second edition of this book. As David highlights, the scope and focus for paediatrics has changed dramatically within a relatively short period of time. New problems and issues within paediatrics have emerged, not least in the field of public health within which there is (still) an unacceptable health inequalities gap between the health of poorer children and young people and their better off peers. There is a pressing need to develop health professionals with the knowledge and expertise to tackle the many issues within children's public health, at both a strategic and policy level as well as in practice and at a practical level. This is a complex enterprise but one of the key challenges facing paediatrics for the future.

Changes have also taken place in the boundaries between the different professions within the field of paediatrics, a trend that is set to continue for the future. The question of which professional group does what has become less important than questions of which individual has the right competencies and who is best placed to lead or deliver care for particular children and their families. Teamwork has always featured in the field of paediatrics and child health which has been a leader in the development of not only inter-professional teamwork but also the inclusion of the patient and their carers within the healthcare team as partners and co-decision makers. Teamwork will become increasingly pivotal to achieving successful future outcomes in paediatrics, since we are likely to see changes and different configurations within the health service in the future with a plethora of healthcare providers. Yet it is well documented that what children and families want and need is seamless care that is tailored to their needs rather than those of professional groups or healthcare institutions.

This book provides a useful basis from which to view new perspectives in paediatrics (such as public health), coupled with its more traditional underpinnings including holistic care for the child and family, and teamwork to provide that care. It will be a valuable learning tool and reference point for the many professionals engaged in paediatric work, including nurses, midwives, health visitors, doctors, physiotherapists and social workers.

Jane Naish
Policy Adviser
Royal College of Nursing
September 2005

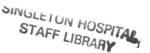
Preface to the second edition

The second edition has further developed the problem-based style which has proved popular with readers and which reflects actual clinical practice. We have made three main changes in the new edition. First, we have emphasised clinical skills, and this is reflected in the new opening chapter. Secondly, we have changed the format of the case studies so that each one is self-contained and can easily be read on its own, while acting as an *aide-mémoire* to the student on common clinical presentations. Thirdly, we have added self-assessment questions at the end of each section for students to use as a means of revision.

All of the chapters have been updated and the coverage of common and important clinical problems has been extended. However, we have retained the original concept of the core curriculum with its focus on common and important conditions, rather than a catalogue of conditions more appropriate to postgraduate reference texts.

Despite reducing the size of the book we have retained the integration of child health and child disease, and our new publishers have maintained the high quality of illustrations and summary features throughout the text.

Tony Waterston
Peter J Helms
Martin Ward Platt
September 2005

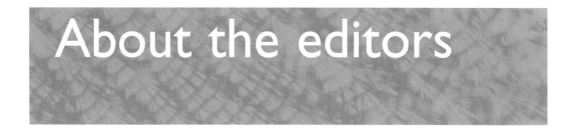
About the editors

Tony Waterston works as a general paediatrician specialising in community child health in inner city Newcastle. He has a special interest in poverty and child health, children's rights and international child health.

Peter J Helms is Professor of Child Health at the University of Aberdeen and Consultant Paediatrician in the Royal Aberdeen Children's Hospital. He has a special interest in respiratory health and disease.

Martin Ward Platt has been a consultant paediatrician in Newcastle upon Tyne since 1990, specialising in neonatal medicine but delivering clinical care to children of all ages; he is also Honorary Senior Lecturer in Child Health at Newcastle University. He has been involved in organising and delivering teaching of paediatrics and child health at all stages of the undergraduate medical curriculum.

List of contributors

Ian Auchterlonie
Consultant Paediatrician
Royal Aberdeen Children's Hospital

Michael Bisset
Consultant Paediatrician
Royal Aberdeen Children's Hospital

Philip Booth
Consultant Neonatologist
Aberdeen Maternity Hospital

William Church
Consultant Ophthalmologist
Aberdeen Royal Infirmary

Gaynor Cole
Consultant Paediatric Neurologist
Robert Jones & Agnes Hunt Hospital
Oswestry

John Dean
Consultant Clinical Geneticist
Royal Aberdeen Children's Hospital

James Ferguson
Consultant in Accident and Emergency
Aberdeen Royal Infirmary

Leonora Harding
Head of Clinical Psychology Services
Stratheden Hospital
Cupar

David Kindley
Consultant Paediatrician
Director, Raeden Centre
Aberdeen

Derek King
Consultant Haematologist/Oncologist
Aberdeen Royal Infirmary

Camille Lazaro
Senior Lecturer in Forensic Paediatrics
University of Newcastle upon Tyne

David Meikle
Consultant ENT Surgeon
Freeman Hospital
Newcastle upon Tyne

Jean Robson
Retired Associate Specialist in
Orthopaedics
Freeman Hospital
Newcastle upon Tyne

Chris Scott
Consultant Ophthalmologist
Aberdeen Royal Infirmary

Peter Smail
Retired Consultant Paediatrician
Royal Aberdeen Children's Hospital

Marion White
Consultant Dermatologist
Aberdeen Royal Infirmary

George Youngson
Professor of Paediatric Surgery
University of Aberdeen
Royal Aberdeen Children's Hospital

1 Clinical skills

- The paediatric consultation: history and examination
- The normal child: development and developmental assessment
- Nutrition: weaning and after
- Early learning
- Children and school
- Children and hospitals
- Ethics and consent

The paediatric consultation: history and examination

Different clinical skills are needed for each of the main epochs of a child's life – neonates, infants, pre-school children, school-age children and adolescents. Common to all of these epochs are the skills of relating to parents.

The word *consultation* is used here to mean any formal meeting between clinician and parent (and usually the child) for the purpose of exchanging clinical information.

For paediatricians, the settings for a consultation may vary widely – an antenatal clinic or delivery room (before a child is born), a paediatric ward, an Accident and Emergency department, a room in a hospital outpatient department, a community clinic or the family's home.

For those without much experience of working with children and families, gaining maximum value from a consultation can be daunting. Some of the main generic issues are set out as 'frequently asked questions' below, followed by those issues that are specific to children of different ages.

Frequently asked questions

Who is a child?

The definition of a child in the United Nations (UN) Convention on the Rights of the Child is anyone from birth to 18 years of age. This definition is used in the UK and is the range used in the Children Act (1989, England and Wales) and its equivalent in Scotland. Adolescence is a developmental phase usually considered to occur from 12 years (or puberty) to 18 years of age, although in some young people (especially boys) it is functionally longer. Whether a young person over 16 years of age is referred with a new medical problem to an adult physician or a paediatrician will largely depend on whether he or she is still at school.

How should I set up the consultation?

Be welcoming and friendly – smiling is important to children because it can defuse fear. You will need to introduce yourself to both parents and to the child. Position the parents and/or child at an angle to the doctor, not with a desk in the way.

Children often want to go off and explore the toys in the room, and there should be plenty available in an outpatient or community clinic. Notice and comment if the child has a toy of their own with them. It is helpful to explain how you intend to structure the discussion. Privacy and confidentiality are important – you may need to go to a room where the door can be closed. If discussions have to take place at a bedside, remember that even when you speak quietly, people on either side can hear everything that is said, and this may not be acceptable for either the child or the parents.

How do I form a relationship?

Active, empathic listening is the key skill. First, let the parent and the child tell their story. Empathy and encouragement can be expressed verbally ('yes', 'right', 'OK', 'Uh-huh'), and non-verbally (by nod or gesture). Always include the child, if only tangentially (a young child may have gone off to play in a corner of the room). Maintaining eye contact is important, otherwise you cannot read the parent's or child's non-verbal signals, so don't write anything down initially. Taking time to get the names (and the spellings) right for all individuals present is a good ice-breaker. Parents and children will only open up if you are warm and friendly in manner, and condescension is to be avoided at all costs. Firing questions at parents and writing down the answers looks superficially efficient, but this approach may well miss key details, and makes it very difficult to build the relationship of clinical trust that is a hallmark of a good consultation. Apart from anything else, it is only when you have listened effectively that you know what supplementary information you need to ask for more specifically in order to flesh out the history.

When two parents are present it is important to include both in the discussion, as the father may well feel left out. Take the chance to address some questions to him so that he feels engaged, too.

How do I obtain the information that I need?

It is best to use open-ended questions, to avoid leading questions, and to use non-technical expressions and language. It is often very helpful to do a reality check: 'If I have heard you right,

what you are telling me is …'. When you need to write things down, it is best to put the consultation on hold while you do that: 'Can we pause for a second while I make a note of what you have just told me?'.

How do I handle personal or delicate issues?

Explain why such information is necessary – this prepares the parent or child for the questions. Unless such a question is necessary, you should not ask it. Don't be afraid to allow the consultation to pause while a reply is being considered – you should not feel uncomfortable with silences.

When should I write it all down?

Writing may take place at intervals during the consultation, after taking the history or doing an examination, or wholly at the end. As writing precludes eye contact and detection of non-verbal leads, it should be minimised while the parent or child is speaking, so create pauses for noting material, and use writing time for further clarification or to summarise.

What then?

Summarise the consultation up to that moment. Do you and the parent perceive the same problems, ranked in the same way? Is there a single, firm diagnosis, a range of possibilities, or simply an undiagnosed problem? Explain to the parent in appropriate language, without condescension, the nature of the diagnoses or problems, and do the same for the child. Recommend or negotiate a suitable plan for their management. If there are to be any investigations, these need to be explained to the child as well. Be sure to check if the parent has any questions that they would like answered or information that they want clarified.

How do I bring it to an end?

Make sure that there is a clearly defined end to the consultation, focusing on any follow-up contact (when, how), or saying what will happen next (e.g. tests), and make a courteous parting statement that includes the child.

What will parents take away?

It is known that parents will only recall a small amount of the information that has been given out at a consultation, especially if there is a high emotional content (e.g. when disclosing a diagnosis of long-term illness or disability). Yet the parents will wish to transmit what you have told them to other members of the family, or to the partner if only one parent is present. There are several ways of handling this. You could write down the salient messages (time consuming), tape record the interview and give the parent the tape (a hassle), or provide an information sheet (useful generic material for complex conditions). However, it is best to send the parents a copy of the letter to the GP, or to write the letter to the parents and copy it to the GP (very powerful, transparent, cheap and easy – one of these should be routine).

Important items of the history, common to all ages

1 To understand family relationships and any family history of illness, it is a good idea to draw a pedigree or genogram (*see* Figure 1.1 for an example). Any family history of illness can be recorded on this. It is sometimes useful to record not only the structure of the extended family, but also who is in the same household as the child, and who is present at the consultation. Important relationships can also be highlighted. In many split families today a child will spend part of the week with each parent, and this situation needs to be known about.

2 The past medical history is conceptually similar to that of an adult (serious illnesses, hospital admissions, visits to Accident and Emergency departments, and surgical operations), but for

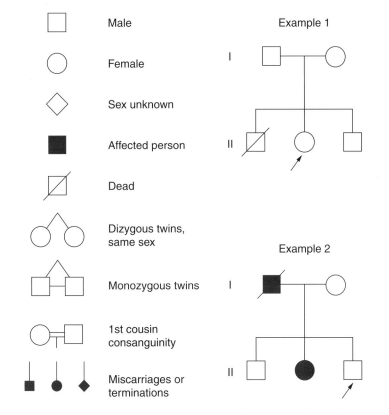

Figure 1.1 Drawing a pedigree. Also see page 154 for additional symbols. The arrow points to the 'proband', i.e. the patient in question.

children an additional enquiry about the common infectious diseases of childhood (e.g. chickenpox) can be helpful.

3 Information about parental employment, state benefits and housing – the 'social history' – should be sought. This should also include parent relationships and supports, caring issues and the involvement of other services with the family.

4 Information on drinking and smoking should be obtained. This is not just parental – children may be exposed to smoking by other relatives, carers or family friends. Many adolescents will be smokers and drinkers themselves, but are unlikely to divulge this in front of their parents.

5 Information about immunisation is needed – not just the primary course but also MMR, pre-school booster and any booster doses of tetanus toxoid given after injury. In certain children, protection against tuberculosis, hepatitis B, pneumococcus, influenza and respiratory syncytial virus may also be a relevant enquiry.

6 Enquire about current prescribed medication, if any, and any over-the-counter or herbal treatments.

7 Ask about allergies, either to medication or to environmental allergens (e.g. pets, pollens, foods).

8 Exposure to pets and recent foreign travel is relevant to all ages – even to some babies under a month old (neonates).

9 The 'systematic enquiry' that is part of the 'adult' history is usually irrelevant in young children, and is rarely relevant in the adolescent. However, you should always ask about eating, toileting and sleeping, as these are common sources of difficulty at all ages.

Items specific to each epoch of childhood are summarised below.

Neonates

The history

The obstetric history of the mother is of immediate relevance and importance. It includes her gravidity (how many pregnancies), parity (how many births, and their gestations at delivery), obstetric diseases (e.g. pregnancy-induced hypertension), and pre-existing medical conditions of relevance to pregnancy (e.g. insulin-dependent diabetes). Related details include the mother's rhesus status, whether she has red-cell antibodies, whether she is rubella immune, and the results of screening for bloodborne viruses (e.g. hepatitis B and C, human immunodeficiency virus).

You need to make a note of maternal medication, including both that taken regularly during the latter part of pregnancy (e.g. anticonvulsants, antihypertensives) and that taken at the beginning of pregnancy, perhaps before the mother realised she was pregnant, as well as medication administered during labour (e.g. opiates), since all of these can affect the neonate directly or indirectly.

There should be a note of the details of the delivery, including the duration of rupture of the membranes, the length of the second stage of labour, and the presentation and mode of delivery, that are the main items of relevance to the newborn.

The name of the baby is also important. Many mothers and fathers have different surnames, and it is important to know in which surname the baby will be registered. Never assume that the baby's name will be the same as that of the mother.

Examining neonates

All newborn babies receive a routine examination, including measurement of their head circumference. The nature of this, and its rationale, are dealt with in Chapter 17.

Examination when a neonate presents with an acute problem is different. The first priority is to see whether the baby is obviously ill (e.g. shocked, in respiratory distress, or centrally blue). In this situation the priority is the resuscitation ABC (airway–breathing–circulation) procedure before doing anything else (and before taking a history).

If the baby is not in such a state, the examination can be more methodical.

1 Observe – look for normal or abnormal facies and morphology, colour (pallor, plethora, jaundice, cyanosis), posture, spontaneous movements, conscious state, breathing effort, precordial impulse, abdominal distension, umbilical flare, integrity of the skin – and listen for moaning or grunting, stridor, and the quality of the cry.

2 Feel – for muscle tone, any restriction of passive movement, the state of the anterior fontanelle and cranial sutures, a precordial impulse, central and peripheral pulses, inguinal hernias, and the abdomen (the neonatal liver should normally be palpable 1 or 2 cm

below the right, and sometimes the left costal margin). Note the response to palpation (for level of consciousness).

3 Listen (with a stethoscope) – to the heart, the chest, and the abdomen if the latter is distended. If there is a cardiac murmur, listen over the left scapula for the radiation of the murmur of a patent arterial duct.

Although this is a completely different approach to the systematic examination of the older child or adult, it should still be recorded in a systematic fashion (i.e. respiratory, cardiovascular, gastrointestinal, musculoskeletal, neurological, etc.).

Infants

The history

As with the neonate, you need information about pregnancy and delivery, but usually in less detail.

Most mothers will know the birth weight – but in pounds and ounces! Fortunately it is usually recorded in kilograms in the personal child health record. Growth can either be plotted on a centile growth chart (for examples, *see* Chapter 14, Figure 14.5 and Chapter 15, Figure 15.5), or the growth rate can be calculated (*see* Box 1.1).

The feeding history (*see* Box 1.2) includes whether or not a baby is being or was breastfed, and for how long. For babies who are currently being formula fed, the number of feeds in the day, the amount given at each feed, and the time it takes for a baby to complete a feed (around 20 minutes, and certainly less than 30 minutes, is normal) need to be asked about and noted down. This allows you to calculate how much food a baby is obtaining in ml/kg/day, and it also identifies babies who take a long time to feed, as these have a feeding problem.

The immunisation history needs to be more thorough than simply asking 'Has she had all her injections?'. Note roughly when each set was given, and whether a complete set was given.

The developmental history entails ascertaining the approximate ages at which particular skills were acquired, and the appropriate questions will depend on the age of the child. Asking about current capabilities in each of the four major domains of development (gross motor, fine motor, language and social; see below) is a good way into this.

Be sure to ask whether the parents have any concerns about development, as sometimes

---

Box 1.1 Calculating growth rate

- Subtract the birth weight from the current weight to give the weight difference.

- Take the age of the child in weeks, and subtract 1 because most babies do not regain their birth weight until around a week of age. This gives the number of 'growing weeks'.

- Divide the weight difference by the number of 'growing weeks'.

- A normal growth rate in the first 2 months is between 150 and 250 grams per 'growing week'.

Box 1.2 Infant feeding history questions

- What milk is being used? (Has the milk been changed frequently?)

- How much is in each feed?

- How often are the feeds given?

- Calculate how many ml/day and ml/kg/day of milk are being fed. You may find gross overfeeding or underfeeding.

- How is the feed made up? (Obtain an exact description.)

- How long does each feed take?

---

they are reluctant to mention seemingly minor anxieties, such as an in-turning eye. Also ask about their views on the child's hearing and vision.

Examining infants

This is similar in structure to the examination of the neonate, but with important differences in emphasis.

1 Begin by developing a relationship with the baby through play. This could start with handing over a toy and showing appreciation of what the infant does with it. This allows you to observe developmental milestones (Is the baby sitting with support? Sitting without support? Interacting normally? Cooing or babbling? Showing strabismus? Moving symmetrically or

with obvious asymmetry? Hypotonic or hypertonic?), and it accounts for most of the neurodevelopmental examination that you need to do. A baby who is too tired, irritable or fractious to play may also be giving you an important message.

2 Next do the things that are least likely to make the child cry. It might be a good moment to listen to the heart, which needs a window of quiet opportunity, and listen to the chest.

3 Look at the baby externally all over, including the genitalia and the back, in order to be sure that you do not miss external signs of physical abuse.

4 Feel the fontanelle, feel for lymph nodes in the neck, axillae and groins, feel the pulses (including those of the lower limbs – their absence suggests aortic coarctation), feel the abdomen and groins (for hernias), and test for neck stiffness in any acutely febrile child.

5 Formal neurodevelopmental examination, when appropriate, includes testing the deep tendon reflexes, looking for abnormal persistence of the neonatal Moro, grasp and stepping reflexes, and assessing head control and truncal posture. It also includes measuring the head circumference and plotting it on a centile chart.

6 Finish with those examinations that babies most dislike, namely the ears (tympanic membranes) and the throat (see Figures 1.2–1.4).

Again, the examination should be recorded system by system even though the information has been obtained in a different order. 'ENT' has become another system heading.

Pre-school children

The history

It is nice, and appreciated by the child, to start off by engaging with the child and forming a relationship. With increasing age of the child, you will gain more and more information from them in addition to the parent. The history should continue to include some birth details, but the emphasis is now on the child's own history. The child may go to a toddler group or playgroup, which is important information in relation to infections and socialisation. Immunisation history should include the MMR. Growth history is important, and so is diet. The child may now have some past medical history of their own.

Development, as for the infant, is important. However, the nature of the questions is different. In part you need to gain an idea of previous developmental achievements (age at walking, age at first words), and you also need to know the child's current skills. Ask about behaviour and toileting, as this is the age when issues of negativism, sleep difficulties and food refusal may begin.

Examining pre-school children

Examining oppositional 2-year-olds and uncooperative 3-year-olds is one of the most challenging aspects of child health and paediatrics. Success is to a large extent dependent on a willingness to compromise in terms of location and position, and on the effectiveness of the 'settling-in' period of the preceding history taking. Rather than separate the child from the mother, do the examination with the child on the mother's lap. Making a game of the examination using distractions and proxies (e.g. dolls and teddies), having warm hands and stethoscope, and doing the examination quickly are the keys to success. Focus the examination on what you really need to know. It is often helpful to explain what you are going to do before you do it. Record it systematically, and record those things that could not be done on that occasion but which may need to be done at some later time.

School-age children

The history

Information about school performance, peer group attitudes and sporting activities is essential for school-age children. This is as important for the child as the world of work is for the adult.

Problems at school (e.g. pressure, bullying) can give rise to somatic symptoms that may look very much like organic illness, and also to psychiatric symptoms that suggest depression. Mood and temperament are therefore important dimensions that may merit enquiry.

If a child is attending mainstream school without special provision, there is rarely any further developmental history that is likely to be relevant. If the child is receiving specialist help, or is not in mainstream school, a developmental history is important, as is an enquiry into the child's current skills and abilities. For a child with manifest disabilities, it is kinder and more positive to focus on what the child can do, rather than on what they cannot.

There may be issues that should not be discussed in front of the child. It can be both hurtful and unnecessary to discuss issues such as behaviour or appearance with a parent while the child is present. It is good practice, particularly in the older child, to say at the outset that both the parents and the child will have an opportunity to speak with you alone and in confidence.

Examining school-age children

Systematic examination, along the lines of the adult model, is usually possible in school-age children so long as they are developmentally appropriate for their chronological age. However, you need to bear the following points in mind.

- Height and weight are still important for the assessment of growth.

- Femoral pulses should still be felt.

- There is an argument for opportunistic blood pressure measurement.

- Examining the ears and throat becomes less relevant in the older child – unless that is where the symptoms are.

Adolescents

The history

There are often issues that should not be discussed in front of the child, and often with a teenager or adolescent there are issues best not talked about in front of the parents. For adolescents there should always be an opportunity to talk to you in private. You may need to know whether the child perceives the same problems as the parent. What are the child's attitudes to the problems? There may be specific questions (e.g. concerning sexual behaviour, substance abuse, attitudes to parents) that can only be addressed without the parents present. When meeting young people on their own, remember to inform them about confidentiality. This means telling them that you will not pass on anything they say to anyone else, unless they are at risk of harm.

School performance and attainments, and activities outside school, may all be relevant.

The examination is in principle similar to that for an adult, but bear in mind that adolescents can be excruciatingly embarrassed by clinical examinations, and you must be sensitive to this. It is also very important to have a chaperone present, whatever the sex of the child. However, under appropriate circumstances you may need specifically to:

- stage puberty (see page 225), especially in a child presenting with delayed or precocious puberty

- measure weight and height and plot these on a centile chart

- examine externally for evidence of physical abuse

- examine the genitalia for evidence of sexual abuse

- bear in mind that a girl may be pregnant.

Remember that the young person is developing autonomy and should be considered a patient in their own right. They will have information needs, will need to take responsibility for their own health, including treatment, and will be expected to give (or withhold) separate consent from their parents.

Case study 1

Emma is 2 years old. She has come to outpatients with minor bowel symptoms. In the waiting area she clings to her mother, who is becoming frustrated.

The most important thing is to spend time introducing yourself to the mother and child, keeping up a patter of small talk as they come into the room. At this age, paying too much immediate attention to the child can be counter-productive, as it is often perceived as a threat. Inviting the mother to let the child do what she wants, rather than confine her to a chair or to the mother's own knee, allows the child to explore the room. She will find the toys in her own time, during which you can observe her developmental progress by watching her play, listening to her talk, and observing her interact from time to time with her mother.

When the time comes to examine her, she may be best on her mother's lap, or she may be confident enough to lie on the examination couch with her mother close by. Either way, it is useful to warm the end of the stethoscope, to make the examination a game, to distract from the examination with toys, and to do peripheral things, such as feeling a radial pulse, before touching the chest or abdomen.

Specific clinical examination skills

The external auditory canal

There are two ways of holding an auroscope for this examination (*see* Figure 1.2(a),(b)). The advantage of the second, with the battery/handle upwards, is that the instrument is stabilised against the child's temporal bone so that it will move with small movements of the child's head. The most important aspect of examining the ears of a young child is that the carer should hold the child still, with the arms and head temporarily immobilised against the adult's body. The less the child moves, the quicker and less uncomfortable the examination will be. The pinna should be gently held upward and backwards to straighten out the ear canal, using your right hand for the child's left ear, and your left hand for their right ear.

The throat

There are two possible techniques for examining the throat. The conventional 'medical' way (*see* Figure 1.3) approaches the child from the front. If the child keeps her mouth tight shut, there is little you can do about this. The second or 'dental' way (*see* Figure 1.4) approaches the child in the opposite fashion and works best for smaller children. The child starts off facing the carer, standing or sitting on their lap. The child is then tilted backwards towards the examiner until she is horizontal, and is usually so surprised to see the examiner above her that she opens her mouth involuntarily, giving an excellent view. Her head

(a)

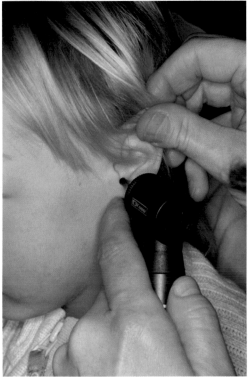

(b)

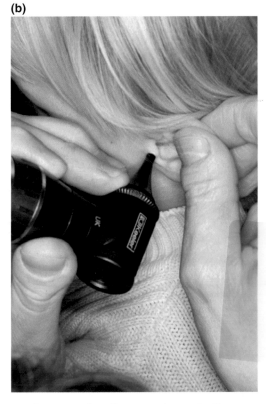

Figure 1.2 (a) and (b)   Two ways of holding an auroscope for external auditory canal examination.

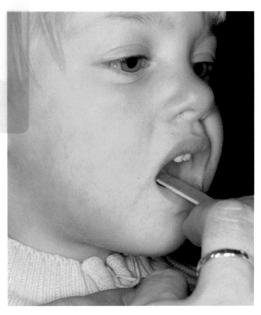

Figure 1.3 Throat examination: the 'medical' way.

can also be stabilised between the examiner's forearms, which is impossible with the conventional approach.

Blood pressure measurement

School-age children and adults tolerate very well the conventional cuff-and-stethoscope technique to determine systolic and diastolic pressures. Younger children can have their systolic pressure measured by the Doppler/cuff technique. In this procedure, the cuff is inflated and deflated in the usual way, but the onset of flow in the brachial artery is detected using a portable Doppler ultrasound device (*see* Figure 1.5). As with any examination, it can be made into a game. The 'whooshing' noise can be likened to the puffing of a steam engine, and your imagination and that of the child can do the rest!

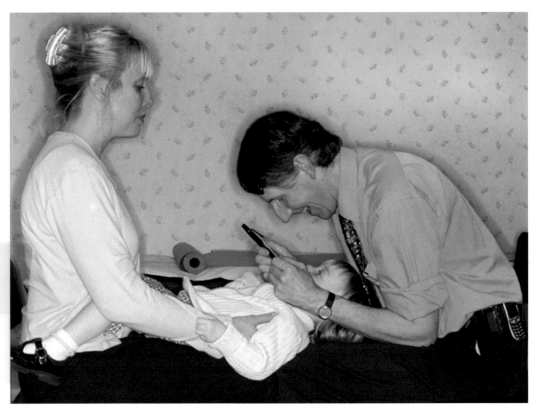

Figure 1.4   Throat examination: the 'dental' way.

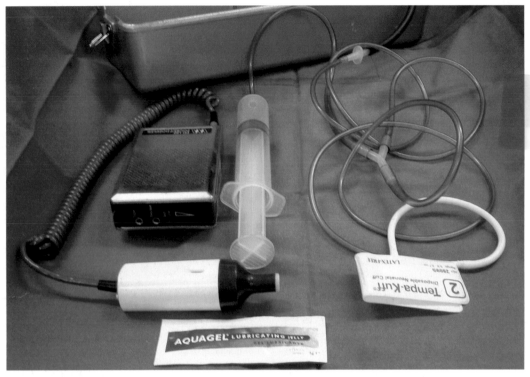

Figure 1.5   Blood pressure measurement: Doppler ultrasound device.

Meningism

Children often resist a simple test of neck stiffness when approached from the front and held behind their head. Asking a child to kiss their knees or to put their chin on their chest is often a more sensible technique: inability to do this is the positive sign. Reflex flexion of the knee and hip when the neck is flexed also suggests meningeal irritation (Babinski's sign).

Tendon stretch reflexes

In the neonate, the deep tendon jerks can often be elicited by percussing the tendon with the middle finger of the examiner's hand. Tendon hammers can be used with almost any child, but it is sometimes easier to tap the tendon through your own finger (*see* Figure 1.6). In part this defends the child from too smart a blow, but it also enables the examiner to seize the moment when the child relaxes the muscle group, and to feel the reflex response to the tap.

Calming the neonate and small infant

If a baby is awake, and certainly if he is fractious, it can be very helpful to let him suck a finger on your non-dominant hand. This enables you to check the palate for obvious clefting, and the infant tends to concentrate on the possibility that there may be food if he sucks hard enough. If the child does not instantly settle to sucking the finger, stroking his cheek with a finger of the other hand

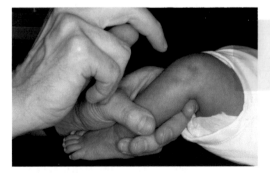

Figure 1.6   Tendon reflexes: tap tendon with own finger.

encourages the rooting reflex, and sucking is almost always established. It is essential for a child not to be crying if any meaningful examination of the chest, heart and abdomen is to be achieved. The dominant hand can then palpate the head, hold an ophthalmoscope to examine the retina, hold a stethoscope on the chest, and palpate the abdomen, groins and testicles. This technique works well until the child has teeth.

The normal child: development and developmental assessment

The child's view of the world is very different to yours and mine. In part, this is physically because of their smaller height. However, children also have profoundly different modes of thinking compared with the adult. It is almost as if children assume that they live in a parallel universe to that of adults, which interconnects, but which is as foreign to adults as the adult world is to the child. From the young child's point of view, the adult world can be bizarre, inexplicable and inconsistent. The child's universe gradually converges with that of the adult as he or she grows up.

The importance of being aware of a child's different world lies in the fact that children have different priorities to adults, and cannot be expected to relate to adult views and needs. In dealing with children we have to rediscover the viewpoint of children (so carefully grown out of in our later schooldays), if we are to be successful in understanding, diagnosing and treating children, preventing them from coming to harm, and encouraging them in habits and behaviours that are conducive to their future health.

There are a number of models of the ontogeny of children's thinking which will not be discussed further here. Of most help to the reader are likely to be those of Piaget and of Eriksson.

What is 'normal' and why do we need to know it?

First, normality is a reference point for abnormality. It is all too easy to assume that a child has an abnormal characteristic, particularly if this is how the parent perceives it, if you do not know what is truly normal and abnormal. Both parents and practitioners need to be able to answer the question 'Is this child normal?'.

Secondly, almost every biological characteristic – including everything measurable about children – varies. The extent of that variation can be ascertained fairly precisely, and a 'range' can be defined, usually corresponding to the 95% of observations centred on the average (the mean or the median). This is a statistical approach to being normal, but it implies neither that all children within the range are necessarily clinically 'normal', nor that all children outside it are necessarily 'abnormal'.

Thirdly, normality may be viewed both as a static phenomenon and as a dynamic process. At any given age a child may have particular characteristics, such as height, weight or developmental progress, which can be related to those of their peers at the same age. However, growth and development are both processes, and their progress, or velocity, may also be either normal or abnormal. Disorders of growth are discussed in Chapter 15 and disorders of development in Chapter 10.

An awareness of normality is also necessary to guide practitioners with regard to the level of expectation of a child's understanding and behaviour, since this has implications for communication, adherence to treatment, and the ability to give consent for procedures or treatment (*see* page 20).

Finally, children only maintain their normal growth and development if their emotional needs are recognised and met – their need for security and love within a family, their social need for stimulation, and the chance to respond to it both inside and outside the family. Security implies a reasonable ability to predict the behaviour of the rest of the world, and requires defined limits on the behaviour of parents and others.

Why are normal children of any concern to paediatricians?

There is a continual challenge in trying to keep children healthy. In part this is the domain of epidemiology (*see* Chapter 2) and prevention (*see* Chapter 22). However, it is also true that growth, development and behaviour influence manifestations of illness, and conversely that illness affects growth, development and behaviour, while a child's family and social environment have an impact on both physical and mental health.

Everyone who deals with children has to be aware of this interconnectedness. Furthermore, parents often become anxious about apparent deviations from normal which in fact are in the normal range (e.g. late walking due to 'shuffling syndrome', or late talking). If the parent asks you about an apparent deviation, you need to know whether this could be anticipated or whether it is a genuine deviation.

Assessing development

All children who come to the attention of a medical practitioner need to have their developmental status taken into account. Part of the initial assessment of any child is a view of the appropriateness or otherwise of their developmental stage relative to their chronological age. To make such a judgement, the clinician must remember how the child might be expected to perform at a given age. You can obtain the information both by asking (from the history) and by observing the child. The latter source is more reliable, but this information is not always easy to obtain, and careful history taking can tell you a great deal about child development.

Development takes place in different domains. Those commonly assessed for clinical purposes

in infancy are as follows:

- *gross motor* – this is about mobility, rolling, crawling and walking
- *fine motor* – this is about delicate movement of the hands, starting with the ability to manipulate small objects and culminating in skills such as tying knots, fastening buttons and writing
- *language* – this is the progression from cooing to babbling, first words, word pairs and sentences
- *social* – this is the reciprocal interaction between child and parent that starts immediately after birth, and proceeds through the development of attachment and interpersonal relationships.

'Milestones' are commonly used to describe developmental progress. However, they can be misleading because they are generally quoted as the average age at which a particular skill is expected to develop, so by definition 50% of all children will achieve the skill later than this. Of much more value in routine practice is knowledge of the normal range of ages for the skill to develop: this might be the time by which different percentages of children have acquired the skill (*see* Figure 1.7).

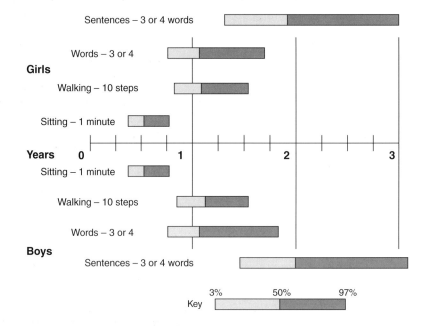

Figure 1.7   Normal ranges for skill acquisition.

Formal developmental assessment is only required if there is a specific reason to believe that a child may be at high risk of developmental delay or cerebral palsy. This may be suspected because of obvious failure to develop normally, or because of specific problems in early life, such as very preterm birth, neonatal convulsions or infant meningitis. Babies born prematurely should be assessed in their early months, with allowance made for their prematurity. However, between 1 and 2 years of chronological age the need to make this allowance fades away.

Quantitative developmental assessment is sometimes needed where detailed multidisciplinary evaluation of a child's needs is being undertaken. Two popular standardised scales for developmental assessment are the Griffiths scale and the Bayley scale. They both yield an overall developmental quotient (DQ) that summarises performance on subscales such as gross motor, fine motor and verbal. The DQ is the ratio of the child's achievement to that predicted for their age. The Griffiths score is standardised to a mean of 100 with a standard deviation of 10. In the early preschool years, these are inevitably weighted towards performance in motor skills and away from cognitive development. Cognitive skills ('intelligence', 'learning ability') can only be assessed with any accuracy after school entry.

Normal development is discontinuous. This means that there will not necessarily be smooth progress from one skill to the next. For example, a toddler who has just learned to walk will frequently do nothing else but explore their world for the next 2 weeks, and ignore skills that require fine motor control. New skills build on previous skills, and a child who is prevented by disease or circumstance from developing one skill will necessarily be retarded in developing those skills that come after it. Multiple or prolonged admissions to hospital also retard the acquisition of new skills.

For some skills there are developmental 'windows' when learning is programmed, so that if the 'window' is missed for any reason, learning the skill is very difficult. An example of this is the difficulty a child may experience with handling food in the mouth if there has been a prolonged requirement for nasogastric tube feeding from birth.

Rates of development are also influenced by other factors. For example, first-born children are more advanced in verbal skills (although not in achieving walking) than subsequent children, and girls are quicker than boys. Children from social class 1 walk later than those in social class 5.

The loss of skills constitutes developmental regression. This is unusual, and can never be regarded as normal. It requires immediate investigation, and is discussed in Chapter 8. Normal ranges are summarised in Figure 1.7 and Table 1.1.

Table 1.1 Child development normal ranges	
Skill	*Age*
Smiling	5–8 weeks
Reaching for objects	5–6 months
Transferring hand to hand	7–9 months
Sitting unsupported	7–10 months
Walking unsupported	15–18 months
Single words with meaning	15–18 months
Speaking in phrases	22–30 months

Nutrition: weaning and after

The initiation of breastfeeding, and comparisons with formula feeding, are covered in Chapter 17. Weaning is the time of changeover from exclusive milk feeding to a diet of mixed solids and milk. In effect, the baby is making a gradual transition from a high-fat food (milk) to a diet that is richer in carbohydrates (solids). Milk continues to be a very important food for babies throughout infancy, but from the moment of introducing solids it increasingly forms just one part of a balanced diet. When to commence weaning is a matter of fashion among parents and health professionals, with relatively little scientific basis. There are several current recommendations (*see* Box 1.3). Figure 1.8 shows the discrepancy between professional recommendations and what mothers have actually done since 1950. The gut of a baby is ready to accept foods other than milk by the age of about 3 months, and exclusive breastfeeding beyond about 6 months places the baby at risk of iron deficiency because most babies' reserves are by then exhausted, and demand for iron exceeds supply unless there is additional dietary provision. It is now officially recommended that

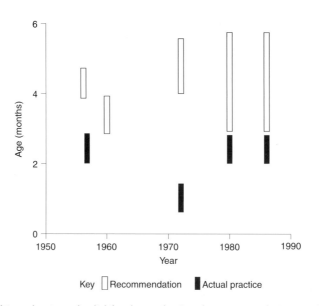

Figure 1.8   Ages of introduction of solid foods: professional recommendations and actual practice.

Box 1.3   Committee on Medical Aspects of Food Policy (COMA) recommendations on weaning 1995: major themes

- The majority of infants should not be given solid foods before the age of 4 months, and should be given them no later than 6 months. (Now altered to start at 6 months.)

- It is stressed that breast milk is the best early nutrition.

- Pasteurised whole cow's milk (not skimmed milk) should only be used as a main drink after 1 year of age, due to its low iron and vitamin content. However, dairy products such as yoghurt, cheese, milk-based sauces and custard may be given from 4 months, and unmodified whole cow's milk can be used on cereal from 6 months.

- Iron deficiency is identified as an important public health problem, and its prevention should be linked to dietary advice. Therefore meat and fish should form an important component of the weaning diet.

- Promotion of fluoridated water and the avoidance of sugar in some meals (backed up by more explicit food labelling) are key recommendations for improving child dental health.

---

exclusively breastfed infants do not need to be offered solids until 6 months of age (*see* Box 1.3).

Weaning diets are often short of iron, so education to encourage the inclusion of meat and fish in babies' diets is an important function of the health visitor. This is especially important in cases where breastfeeding is likely to be the baby's main source of milk for the next few months, or in families who choose to ignore the advice not to use unmodified cow's milk as the main milk source. Babies who continue to receive infant formula (or a 'follow-on' formula)

as their main milk source are at little risk of iron deficiency at this time. Vitamin C or orange juice given with food increases the absorption of iron. Iron-deficiency anaemia is discussed in Chapter 16.

At around the time when solid food is becoming an important part of a baby's diet, the first teeth (commonly the lower incisors) appear. Much lay significance is attached to teething, which is blamed for every kind of minor ailment that may coincide with it (*see* Box 1.4).

Box 1.4   Minor ailments that may coincide with teething

- Chewing fingers
- Copious salivation
- Discomfort relieved by paracetamol
- Waning humoral immunity, exposure to pathogens
- Upper respiratory and gastrointestinal infections

From the end of the first year, it is reasonable to allow babies to have unmodified (but not unpasteurised!) cow's milk. This should always be whole milk – semi-skimmed or skimmed milk is only suitable for health-conscious adults, as young children need the fat.

Control of diet is initially entirely the parents' responsibility. However, even the introduction of a limited range of solids allows the infant to express likes and dislikes for each new taste as it is presented, and gradually these preferences modulate what the parent offers in the way of diet. Young toddlers are notorious for their apparent ability to thrive on very little food, and an apparently low food intake is quite a common reason for bringing a child to the GP or asking advice from a health visitor. Box 1.5 summarises the key issues for weaning.

On a population basis, the most common *dietary deficiencies* in the UK are iron and vitamin D, but the most common *dietary problem* is obesity (*see* Box 1.6).

Early learning (*see* Box 1.7)

The newborn baby has a much wider repertoire of sensation, expression and comprehension than she is generally credited with, and the process of learning probably starts before birth. She can recognise her own mother's voice from others, and her own mother's milk by its smell, within 2 or 3 days of birth. The newborn preferentially responds to higher-pitched sounds, corresponding to the frequency content of a female voice. She prefers oval shapes to other shapes, and responds best at a distance of 20 to 30 centimetres, corresponding to the distance

from her mother's face to her own when she is feeding. The effects of fetal learning can be demonstrated postnatally. The newborn can vary her cry to express different needs, and her mother quickly learns to interpret this simple 'language'.

The world of the infant gradually expands so that within a few months the activities of other people in the same room will often capture her attention. At around 3 to 4 months she starts to coo, and this encourages her carers to talk to her even more, and to start to create pretend conversations. As she starts to babble, this pattern develops, and it is a necessary precursor to the start of real language.

Learning abilities expand dramatically with the development of an upright posture, and with walking. At around the age of 1 year the twin abilities of enormously increased potential for

Box 1.5   Weaning: summary

- Weaning diets are often short of iron.
- The best iron source is meat and fish.
- Babies who are fed on formula are at least risk of iron deficiency.
- Milk remains the main source of calcium.

Box 1.6   Dietary deficiencies: summary

- These are most prevalent where there is socio-economic deprivation.
- Deficiencies of iron and vitamin D are commonest.
- Vitamin D deficiency is a hazard for dark-skinned children.

Box 1.7   Early learning: summary

- Starts in fetal life.
- Occurs through the interaction of baby and parent.
- Is impaired by maternal depression.
- Is impaired in deprived families.
- Is enhanced by nursery education.

communication and physical movement together transform the world of the child, because this world becomes susceptible to manipulation and exploration. A child's constant fascination with experimentation in this expanding world is what adults call 'play'. (Adults do this as well, of course, but commonly give it less pejorative names!)

Pre-school children can benefit from attending a playgroup. Some playgroups are formally attached to the primary school which most of the children will subsequently attend. Children who attend a well-structured nursery make more rapid progress in school than those who do not.

Children and school

School dominates the life of children, just as work (when it is available) dominates that of adults. For the child it is the main source of friends outside the family, and a major source of praise and criticism, success or failure. School is not just about the teaching in the classroom. It is a community, and children learn many things about socialising, making and keeping friends, having activities and interests in common, and relating to adults who are in authority but who are not their parents.

Paediatricians, general practitioners and other primary care professionals have to relate to children and their schooling in a variety of ways.

A child who is identified in the pre-school years as having special needs (e.g. cerebral palsy, learning difficulty, hearing loss, visual impairment) may or may not manage in mainstream school. Such children need a 'statement of educational needs' so that their schooling is minimally disadvantaged by their other problems. The statement is prepared with input from all of the relevant professionals, and the parents also have a substantial say in the recommendations of the statement. Paediatricians commonly make an important contribution to this process, and have to work closely with professionals from other disciplines and agencies.

The school may be a source of problems such as bullying for a child. Children often conceal their problems and distress, and the result may be 'somatisation' – the development of physical symptoms that relate to the child's inner unhappiness. Examples of somatisation include pain (abdominal, headache), enuresis and

'difficult' behaviour. Bullied children can also become depressed, and this condition may coexist with these symptoms.

Many chronic illnesses have an impact on school life, and can be particularly hard to deal with in mainstream school, where most children are by definition free of significant illness. Important examples include diabetes, asthma and epilepsy. Children on regular medication who require a dose during school hours may need special arrangements to be negotiated. Serious but rare illnesses such as cystic fibrosis, leukaemia and cancer can result in considerable spells of school absence, and close liaison is required between the hospital teaching service, the parents and the school to minimise the educational effects of such serious illnesses.

Box 1.8 Additional information: other health functions of school

- Schools are a useful place for organising mass immunisation with BCG for tuberculosis at around the age of 12 years.

- There was a mass measles/rubella immunisation programme for school-age children in 1994 to prevent a predicted epidemic of measles in 1995 (*see* Chapter 22).

- Teaching on healthy eating, sexual health, smoking, and drug and alcohol abuse takes place in most secondary schools. Means of making this more effective remain controversial (*see* Chapter 22).

Children and hospitals

Much has been learned in recent years about how to make the hospital less of a hostile environment for children, but much of the credit for this must go to the lay groups, such as Action for Sick Children, which helped to revolutionise medical and nursing thinking.

Some of the principles which underpin the healthcare of children both in hospital and in primary care environments are as follows.

Appropriate design and furnishing to cater for the relevant age groups

Getting away from dour functionality is not only pleasant for staff, but also signals to children and their parents that the institution is trying to be *child-friendly*. This means lively artwork, perhaps including recent work by children attending that department, small chairs for young children, and carpet on the floor.

Provision of toys, activities and play areas (*see Figure 1.9*)

Outpatient and clinic visits always mean waiting, and waiting means boredom. This is greatly helped by toys appropriate to a child's developmental stage. In hospital, the older children need an area to themselves, and can often use a pool table or watch videos rather than daytime children's television, which is mostly aimed at younger children. Play specialists can not only help to entertain the children, but can also help them to work through hospital- or illness-related anxieties by means of play.

Young children admitted to hospital should, whenever possible, be accompanied by a parent or relative

This simple principle, first adopted in the Newcastle Babies' Hospital after World War Two, took around three decades to achieve universal acceptance. It is now recognised that hospital admission, where illness is accompanied by enforced separation of children from their parents, can be immensely damaging psychologically, and the corollary to this is the need to avoid admitting children whenever possible, and to keep hospital lengths of stay as short as possible. 'Visiting' by parents has itself become an obsolete concept – they come and go as they and their child feel they need.

Relaxed clothing for staff

It is now commonplace for child health doctors not to wear white coats, and for nurses to be less formal, often with colourful tabards over their hospital uniform. Interestingly, surveys of children's interpretation of clothing have shown, at least for

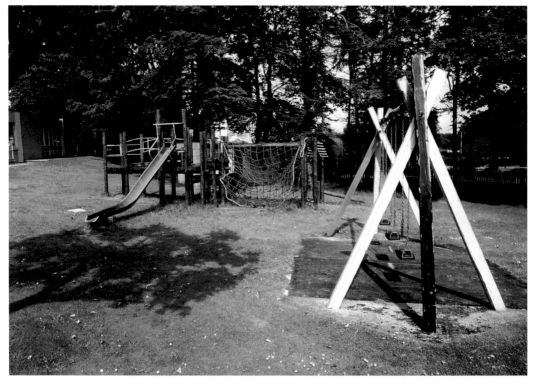

Figure 1.9   Outside play area at a hospital.

doctors, that while the less formal look is appreciated as friendlier, the white coat is still associated with greater competence!

Awareness that it is inappropriate, unnecessary and sometimes counter-productive to separate children from their parents, even for short lengths of time or for minor procedures

It can be a major professional hurdle for staff to overcome their discomfort at having to work with parents present. Appropriate training, experience and professional role models have all contributed to the recognition that parents can play a useful role in helping their children to cope with procedures, including accompanying them to the anaesthetic room prior to induction of anaesthesia for surgery.

Recognition that children have different coping strategies for painful or uncomfortable procedures, and that these need to be understood and respected

Whether it is an immunisation or changing a dressing, some children cope better with distraction, and others with attention. It does not help children to cope with a short-lived adverse experience if staff carry preconceptions (from their own childhood or their own children) of how a particular child should manage. Children, like adults, need an individualised approach to coping with pain and discomfort.

Attention to strategies of pain prevention and analgesia

The development of skin anaesthesia with eutectic mixture of local anaesthetic (EMLA) cream (*see* Figure 1.10) has revolutionised procedures such as insertion of intravenous lines and drawing blood samples. At the same time, reliable methods for assessing pain in children are beginning to refine the process of giving optimum pain control after surgery. Intramuscular injection (a source of great fear for many children) for analgesia or any other purpose has become virtually obsolete.

Patient-centred (as opposed to task-centred) nursing care

It was in paediatric nursing that the concept of patient-centred nursing first appeared, spreading rapidly to other specialties. It is a professional model which attaches nurses to groups of patients, the emphasis being on all the nursing needs of the children, rather than a concentration on tasks such as changing beds, doing drug rounds and checking infusions.

Child-centred therapeutics

Young children cannot manage inhalers, pills or tablets. They may cope with liquid medicines, but refuse them if the taste is unpleasant. Therapeutics

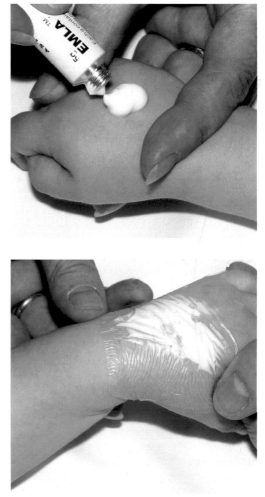

Figure 1.10 Applying local anaesthetic cream.

is always the art of the possible, and drug delivery systems and paediatric prescribing must take account of this. Syringes are now often used for administering oral liquid medicines, as they are more convenient and accurate than the traditional 5 ml spoon. Dosage is generally calculated on the basis of body weight (which is easy to measure), although under certain circumstances surface area (calculated using a nomogram based on weight and height) is used in preference. Intramuscular injection is generally avoided, as few drugs need to be given by this route in preference to the oral or intravenous route (immunisations being the unfortunate exception). Oral drugs should taste pleasant, but it is important to avoid sucrose because severe caries can result if a child is on long-term treatment with a sucrose-containing liquid.

Impaired renal or hepatic function may alter the rate of disposal of drugs in children just as in adults. The immature neonate is an extreme example of this, but awareness of the routes of disposal of drugs is important throughout paediatric therapeutics. Allowance should be made for immature function, and alternative drugs should be considered (e.g. cephalosporins instead of aminoglycosides in a child with renal impairment). Conversely, drugs used in epilepsy, a relatively common area of paediatric practice, may induce enzyme activity or interact with each other or with other drugs. Measuring the levels of these drugs (sometimes possible in saliva) can assist in prescribing and can be used to assess adherence to treatment.

Adherence to a prescribed treatment is generally the responsibility of parents, but must become the responsibility of the child as he or she gets older. Particular difficulties in ensuring adherence arise in adolescence with the management of chronic conditions that require continuous treatment, such as diabetes, asthma and epilepsy.

Preparing a child for admission to hospital

Most children with medical conditions are admitted as emergencies, but for surgery most come electively. For elective admissions there is an opportunity to bring the child for a visit prior to admission, when staff can meet the family, and the family can become familiar with the staff and the environment. Most children have fears about

hospital, and any opportunity to alleviate these helps both the child and the family to cope with what is always a stressful experience.

Hospital teaching services

Median lengths of stay for children with medical conditions are very short – of the order of 2 days or less. However, there are still some children who may stay for many days or even weeks (e.g. those with orthopaedic conditions, children with rare illnesses such as cancer, leukaemia, cystic fibrosis, inflammatory bowel disease or osteomyelitis, and some with psychiatric disorders such as anorexia nervosa). School-age children may have their education seriously disrupted by prolonged periods in hospital, and continuing their school work is potentially therapeutic for these children, mimicking to some extent the reality of the outside world, and preventing boredom. The hospital teaching service exists to provide liaison with the child's school, and to maintain some measure of educational input. Occasionally the hospital teachers find themselves invigilating for a public examination.

Parents of the ill child

Having a sick child in hospital is inherently stressful, no matter how 'child-friendly' and 'parent-friendly' the environment may be. Under such conditions, explanations can easily be forgotten, or scarcely heard in the first place. It is vital to remember basic courtesies, such as introducing yourself clearly, and to spend a little time sympathising with the experience that the parent has undergone. Most of what you say to a parent will need to be repeated later, and carefully written fact sheets can assist this (but can never substitute for a personal discussion).

When serious or life-threatening illness occurs, a great deal of time is needed for explanation, counselling, and helping the parents to come to terms with the situation. They often need assistance with finding the most appropriate way to help and support their child. Nomination of particular members of the nursing and medical team to provide continuing support for families is helpful, and close liaison and outreach with community services, primary care and school are vital. Formal or informal parent support groups can also be valuable for some families.

The adolescent in hospital

Adolescents do not mix easily with younger children. They may be very sensitive about their bodies, they need privacy, and the occupations that may interest them are different to those appropriate for younger children. Providing either a separate ward (this is only possible in a large children's hospital) or a dedicated bay within a children's ward are important ways of catering for their needs.

Ethics and consent

It is important to distinguish between legal requirements and ethical practices. While it is unlikely that an illegal act is ethically justifiable, an unethical situation may nevertheless be perfectly legal. As practitioners, we have a civic duty to remain within the law, and to work to change bad or anomalous laws, and we have a professional duty to practise ethically. All professionals who deal with children need to be aware of children's rights as defined by the United Nations Convention on the Rights of the Child (1989, www.unicef.org/crc/crc.htm). *See* Chapter 23.

The legal framework for child health revolves around the Children Act (1989), all legislation involving primary and secondary education, the Infant Life Preservation Act (1929), the Human Embryology and Fertilization Act (1994), and a variety of other measures in relation to road traffic law, employment law and much else.

Some *cardinal principles* of ethics are set out in Box 1.9.

Box 1.9   Cardinal principles that underpin ethical considerations

- *Autonomy*: respect for the individual's right to determine his or her own destiny.

- *Beneficence*: the intention to do good.

- *Non-maleficence*: the intention not to do any harm.

- *Justice*: the requirement to be fair. Some authors separately distinguish the need for *equity*.

Case study 2

Mary, a 4-year-old girl, is admitted for insertion of grommets for refractory otitis media with effusion and bilateral hearing loss. The operation is explained to her parents, who then sign the hospital's 'consent' form.

Difficulties arise in child health because the younger the child, the less *autonomy* he or she has. While an adult or an older child can give informed *consent* for a treatment or procedure, for the young child or baby the parents can only *assent* on their child's behalf. There is no clearly defined cut-off point between the dependent younger child and the independent older child. For children under 16 years of age, the Gillick principle applies – that is, they can give legally effective consent to surgical or medical treatment, independent of their parents' wishes, provided that they have sufficient understanding of their condition and what is proposed. However, the issue of refusal of consent, especially for life-saving treatment, by a 'Gillick-competent' child under 16 years of age becomes complicated, and usually has to be determined by a court.

Case study 3

Kylie has been on the 'at-risk' register for 2 years. Now 3 years old, she is failing to thrive and is showing signs of emotional abuse and physical neglect. She is in and out of hospital for relatively minor illnesses that invariably present in the late hours of weekend nights. At a case conference, the paediatrician forcibly argues for Kylie's removal from the family. The health visitor argues for further work with the family for another few months to try to improve the mother's parenting skills.

The conflict here is between the *autonomy* of the parents to bring up Kylie as they think fit (championed by the health visitor), *beneficence* towards Kylie (championed by the paediatrician), and the very real issue of *non-maleficence* (would Kylie be more harmed, at the age of 3 years, by removal from the family she knows, first to a foster home, and then perhaps for adoption, and the prolonged uncertainty which could arise from the inevitable legal wrangling?). The legal framework is that of the Children Act (1989), whose cardinal principle is that the child's interests are paramount. The issue here is how to translate this into practice – that is, what are Kylie's 'best interests'?

Serious ethical debates need to be informed by accurate facts whenever these can be obtained. For instance, legitimate concerns about the ethics of resuscitating very premature babies must be based on the facts of neonatal outcome among the survivors.

Case study 4

Sam is born with Down syndrome to a low-risk mother, and the family is devastated. Within hours, it is clear that Sam cannot tolerate feeds, and the diagnosis of duodenal atresia is made. Resection of a duodenal atresia is a well-established operation with very low morbidity and mortality. Sam's parents readily assent to this, and he has the operation and does well thereafter. Two days postoperatively, Sam's colour becomes a little dusky. Echocardiography reveals a large atrioventricular septal defect, which is a well-known complication of Down syndrome. His parents wonder whether they can justify putting him through an operation for this as well.

Could Sam's parents reasonably have refused him correction of his duodenal atresia? Two decades ago, not all babies with Down syndrome would have been offered this operation. Yet the procedure is safe, it is certainly life-saving, and without it Sam would have died of dehydration, modulated only by sedation (which would have had to be given parenterally). It would be very difficult to counter the argument of *beneficence*

towards Sam with the suggestion that his parents have the *autonomy* to refuse him a simple and life-saving operation. With the prospect of cardiac surgery, the decisions can be delayed. An atrioventricular septal defect, if not repaired, usually results in irreversible pulmonary hypertension, which might be expected to limit Sam's life to his teens or twenties. A repair, if undertaken, would normally be done at the age of a few months. Clearly, if the mortality for this procedure was around 40%, a good case on the grounds of *non-maleficence* could be made for not undertaking it. However, if the mortality was only 4%, how might we view the parents' reluctance then? They could still argue that major cardiac surgery, with even a small chance of a poor outcome, would not alter Sam's quality of life for many years, and much else might have happened to him during that time. This would be the same argument of *non-maleficence*. The paediatrician might counter this by saying that any procedure offered to a normal child should be equally available to one with special needs. This is an argument on the grounds of *equity*.

Difficult ethical questions cannot have easy answers. For clinicians, the important thing is to be able to consider the issues within a conceptual framework, and the principles and examples given above provide a way into this.

Further reading

- Eriksson EH (1950) *Childhood and Society.* Norton, New York.

- Hall DMB, Hill P and Elliman D (1999) *The Child Surveillance Handbook* (revised 2e). Radcliffe Medical Press, Oxford.

- Illingworth RS (1991) *The Normal Child: some problems of the early years and their treatment* (10e). Churchill Livingstone, Edinburgh.

- Piaget J (1926) *The Language and Thought of the Child.* Harcourt Brace, New York.

2 Causes of child death and ill health

- Causes of child deaths
- Breakdown by age
- Trends in child deaths over recent years
- Causes of child illness
- Changes in society and their influence on children's health

Causes of child deaths

Fortunately, child death is now uncommon in the UK. However, this makes it all the more tragic for parents when it does happen. Table 2.1 lists the causes of death in childhood.

The most common cause overall is accidental injuries. The main cause of injury or death in the UK is a collision between a child who is walking or playing on the street and a motor vehicle. There is a marked social gradient in accidents in the UK, with deaths in social class 5 being much commoner than deaths in social class 1. This gradient is discussed further below.

Breakdown by age

Table 2.1 shows the causes of death at various ages.

Trends in child deaths over recent years

Infections are still important causes of death, in particular respiratory infections. Fortunately, there has been a significant fall in certain types of infection, due to immunisation. The trend in measles and *Haemophilus* infections is shown in Figures 2.1 and 2.2.

As infectious disease and accidents become less common, the relative importance of cancer as a cause of death increases. As treatments for cancer improve, death becomes less common. In the UK today, fewer children die but more suffer chronic illness and disability from the same conditions that used to kill them.

It is usual to look at the causes of death by age of the child, as the causes are very different at different ages. Table 2.1 (see overleaf) shows a breakdown of causes in the first year of life.

Table 2.1   Main causes of child mortality at 1–19 years in England and Wales

Injury and poisoning	47%	Mortality at 1–4 years	
Cancer	14%	Injury and poisoning	24%
Nervous system	10%	Congenital anomaly	21%
Congenital anomaly	9%	Nervous system	11%
Respiratory cause	7%	Cancer	11%
Other	13%	Respiratory cause	9%
		Infectious disease	7%
Mortality at 28 days to 1 year		Other	17%
Perinatal causes	44%		
Congenital anomaly	24%	Mortality at 15–19 years	
Sudden infant death	19%	Injury and poisoning	60%
Respiratory cause	4%	Cancer	9%
		Nervous system	9%
		Heart and circulation	4%
		Drug abuse	4%
		Respiratory cause	4%
		Other	11%

Source: Office for National Statistics.

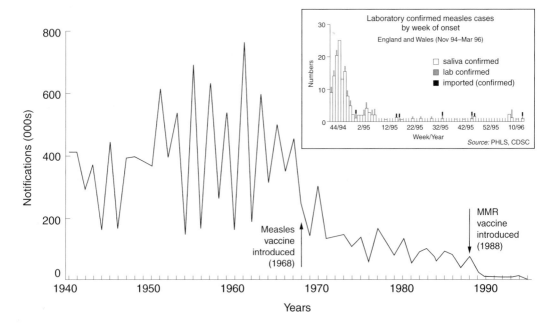

Figure 2.1   Notification of measles to ONS, England and Wales, 1940–1995.

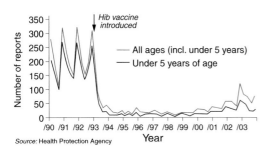

Source: Health Protection Agency

Figure 2.2 Laboratory reports of Hib disease in England and Wales, 1990–2003. (Hib = *Haemophilus influenzae* type b.)
Source: Health Protection Agency.

These reflect the vulnerability of infants and the effect of traumatic labour. The first year of life is when the child is most at risk of death, and there is also a considerable social class gradient at this age. The reasons for the gradient are discussed below. Note that sudden infant death syndrome (SIDS) is the commonest cause of death after the first week of life. The incidence of SIDS has dropped considerably in recent years, and the reasons for this are important. Until quite recently, medical advice to parents was that an infant should be laid to sleep on their stomach – to prevent inhalation of regurgitated milk and to encourage muscle development. This position is now known to be a contributing factor in SIDS. It was noted that in countries with a low incidence of SIDS, the custom of babies sleeping on their back prevails. The guidance to parents was altered in the UK through the 'Back to Sleep' campaign, and this led to a remarkable reduction in the rate of SIDS. The cause of this condition is not yet entirely understood, but the lesson is that advice should not be given to the general public without good evidence that it is of benefit and does not cause harm.

After the age of 1 year the causes of death reflect the development of the child, exposure to infections and risk-taking activity. Accidental injuries are the main cause of death among teenagers, but it should be noted that suicide is a significant cause in young men. This reflects the increasing prevalence of mental health problems in this age group.

What illnesses do children have?

Now that fewer children die, parents attach greater importance to being healthy, and become more anxious when their child is unwell. Yet the burden of chronic illness is now more common than ever, due to earlier diagnosis and better treatment.

The burden of chronic ill health and disability is described as *morbidity*. However, this term covers many different conditions, and we need to consider here the definition of health, which is not just the converse of disease. Box 2.1 lists several definitions of health that are in current usage. To measure health status, we need to ask children about their health as well as define what illness they are suffering from. Boxes 2.2, 2.3 and 2.4 indicate the sources of information that tell us about children's health.

There is often confusion about the use of terms in epidemiology, especially the terms *prevalence* and *incidence*. These are defined in Box 2.5.

Box 2.1 Definitions of health

• World Health Organization:

'A state of complete physical, mental and social well-being, and not merely the absence of disease or infirmity.'

• The Ottawa Charter for Health Promotion 1986:

'Health is a resource for living, not the object of living. It is a positive concept emphasising social and personal resources as well as physical capabilities.'

• World Health Assembly at Alma Ata in 1977:

'The main social target of governments and of the World Health Organization in the coming decades should be the attainment by all citizens of the world ... of a level of health that will permit them to lead socially and economically productive lives.'

Box 2.2 How children in England have described what health means

- Being myself
- Absence of illness
- Body working well
- Behaviours that promote health (e.g. cleaning teeth, eating well, running)
- Positive feelings
- Absence of negative feelings
- Being normal
- Being involved – having opportunities and experiences
- Achievement
- Independence and choice
- A sense of security
- Good relationships with others (parents, friends, siblings)

Box 2.3 Sources of information on children's health

- Registration of Births, Marriages and Deaths
- National Census data: numbers, ethnic origin, occupation of parent
- Notification of congenital anomalies
- Hospital episode statistics
- Routine data collection on weight and height at specified ages, data from child health surveillance, immunisation rates
- Annual health survey for England: questionnaire and physical measurement
- GP consultations
- Notification of infectious disease
- Specific survey data (e.g. health-related behaviour, regular infant feeding surveys)

Box 2.4 Data which can inform on children's health status

- Birth weight and local/socio-economic variation
- Breastfeeding rates at birth and at 6 weeks
- Weight at various ages
- Frequency of congenital malformations
- Immunisation uptake at various ages
- Infectious disease incidence
- Accidental injury prevalence
- Disability and chronic illness prevalence
- Teenage pregnancy rate
- Rates of smoking, alcohol intake and drug use

Box 2.5 Definitions of prevalence and incidence

Incidence: the rate of acquiring a disease or a characteristic thereof. The *numerator* consists of new cases developing the disease in a specified time period. The *denominator* is the population or sample from which this information was collected.

Prevalence: the risk of having the disease or a characteristic thereof at any given point or within a given time period. The former is called *point prevalence* and the latter is termed *period prevalence*.

Causes of child illness

In this section we shall look at the main causes of ill health in the UK, under the headings acute illness, chronic illness, disability, injury, nutritional disorders and mental health disorders.

Acute illness

Most acute illness in children is short and self-limiting, and is managed at home by the parents. However, severe acute illness still occurs, and is devastating for the child's family. Table 2.2 shows the commonest causes of GP presentations in under-fours in the UK. The majority of these are managed by the parents without outside assistance. A small number are treated by primary care staff (a GP or practice nurse), and a small proportion reach hospital and are admitted. However, even the most minor illness may cause the parents considerable distress, especially if there is fever, vomiting or pain. Such illness can also lead to behavioural disturbance with poor sleeping.

Table 2.2 Acute illness: reasons for GP consultations at 0–4 years in England and Wales over a 12-month period: episodes per 1000 population

Respiratory causes	1188
Nervous system and sense organs	566
Infectious disease	447
Signs and symptoms	390
Injuries	124
Other	498

Source: Office for National Statistics.

The more serious types of acute illness are meningitis, urinary tract infections, pneumonia, gastroenteritis, septicaemia and trauma.

Chronic illness

The common chronic illnesses are listed in Box 2.6, together with their prevalence. Asthma is by far the most common, and is increasing in frequency, as is eczema, which is also common and debilitating due to the constant itching and the disfiguring effects on appearance.

Box 2.6 Chronic illness

Diabetes	1%
Epilepsy	2%
Asthma	25%
Cancer/tumour	1%
Heart disease	3%
Skin conditions	8%
Musculoskeletal disorders	5%

Diabetes and asthma are both increasing in prevalence, the former due to changes in nutrition and the latter for reasons perhaps related to a reduced risk of infection in early life as well as to increased levels of atmospheric pollution. In these conditions, the life of the child may be relatively normal owing to the development of modern drugs and treatment regimens. Diabetes is distinctive because the child is usually required to have injections, and this makes a considerable difference to their lifestyle, although children adjust to this remarkably quickly. Epilepsy still carries a stigma which means that children may hide their condition from their peers, although effective information provision can help to reduce this problem. In all chronic conditions there is a need for the child to develop autonomy and to learn to understand and manage the condition him- or herself. Parents often find this difficult to appreciate because of their wish to protect their child. It is important that health professionals understand the provisions of the UN Convention on the Rights of the Child (*see* Box 23.3, page 348), and that they provide the child or young person with information at a level they can understand, ensure confidentiality and obtain the young person's consent to any new intervention.

Disability (also see Chapter 10, page 136)

> **Box 2.7** Definitions
>
> *Impairment*: an injurious weakening – any loss or abnormality of physiological or anatomical structure.
>
> *Disability*: a want of ability – any restriction or loss of ability due to an impairment in performing an activity in a manner or range considered normal for a human being of that developmental stage.
>
> *Handicap*: a disability that makes success more difficult – a disadvantage for an individual arising from a disability that limits or prevents the achievement of desired goals (an uncompensated disability).

Disability may affect mental development (learning disability), sensory development (hearing loss or visual impairment) or motor development (cerebral palsy or muscular dystrophy), or a combination of these.

The prevalence of different forms of disability in the UK is shown in Box 2.8.

> **Box 2.8** Prevalence of disability
>
> | | |
> |---|---|
> | Severe learning difficulties | 3% |
> | Moderate learning difficulties | 3% |
> | Physical disability | 3% |
> | Visual impairment | 0.3% |
> | Moderate hearing impairment | 2% |

The most common causes of disability in the UK are cerebral palsy, prematurity, congenital anomaly (e.g. Down syndrome, muscular dystrophy), visual defect, sensorineural hearing loss, trauma and infections.

There is still considerable discrimination against children with disability in terms of both attitudes of society and access to services such as education, although major efforts are being made to reduce this. These issues are dealt with further in Chapter 10.

Injury

Injuries may be accidental or non-accidental, the term *non-accidental injury* sometimes being used for child abuse. Accidental injuries remain the main cause of childhood deaths, and are highly preventable. Children will always be prone to accidents, but the extent of injury resulting from them can be reduced to a minimum by appropriate environmental measures. Table 2.3 gives a breakdown of the causes of accidental injury in the UK at different ages and Figure 2.3 illustrates some of them. It can be seen in Figure 2.4 that there is a very significant social class divide with regard to accidental injury. This is mainly due to the different environmental conditions to which children are subject according to their parents' income category. Health professionals need to recognise that 'accidental' injuries are often far from accidental. If a child grows up in a house

Table 2.3 Causes of accidental injury in England and Wales

Under 1 year	(Average 67 deaths/year)
Suffocation	44%
Road accident	20%
Fire	12%
Drowning	6%
Falls	6%
5–9 years	(Average 188 deaths/year)
Road accident	64%
Fire	11%
Drowning	8%
Falls	4%
15–19 years	(Average 829 deaths/year)
Road accident	81%
Poisoning	4%
Drowning	3%
Falls	3%

Source: Office for National Statistics.

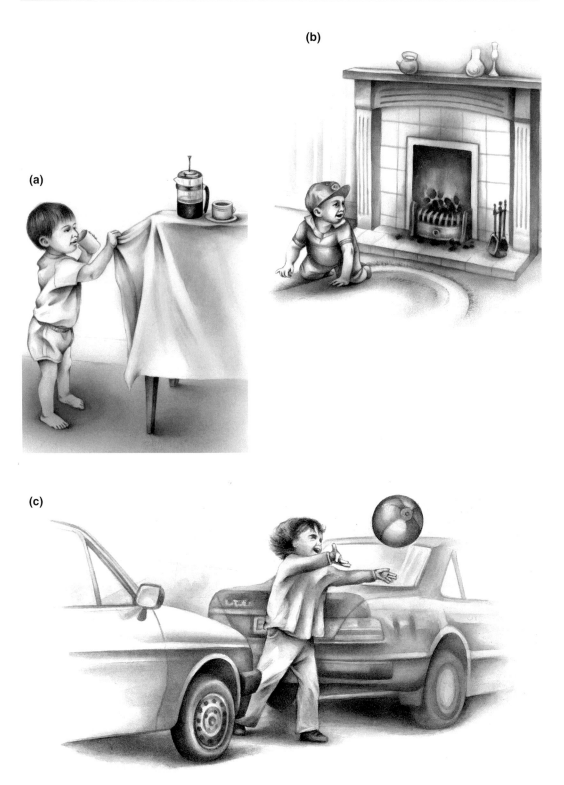

Figure 2.3 (a), (b) and (c)   Accidents waiting to happen.

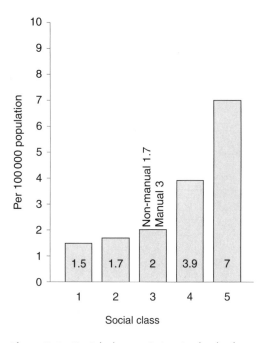

Figure 2.4 Social class variation in deaths from traffic collisions with pedestrian, age 1–14 years.

Box 2.9 Definitions of non-accidental injury

- *Physical abuse*: any physical assault which results in injury.

- *Sexual abuse*: actual or likely sexual exploitation of a child or adolescent.

- *Emotional abuse*: the habitual verbal harassment of a child by disparagement, criticism, threat and ridicule, and the inversion of love; by verbal and non-verbal means, rejection and withdrawal are substituted.

- *Neglect*: the persistent or severe neglect of a child, or the failure to protect a child from exposure to any kind of danger, including cold or starvation, or failure to carry out important aspects of care, resulting in the significant impairment of the child's health or development, including non-organic failure to thrive.

---

without window guards or smoke alarms, with no safe play area nearby and with broken glass in the street, accidental injury is predictable.

Non-accidental injury

Non-accidental injury has been recognised since the 1960s and occurs in all realms of society, although it is more common in families afflicted by poverty and stress. Four types of non-accidental injury are recognised, and these and their definitions are listed in Box 2.9. Child abuse is discussed further in Chapter 14. At present it is thought that physical abuse is becoming less common, whereas the incidence of the other types has remained the same, although measuring their prevalence is anything but an exact science. Emotional abuse in particular is rather like an iceberg – what presents is much less than what lies beneath the surface. For the health professional, managing a case of emotional abuse is one of the most disturbing and challenging experiences they can encounter, yet one of the most satisfying to rectify.

Nutritional disorders

Malnutrition is still a significant phenomenon in UK society, but the situation today is very different from the recent past. Undernutrition is now uncommon, and rickets and scurvy are rarely seen except in metabolic disorders, although certain groups in the community are at higher risk for micronutrient deficiency. However, obesity is occurring in epidemic proportions, with serious implications for adult health. Box 2.11 summarises the current thinking on obesity.

Box 2.10 Commoner types of nutritional disorder in the UK

Iron-deficiency anaemia

Dental caries

Growth faltering in infancy

Obesity

Mental health is defined in Box 2.12.

Box 2.11   Current prevalence of and reasons for obesity

- There was a 60% increase in overweight and 70% increase in obesity in 3- to 4-year-olds between 1989 and 1998.

- Obesity leads to low self-image, type 2 diabetes in childhood, arthritis and back pain, and to cardiovascular disease in later life.

- The current epidemic is due to increasing inactivity and the culture of snacking on high-fat, high-sugar foods plus soft drinks.

- A population approach is needed, as treatment of the individual is very difficult.

- Public health measures should include nutritional labelling of foods, curbing the marketing of convenience foods aimed at children, making fruit and vegetables available at lower cost, improved school meals and nutrition education, and education on restricting television use. In relation to exercise, sports facilities at school and in the community should be improved and made more readily available.

Box 2.12   Definition of mental health

Good mental health is indicated by:

- a capacity to enter into and sustain mutually satisfying personal relationships

- continuing progression of development

- an ability to play and learn so that attainments are appropriate for age and intellectual level

- a developing moral sense of right and wrong

- the degree of psychological distress and maladaptive behaviour being within normal limits for the child's age and context.

Source: Hill P (1995), cited in Williams R and Richardson G (eds) (1995) *Together We Stand*. Health Advisory Service, HMSO, London.

Mental health disorders

Mental health disorders are extremely common in UK children, and should not be considered separately from physical conditions. Their prevalence is increasing and they have a major impact on other areas of children's lives, in particular education.

The main presenting mental health problems in children, and their current prevalence, are listed in Box 2.13. The figures are estimates, as accurate collection of data is very difficult.

Mental health problems in children are extremely common, and most are related to parenting factors. Parenting is covered in greater detail below. These problems are of considerable importance because of their consequences in adult life. Behavioural difficulties, which are the commonest of the above conditions, can lead to relationship difficulties, marital conflict, failure in terms of school achievement, dropping out of school, risk-taking behaviour and conflict with the law. Their antecedents lie in the first 3 years of life, and therefore interventions targeted at this period have the greatest likelihood of success. It is particularly important to break the cycle of disadvantage which allows the poor parenting style of one generation to be passed on to the next. There are certain endogenous factors which

Box 2.13 Mental health problems in children

Sleep disorder	Up to 1 in 10 pre-school children
Oppositional behaviour	5–10%
Enuresis	980/10 000 at age 7 years
Encopresis	150/10 000 at age 7 years
Attention deficit hyperactivity disorder	1%
Conduct disorder	5%
Depression	200/10 000 school-aged children
Anxiety	4%
Learning difficulty	1%
Autism	4.5–20/10 000

Box 2.14 Endogenous factors in the child which lead to behavioural difficulties

Temperament and gender (male)

Developmental delay

Learning difficulties

Attention deficit hyperactivity disorder

Hearing loss

Physical illness

Pervasive developmental disorder (autistic spectrum)

Certain congenital syndromes (e.g. Tourette's syndrome)

may contribute to behavioural difficulties by affecting the way in which the child responds in social situations. These are listed in Box 2.14.

High-risk behaviour

This term is used for behaviour which is likely to lead to ill health (e.g. smoking and alcohol abuse). Such behaviour is extremely common in adolescents, and most young people pass through such a phase, but if the behaviour is continued or taken to extremes the consequences may be very serious. Box 2.15 shows the common types of risk-taking behaviour and their prevalence at different ages.

Box 2.15 Risk-taking behaviour

	Male	*Female*
Smoking	24% at age 15 years	36% at age 15 years
Alcohol use (> 8 units week)	26% at age 16–17 years	18% at age 16–17 years
Drug taking (cannabis)	16% had used at some time (sex unspecified)	
Sexual intercourse	28% before 16 years	19% before 16 years
Victim of violence	20% at age 16–24 years	8% at age 16–24 years
Bullied	23% at age 11–15 years	31% at age 11–15 years

Source: Coleman and Schofield (2001).

Changes in society and their influence on children's health

What causes child illnesses?

For some conditions the answer is obvious (e.g. streptococcal infection for tonsillitis and a gene defect for cystic fibrosis). But what are the causes of child abuse, child pedestrian accidents and obesity? For these conditions there are a number of different causes, and some of these are deeply implicated with the changes under way in society. One useful way of looking at causes of illness and ill health is to consider a hierarchy of causes as follows (*see also* Box 2.16):

- determinants in society – these include the increase in car traffic and changes in the built environment, marketing of fast foods, the increasing influence of television and computer games, changes in the nuclear family, and the widening of the income gap between rich and poor

- risk factors in the family – these include single-parent families, low income, unemployment, alcoholism, parents with learning difficulties, and preterm birth (*see* Figures 2.5–2.7)

- immediate causes – these include congenital disorders, infective agents and accidental injury.

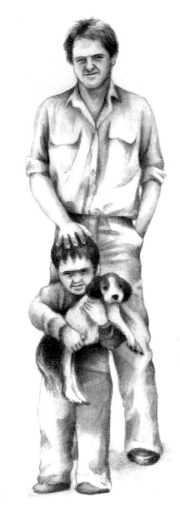

Figure 2.5   A single-parent family.

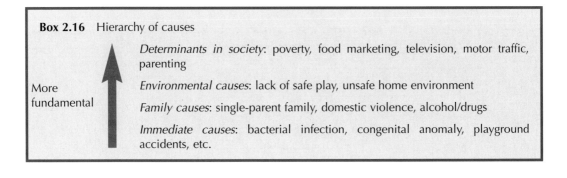

Box 2.16   Hierarchy of causes

More fundamental ↑

Determinants in society: poverty, food marketing, television, motor traffic, parenting

Environmental causes: lack of safe play, unsafe home environment

Family causes: single-parent family, domestic violence, alcohol/drugs

Immediate causes: bacterial infection, congenital anomaly, playground accidents, etc.

Figure 2.6 A two-parent family.

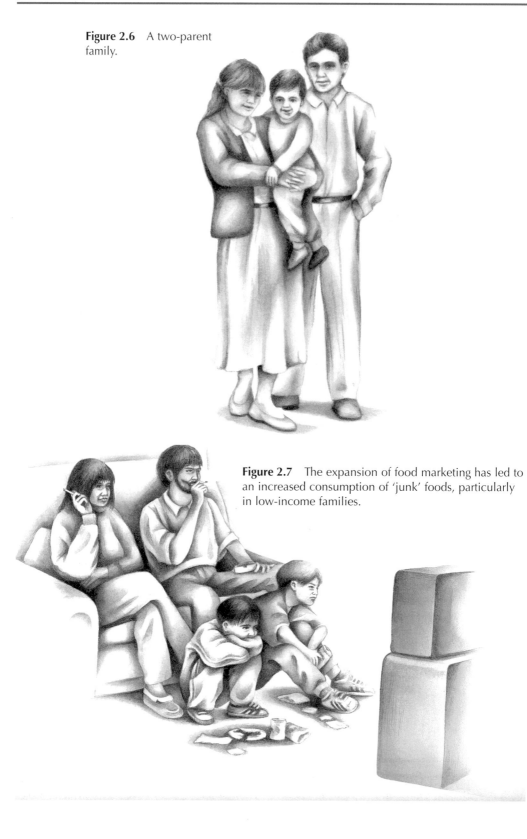

Figure 2.7 The expansion of food marketing has led to an increased consumption of 'junk' foods, particularly in low-income families.

Determinants

This section takes three important determinants, namely poverty/income inequality, parenting and nutrition, and examines them in more detail. These are thought to be of particular importance and can all be modified by intervention at either local or national level.

Poverty/inequality

Poverty can be considered either as an absolute condition or as a relative factor in society. Absolute poverty would mean not having enough to eat, inadequate housing, no fuel for heating and lighting, and very few possessions. This condition is present in many developing countries, but affects only small numbers of individuals in the UK. On the other hand, relative poverty – that is, being poor in relation to the norm in society – is certainly present in the UK. Figure 2.8 shows the position of the UK in relation to other industrialised countries, in terms of the proportion of children living in families who earn less than half the national average income.

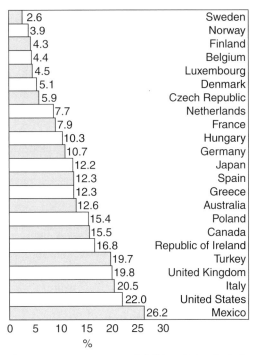

%	Country
2.6	Sweden
3.9	Norway
4.3	Finland
4.4	Belgium
4.5	Luxembourg
5.1	Denmark
5.9	Czech Republic
7.7	Netherlands
7.9	France
10.3	Hungary
10.7	Germany
12.2	Japan
12.3	Spain
12.3	Greece
12.6	Australia
15.4	Poland
15.5	Canada
16.8	Republic of Ireland
19.7	Turkey
19.8	United Kingdom
20.5	Italy
22.0	United States
26.2	Mexico

0   5   10   15   20   25   30
%

Figure 2.8 Percentage of children living in 'relative' poverty (households with income below 50% of national median) (*BMJ* (2000) **320**: 1621).

Children's health is worse in countries with a high level of relative poverty, and this is thought to be due to the feeling of social exclusion in the families at the lower end of the socio-economic spectrum. They do not have access to the material goods and possessions which are so widely available in society, and this material deprivation has wide effects on mental health.

Parenting

Parenting is as important a determinant of children's health as poverty, and is closely related, in that parenting ability is restricted in low-income families. The term *parenting* means the nurturing of and provision of food, love and security for the growing child. When parenting is deficient, the consequences for the child can be poor nutrition, emotional and behavioural problems and accidental injury. Behavioural disorders are becoming increasingly prevalent in our society, and this is likely to be due to the problems that affect parents (e.g. teenage pregnancy, single parenthood, parental conflict and split families). There is much that can be done both by the state and by local services to support parents in their difficult task, and health professionals have a major part to play in this.

Nutrition

The significance of poor nutrition in children is being increasingly recognised, particularly as the Barker hypothesis (concerning the links between fetal and early infant nutrition and health in later life) becomes better known. Why is children's nutrition still a problem in our wealthy and highly developed society when every kind of food is available within easy reach?

The main reasons are shown in Box 2.17.

In the UK the consequences of poor nutrition are twofold, namely undernutrition in infancy (children who fail to thrive due to lack of calories) and malnutrition affecting older children (obesity due to excess intake of calories over expenditure, and high sugar and fat intake). Undernutrition mainly affects low-income families, while obesity affects all social classes. A recent study showed a 3.3% prevalence of undernutrition and an 8.5% prevalence of obesity in 3-year-olds in Scotland, with a significant social class bias towards the deprived. It is understandable that poor families provide their children with an unbalanced diet,

> **Box 2.17** Reasons why poor nutrition is still common in the UK
>
> - It is cheaper to feed children on an unhealthy diet than on a healthy one.
> - Nutritional awareness of the content of processed food is limited.
> - Many processed foods contain 'hidden' salt and sugar.
> - Foods with a high sugar and fat content are heavily marketed to children.
> - Fewer families cook meals regularly and more rely on convenience foods.
> - Exercise levels in children have decreased markedly.

as foods such as pies, sausages and crisps, which are nutritionally unbalanced, are the cheapest source of calories. Moreover, parents in low-income families are unwilling to risk offering their children new varieties of food, since if they will not eat it the food will have to be discarded. In low-income families, food costs are a higher proportion of the total budget than in moderate-to high-income families, and consequently these parents are more anxious not to waste food.

The various means of tackling this problem were summarised in Box 2.11.

Further reading

- Bellman M and Kennedy N (2000) *Paediatrics and Child Health: a textbook for the DCH.* Churchill Livingstone, Edinburgh.
- Blair M, Stewart Brown S, Waterston T and Crowther R (2003) *Child Public Health.* Oxford University Press, Oxford.
- Coleman J and Schofield J (2001) *Key Data on Adolescence.* Trust for the Study of Adolescence, Brighton.

Self-assessment questions

1 In relation to child deaths:
(a) the commonest cause is accidental injury — True/False
(b) the commonest cause during the first year is sudden infant death syndrome — True/False
(c) the biggest socio-economic difference occurs in accidental injury — True/False
(d) the commonest cause worldwide is diarrhoeal disease. — True/False

2 In relation to child illnesses:
(a) mumps is becoming more common — True/False
(b) meningococcal meningitis is becoming less common — True/False
(c) asthma is becoming more common owing to pet ownership — True/False
(d) child abuse is more common in ethnic-minority families. — True/False

3 Poverty in the UK:
(a) is defined as relative to national income — True/False
(b) currently affects over 30% of children — True/False
(c) affects children's health more than adult health — True/False
(d) is worse in the south of the country than in the north. — True/False

4 Risk-taking behaviour:
(a) is a normal part of growing up — True/False
(b) is more prevalent in young people from low-income families — True/False
(c) includes tattooing and body piercing — True/False
(d) can be reduced by school-based interventions. — True/False

3 Infectious disease and immunology

- Background
- Fever
- Common childhood infections
- Immune deficiency
- Fetal infections
- Meningitis
- Kawasaki disease

Background

Throughout human history infectious diseases have been responsible for more death and morbidity in childhood than any other single cause. Pathogens interact with deprivation, malnutrition, overcrowding and poor sanitation to give rise to human disease. Consequently, economic improvement, planned housing, clean water and sewage disposal are as critical to controlling these diseases as immunisation and antibiotics.

The eradication of smallpox in the 1970s remains the only complete victory of humans over a specific infectious agent. Against this solitary triumph have to be placed the rise in antibiotic-resistant organisms and the emergence of new infections (most notably the human immunodeficiency virus, HIV), as well as the reappearance of conditions such as polio and diphtheria when immunisation rates have fallen. In addition, infections such as gastroenteritis, measles, pneumonia and tuberculosis, which are rarely fatal in Europe or North America, still have high mortality rates in parts of the developing world. Measles has a mortality rate of 30% or more in some areas of Africa.

In the UK, infectious diseases are the commonest reason for a child consulting a primary care physician or being admitted as an emergency to hospital (see Figure 3.1a, b and c). Many such cases are relatively minor viral infections, but they may cause both misery to the child and great anxiety in some families. Serious infections such as bacterial meningitis, herpetic encephalitis or staphylococcal pneumonia occur rarely, but can be fatal or lead to significant disability.

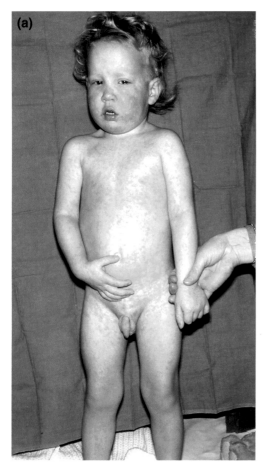

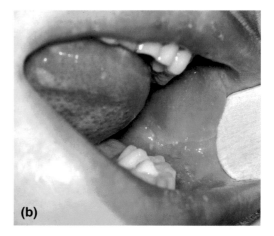

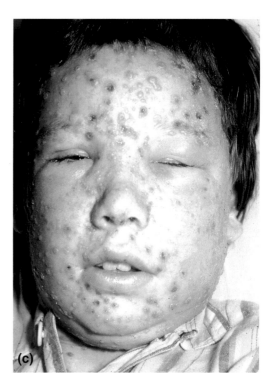

Figure 3.1 Characteristic features of rashes in two infectious diseases. (a) Measles. Note the generalised maculopapular rash with bleary facial appearance and conjunctivitis. (b) Koplik's spots are typically seen inside the mouth, and are described as 'grains of salt'. (c) Chickenpox (varicella). Note the vesicles and the different stages of evolution in the rash, with crusting in some lesions and vesicle formation in others, described as 'cropping'.

Recognition and early aggressive treatment of the child with a serious infection are essential to prevent the rapid deterioration which may occur in such cases. Box 3.1 lists the infectious diseases which must be notified to the Registrar General in the UK.

Fever

Fever is the commonest manifestation of infection, and infection is the commonest cause of fever. Key items in the history are shown in Box 3.2.

The examination starts with inspection. Use the least threatening manoeuvres and watch the reaction. Seriously ill children tend to be pale, floppy

Box 3.1 Notifiable diseases (in the UK)

- Typhoid
- Paratyphoid
- Dysentery
- Food poisoning
- Tuberculosis
- Whooping cough
- Scarlet fever
- Meningitis
- Meningococcal septicaemia

- Tetanus
- Measles
- Mumps
- Rubella
- Viral hepatitis
- Malaria
- Leptospirosis
- Acute encephalitis
- Ophthalmia neonatorum

Box 3.2 History for fever

Symptoms

- Rashes
- Diarrhoea
- Vomiting
- Cough
- Nasal discharge

Background

- Contacts
- Immunisations
- Pets
- Overseas travel
- Malaria prophylaxis

and uninterested, but irritability is important, too. Other important signs are shown in Box 3.3.

Observe whether there is discomfort when some limbs are moved but not others, suggesting a possible local infection in soft tissue, bone or

Box 3.3 Examination for fever

- Posture
- Colour
- Rash
- Respiration
- Ears, nose and throat
- Lymphadenopathy
- Hepatomegaly
- Splenomegaly
- Meningism

joint, and whether the abdomen is soft or if there are areas of guarding. When listening to the chest, remember that in young children, and sometimes in older ones, pneumonia may have no abnormal sounds. When examining the ears for infected tympanic membranes, remember that a crying child will often have infected ears without underlying infection. No examination is complete without seeking signs of meningitis (neck stiffness and photophobia). If there are no focal signs, consider other causes of fever, such as urinary tract infection.

Because serious infections, such as meningitis, may not be easily diagnosed at an early stage, and children can deteriorate rapidly, be prepared to reassess after a short time. Make sure that the family knows who to contact again if they are concerned, and that they are aware of the types of symptoms which they should look out for, such as poor feeding or increasing drowsiness.

Distinctive features of the main viral infections are shown in Table 3.1.

Table 3.1 Features of viral infections

Virus	Features
Measles	Incubation 10–14 days
	Koplik's spots in mouth
	Generalised rash and fever
	Conjunctivitis
	Cough
Mumps	Incubation 14–21 days
	Fever
	Parotid swelling
	May affect pancreas and testes
Rubella	Incubation 14–21 days
	Low-grade fever
	Generalised rash
	Occipital lymph nodes
Herpes simplex	Gingivostomatitis
	Conjunctivitis
	Encephalitis
Varicella (chickenpox)	Incubation 10–21 days
	Generalised itchy rash
	May become infected

All of these infections are very severe in individuals with depressed immunity. Measles, mumps and rubella are now rare in the UK following the introduction of the MMR vaccine.

Case study 1

Fiona, aged 18 months, is the only child of healthy parents in their early thirties. Her father is an engineer in the oil industry who has moved back to the UK after working for 12 months in Abu Dhabi in the Middle East. Apart from uncomplicated chickenpox at the age of 10 months, Fiona has been previously well and is up to date with her immunisations, including BCG. Three weeks after returning to the UK she woke one morning with fever and was much quieter than normal. Her parents were anxious and contacted their new GP. In this case, because she had recently returned from overseas, the history should also include where the family were living and when they returned.

Fiona was not lying with her head retracted suggesting meningismus, nor with her legs pulled over her abdomen suggesting abdominal pain. She was not distressed. There were no rashes, no obvious swellings to suggest a local infection or lymphadenopathy, and no joint swelling. On examination she had a fever of 38°C, and a marked nasal discharge with infected tonsils but no pustules.

Since the examination suggested a viral nasopharyngitis, antibiotics were not prescribed. Fiona was treated with paracetamol, and on review the following day was much recovered.

In this family there was also the question of travel abroad. Abu Dhabi is a very low-risk area for malaria, for which prophylaxis is not routinely recommended. However, malaria should always be considered in anyone with a fever in the first few months after returning from a malarial area. It can present as a flu-like illness, and missing the diagnosis can be lethal. Malaria may not show in the first blood sample, so be prepared to repeat it when the child is febrile if the diagnosis remains uncertain. Another disease which has to be remembered in any child coming from a developing country is tuberculosis, although the onset tends to be rather more insidious than in the case described here, and is also unlikely because the child has had BCG immunisation.

Common childhood infections

Measles

Measles is no longer the common plague in the UK that it was until quite recently. Immunisation has brought the numbers to a low level, although there is always a risk of an epidemic as parents decline the injection due to fear of autism (*see* Chapter 22). In the Third World measles is still a killer, probably because of the high infective dose in an overcrowded environment.

The main features of measles are inflammation of mucous membranes in the mouth, ears, eyes and gastrointestinal tract. Conjunctivitis can be severe, as can diarrhoea, and there is a high level of misery in affected children. Because it is a viral infection, only symptomatic treatment is possible. The most severe complication in this country is encephalitis. Measles is still a killer in immuno-suppressed children in the UK.

Rubella

Rubella (or German measles as it is commonly known) is also much less common than it used to be, due to immunisation. A mild disease in children, the major impact is on the unborn fetus, which may be severely damaged if the mother contracts the disease in pregnancy. Arthritis and encephalitis are possible complications in infected children.

Mumps

This is another viral infection which causes parotid enlargement and pain, which may be uni- or bilateral. Orchitis (inflammation of the testicles) is a possible complication, although it is uncommon. Meningitis occurs in a proportion of cases and is self-limiting.

Varicella (chickenpox)

Chickenpox is characterised by an itchy rash which starts on the scalp or trunk and spreads across the body. There is not usually much systemic upset. The condition is highly infectious until the scabs have dropped off. Encephalitis is a possible complication, and the disease is severe in immuno-suppressed individuals. An effective varicella vaccine is available but is not used routinely.

Herpes simplex

Neonatal herpes is caused by herpes simplex virus (HSV) type 2 as a result of direct contact with maternal genital herpes during delivery.

Later in childhood the agent is HSV type 1, which leads to gingivo-stomatitis. This can be very painful and interferes with eating and drinking. Cold sores are recurrent HSV1 infections. Eye and CNS disease also occurs. Acyclovir administered either topically or systemically is used to treat severe cases.

Infectious mononucleosis (glandular fever)

This is another common viral infection, caused by Epstein–Barr virus, which leads to lymphadenopathy (predominantly cervical), fever, tonsillitis, splenomegaly and sometimes jaundice. Atypical lymphocytes are seen on the blood film, the Monospot test is positive, and there may be persistent fatigue after the acute infection resolves. Treatment is symptomatic.

Impetigo

This is one of the commonest bacterial infections in childhood, caused by *Streptococcus* or *Staphylococcus*. Lesions are usually on the face or hands and become crusted with satellite lesions. It is highly infectious and can spread to other parts of the body. Topical antibiotics are effective, but in severe infections a systemic antibiotic is needed.

Immune deficiency

When a child has recurrent infections, perhaps missing many days of school, parents commonly express concern and feel that 'something must be wrong'. It is always worth exploring what particular 'something' may be worrying the parents. It is not uncommon for parents' true fear to be that their child may have leukaemia, or a condition such as diabetes mellitus, because they have heard that these conditions may present with repeated infections or fever.

A history of uncomplicated chickenpox strongly suggests that cellular immunodeficiency can be ruled out, since varicella can be life-threatening in the presence of immunodeficiency states. The parents can be reassured that the infections are occurring with a normal frequency.

Recurrent upper respiratory tract infections are common in pre-school children, especially those who attend playgroups or the equivalents. Studies have suggested that normal children under the age of 5 years may have at least 6 infections per year, and some as many as 12. Thus it is common to see children who appear to have a permanent 'cold', so short are the gaps between infections. Some children described as having frequent coryzal infections in fact have an allergic rhinitis, but typically they do not have fever.

> **Box 3.4** AIDS (acquired immunodeficiency syndrome)
>
> - Caused by HIV (human immunodeficiency virus).
> - In children there is usually vertical transmission (intrauterine or via breastfeeding).
> - Vertical transmission is minimised by aggressive treatment of the pregnant mother, Caesarean delivery, prophylactic treatment of the baby and avoidance of breastfeeding.
> - HIV seropositivity does not indicate infection < 18/12 due to circulating maternal antibody.
> - Diagnosis is by direct detection of viral genome.
> - Clinical presentation is with lymphadenopathy, recurrent infection and pneumocystis pneumonia.

Given the number of infections in normal children, who should be investigated? A reasonable approach is to reserve investigations for:

- dramatic and very rare situations, such as vaccine-induced polio
- children with two episodes of invasive meningococcal infection or more than one episode of pneumonia within a 12-month period
- any child with recurrent staphylococcal infections such as discharging ears, lymph-node abscesses, skin or other local infections
- infants with intractable diarrhoea, failure to thrive and erythroderma. They may have a severe deficiency of both B- and T-lymphocytes (severe combined immune deficiency syndrome, SCIDS), which can be fatal, but which can be cured by bone-marrow transplantation.

A very severe form of immunodeficiency seen increasingly in children is HIV infection, usually associated with transmission from the mother. The features of AIDS are shown in Box 3.4.

Immunodeficiency states may be primary or secondary. Primary immunodeficiency syndromes vary in incidence from the relatively common (e.g. selective IgA deficiency, with a prevalence of about 1 per 600 of the population) to the extremely rare. The main components of the immune system that need to be considered when planning investigations are shown in Box 3.5.

Box 3.5   Main components of the immune system

- Phagocytosis (both granulocytes and macrophages)
- Immunoglobulins
- Cellular immunity
- The complement system

The specific tests depend on the type of infections being investigated. One of the commonest deficiencies relates to IgG subclasses. For example, in a child with recurrent pneumonia due to *Streptococcus pneumoniae*, the possibility of IgG_2 deficiency should be considered because the bacterial wall of these organisms generates antibodies in the IgG_2 subclass. Measurement of total immunoglobulin levels alone will often not show up a subclass deficiency. Some of the main primary and secondary immune deficiency states are listed in Box 3.6.

Box 3.6   Some immunodeficiency states

Primary

- Selective IgA deficiency
- IgG subclass deficiencies
- Cyclic neutropenia
- Agammaglobulinaemia (X-linked)
- Severe combined immune deficiency syndrome (SCIDS)
- Deficiency of complement

Secondary

- Acquired immunodeficiency syndrome (AIDS) (*see* Box 3.4)
- Chemotherapy for cancer
- Anti-rejection treatment for transplants
- Steroid treatment

Fetal infections

Fevers with rash are common in childhood, and the main concern is whether the organism might be capable of affecting the fetus if the child's pregnant mother contracts the infection. The acronym *TORCH* (*see* Box 3.7) covers many of the important pathogens that may affect the fetus. The range of effects varies widely between infections, and the timing of infection during pregnancy is also important in determining the outcome.

Box 3.7   Organisms that can affect the fetus (TORCH)

- **T**oxoplasma
- **O**ther (syphilis)
- **R**ubella
- **C**ytomegalovirus
- **H**erpes

also

- Parvovirus B19

Cytomegalovirus (CMV) is the most important pathogen in public health terms, because it is a common pathogen among children and there is no effective immunisation. The hazard is greatest for pregnant workers in day-nurseries and healthcare, since they may be exposed to droplet spread from young children who are experiencing their first CMV infection, which is commonly coryzal.

It is the possibility of rubella that causes most concern and diagnostic problems, but with near universal vaccination, congenital rubella is now very rare indeed in the UK except in populations such as refugees. The clinical diagnosis of rubella is unreliable and must be confirmed by serology.

Toxoplasmosis is also rare. Other pathogens that seldom infect the fetus, but which may be transmitted perinatally, are HIV, hepatitis B and hepatitis C (*see* Chapter 17).

Meningitis

The onset of meningitis does not discriminate it from other infections. Altered level of consciousness, irritability, presentation with a seizure and the presence of a rash are all pointers to the need to consider meningitis as a possible diagnosis (*see* Box 3.8 and Case study 2). Neck stiffness is the classical sign in meningitis, but may be absent in early infancy or masked by anti-convulsant medication. Inability to straight leg raise is rarely helpful under the age of 18 months. Although meningismus without meningitis may be found in some children with other infections (e.g. tonsillitis), a lumbar puncture must be performed. The arguments for delaying or even omitting lumbar puncture are covered in Chapter 8. The different types of meningitis that occur in children are shown in Box 3.9, and CSF findings in Table 3.2.

As well as examination of the cerebrospinal fluid (CSF), it is important to culture blood and urine. If there is a purpuric rash (*see* Figure 3.2), it is possible to prick the lesion with a lancet or needle to produce a small blob of serum or blood

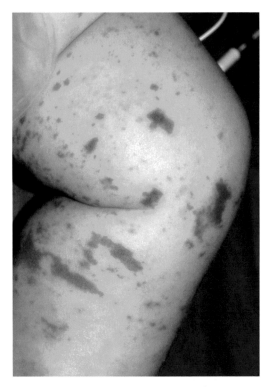

Figure 3.2 Typical purpuric rash of meningo-coccal septicaemia.

Box 3.8 Meningococcal infection: summary

- Rapid onset.
- High case fatality rate.
- Purpuric rash.
- Decreased level of consciousness.
- Septicaemia without meningitis has the highest mortality.
- Thrombotic complications compromise digits and limbs.
- Pre-hospital penicillin may be life-saving.
- Meningitic cases need audiological follow-up.

Box 3.9 Types of bacterial meningitis

Age	Types
Under 3 months	Group B streptococcus *Escherichia coli* *Listeria monocytogenes*
1 month–6 years	*Neisseria meningitidis* (*see* Box 3.8) *Streptococcus pneumoniae*
Over 6 years	*Streptococcus pneumoniae* *Neisseria meningitidis*

Haemophilus influenzae type b and *Neisseria meningitidis* group C are rare causes since the introduction of immunisation. Viral meningitis is usually caused by an enterovirus or Epstein–Barr virus. It can occur at any age and is usually less severe than bacterial meningitis.

which can be both cultured and examined with a Gram stain for meningococci.

Urinary tract infections should always be considered, and at this age are more common in boys than in girls, sometimes presenting as a severely ill infant with septicaemia. Urine culture is important, and to avoid delays in starting treatment or missing the diagnosis a suprapubic bladder tap is sometimes indicated in children under 1 year of age.

Since the only sign of pneumonia may be fever, a chest X-ray is also indicated. Additional investigations might include a full blood count with white cell differential, electrolytes (for biochemical evidence of dehydration), blood glucose (to check for hypoglycaemia and to compare with the value in the cerebrospinal fluid) and blood gases (if there is a possibility of respiratory failure). C-reactive protein (CRP) or erythrocyte sedimentation rate (ESR) may be measured as markers of an inflammatory process, but of the two the ESR is slower to rise. Neither CRP nor ESR should be elevated in a viral infection.

The length of the antibiotic course in meningitis depends on the organism, but in the case of meningococcal infection is usually about 7 days. It should be followed by rifampicin to clear carriage because:

- the infection does not confer immunity

- the treatment itself may not clear carriage

- re-infection can occur even in immunologically normal children.

Dexamethasone is given to reduce the risk of complications such as deafness, but it has to be given immediately before the antibiotics to be effective.

Close contacts also need rifampicin to try to clear carriage of the organism, and this is normally the responsibility of public health authorities. Rifampicin in four doses is currently the most widely used prophylaxis, but a single dose of ceftriaxone is an effective alternative. Penicillin is not effective in clearing carriage.

Meningococcal infection has a significant mortality rate. Meningococcal septicaemia in the absence of meningitis carries a worse prognosis than when it coexists with meningitis. In this situation, the virulence of the infection is such that the patient presents during the initial septicaemic phase before the organism has penetrated the CSF. Additional poor prognostic features are low white cell count and thrombocytopenia.

In a serious life-threatening situation, such as bacterial meningitis, communication with the parents is of central importance. Parents cope better when they have some understanding of what meningitis means, the nature of the treatment, and the most common short- and long-term complications. Individual parents often have different ways of coping and different requirements from their respective partner, so it is important to speak to both parents and answer their very different questions and concerns. It is also helpful to provide written information.

Hearing impairment is an important complication. Transient deafness may occur during the initial few weeks, or there may be permanent sensorineural loss. Children should therefore undergo formal audiological assessment.

Table 3.2 Cerebrospinal fluid findings in meningitis

	Cells	Protein	Glucose
Normal	$< 2 \times 10^6/l$	< 0.05 g/l	> 40% blood glucose
Bacterial meningitis	Neutrophils	Raised	< 40% blood glucose
Viral meningitis	Lymphocytes	Normal	Normal

Case study 2

Fiona's baby brother is christened James at 3 months of age. A few hours after the service he is noted to be febrile and he vomits his evening feed. He is unsettled and remains feverish overnight. The following morning he vomits twice further and refuses all feeds. When the GP comes to see him she notes a rectal temperature of 39°C but is unable to find any focus of infection. While she is in the home James has a generalised clonic-tonic seizure that lasts approximately 2 minutes. He is given rectal diazepam and referred as an emergency to the local paediatric department.

James has had a fit in association with a fever. It is not a simple febrile convulsion because he is too young (*see* Chapter 8), and other diagnoses must be sought. On arrival at the Accident and Emergency department he is febrile, pale, hypotonic, and irritable on handling. He is now an ill, infected infant who needs urgent examination, investigation and treatment. The history is focused on the presenting condition – details of the family history and social background can wait.

Examination is directed towards confirming or excluding meningitis. Are there signs of meningismus or the presence of purpura (*see* Figure 3.2)? Is the fontanelle open and, if so, is it full or tense? One has to be cautious with this, as the fontanelle may bulge if the infant is crying. A high-pitched cry and irritability on handling may be the only signs suggesting meningitis.

After a rapid examination, an intravenous bolus of saline is given, together with dexamethasone and the first dose of antibiotics. As James stabilises quickly, a lumbar puncture is performed, which shows turbid fluid. A few purpuric lesions appear on the foot prior to lumbar puncture.

The cerebrospinal fluid (CSF) shows a white cell count of 500×10^6/l (all neutrophils with no red cells). The CSF glucose concentration is 0.8 mmol/l (blood glucose 4.1 mmol/l), and the protein concentration is 9.1 g/l. Gram staining shows Gram-negative diplococci, but the antigen test is negative for meningococcus. The circulating neutrophil count is 23.4×10^9/l with a platelet count of 560×10^9/l.

The diagnosis was *meningococcal meningitis* on the basis of the culture of CSF and blood. The antigen test is often negative. The differentiation of bacterial and viral meningitis is usually possible on the basis of the cell count together with protein and glucose levels (*see* Table 3.2). If there is any doubt, it is safer to treat the condition as a bacterial meningitis.

James is treated with an intravenous third-generation cephalosporin for 7 days, and with dexamethasone for 2 days.

Three months later, he is reviewed for neurodevelopmental progress, which is normal. His parents want to know whether he could contract meningitis again. There can be no guarantee that he will not get meningitis again, even with the same organism, although probably not within *Haemophilus influenzae*, against which he has had routine immunisation (*see* Chapter 22, page 334). However, meningitis of any cause is rare.

Kawasaki disease

This unusual but distinctive infection affects children from 6 months to 4 years of age. It is more common in children of Asian background than in Caucasians. It is thought to be caused by a bacterial toxin that acts as a superantigen. The disease leads to a vasculitis which affects small vessels, including the coronary arteries, leading to aneurysms. These are visible on echocardiography. There may also be gastrointestinal symptoms and meningitis. *See* Box 3.10 for other clinical features. Treatment is with intravenous immunoglobulin and with aspirin to reduce the risk of thrombosis.

Further reading

- Davies EG, Elliman DAC, Hart CA, Nicoll A and Rudd PT (2001) *Manual of Childhood Infections*. WB Saunders, London.

- Health Protection Agency www.hpa.org.uk

- NHS Immunisation www.immunisation.nhs.uk

Box 3.10 Clinical features of Kawasaki disease: summary

- Persistent high fever for over 5 days
- Sterile conjunctivitis
- Macular rash
- Hands and feet may be swollen and red
- Inflamed mouth and tongue
- Cervical lymph node enlargement
- Peeling of skin of fingers and toes during resolution

Self-assessment questions

1 Meningitis:
(a) in early infancy is usually caused by *Neisseria* species   True/False
(b) *Haemophilus influenzae* causes most cases in early childhood   True/False
(c) may be accompanied by a purpuric rash   True/False
(d) may lead to sensorineural deafness   True/False
(e) leads to a low level of glucose in the cerebrospinal fluid.   True/False

2 Among infectious diseases:
(a) whooping cough is notifiable   True/False
(b) rubella is common   True/False
(c) varicella is treatable   True/False
(d) cytomegalovirus can infect the fetus   True/False
(e) *Toxoplasma* is a bacterium.   True/False

3 Measles:
(a) is an important cause of death in developing countries   True/False
(b) is curable with antibiotics   True/False
(c) has been eradicated in the UK   True/False
(d) is associated with eye disease   True/False
(e) is effectively prevented by vaccination.   True/False

4 In a child with fever:
(a) convulsions are common over the age of 5 years   True/False
(b) paracetamol is effective in reducing temperature   True/False
(c) the commonest cause is a viral infection   True/False
(d) temperature reduction will reduce the chance of a convulsion   True/False
(e) malaria could not be the cause in the UK.   True/False

4 Gastrointestinal disorders and nutrition

- Development and structure of the gut
- Function of the gut
- Gastrointestinal symptoms: history and examination
- Nutritional requirements in childhood
- Acute infective diarrhoea
- Chronic diarrhoea
- Inflammatory bowel disease
- Vomiting in infancy
- Recurrent abdominal pain
- Persistent neonatal jaundice
- Growth faltering
- Malnutrition
- Constipation and faecal soiling
- Hirschsprung's disease

Gastrointestinal problems are among the most common seen both in general practice and in hospital. Enteric infections are not only a major cause of morbidity in the UK, but worldwide may cause approximately 2.5 million deaths in children under 5 years old each year. This enormous mortality is entirely preventable, as it is caused by a lack of clean drinking water and inadequate sewage disposal.

Problems such as recurrent abdominal pain, chronic diarrhoea and constipation, and failure to thrive, although rarely life-threatening, occur very commonly in children and form a major part of the workload of paediatricians.

Disease of the gastrointestinal tract and the ability of the child to digest and absorb nutrients and grow normally are very closely linked. Therefore the assessment of any child with

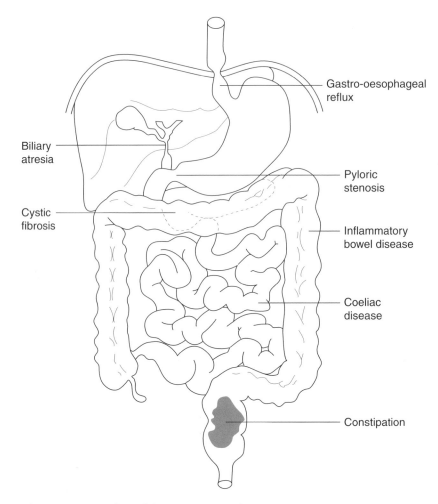

Figure 4.1   Disorders of the gastrointestinal tract.

gastrointestinal disease requires a knowledge both of their nutritional intake and of their growth (*see* Figure 4.1).

Development and structure of the gut

The embryonic foregut gives rise to the oesophagus, stomach, upper duodenum, liver and pancreas. The mid-gut extends from the lower duodenum to the distal third of the transverse colon, and the hind gut extends from there to the anus. The primitive gut undergoes rapid elongation and extension through the umbilical orifice between 5 and 10 weeks, and subsequently between 10 and 12 weeks the gut returns to the abdominal cavity. Failure of this process results in exomphalos (*see* Chapter 17). The gut undergoes a counter-clockwise rotation through 270 degrees, which leaves the small intestine positioned centrally with the caecum in the right iliac fossa and the colon lying in a lateral position. The failure of this process, called *malrotation*, can lead to torsion or obstruction of the gut in the neonatal period or infancy, and presents as a surgical emergency (*see* Chapter 18).

Function of the gut

Digestion occurs in two phases. There is an initial intraluminal phase during which pancreatic enzymes break down large macromolecules into smaller units which are further digested by brush-border enzymes into small molecules that can be directly absorbed. Most nutrients can be absorbed anywhere along the length of the small intestine, although vitamin B_{12} and bile salts can only be absorbed from the terminal ileum. Food which is not digested passes into the colon, where excess fluid is reabsorbed, and the semi-solid waste is passed as stool through the anus. When digestion is impaired for any reason, the clinical presentation usually includes diarrhoea and poor growth.

Disturbances of the normal movement of food through the gastrointestinal tract may also occur if there is disordered nervous and muscular control of intestinal function, as in the immature preterm infant, or in children with cerebral palsy or other severe brain insult. Problems include difficulty with swallowing, regurgitation of food from the stomach, and constipation.

The gastrointestinal tract also has a very important immune function. It protects the body from the passage of bacteria and viruses through the wall of the gut, and develops tolerance to foreign proteins which are commonly found in ingested food. Failure of these mechanisms can lead to chronic intestinal infection or the development of food intolerance.

There is a link between 'psyche' and 'soma' in gut function, and this is as true in children as it is in adults. The commonest manifestation is with recurrent abdominal pain, sometimes associated with vomiting ('periodic syndrome'), which occurs in school-age children in association with emotional triggers such as bullying, anxiety over parental stress, or exams.

In young children, food refusal or oppositional behaviour with toilet training may be used as a means of asserting independence, and can cause significant degrees of family disruption.

Gastrointestinal symptoms: history and examination

Common gastrointestinal symptoms are listed in Table 4.1. The likely cause of each symptom will depend on the age of the child. An accurate history of the timing of symptoms relative to the ingestion of food is very important. Symptoms apparently related to the gastrointestinal tract may arise from disease elsewhere. For example, vomiting may be a symptom of infection, poisoning or head injury, and abdominal pain may occur in a child with pneumonia or diabetic ketoacidosis.

Accurate assessment of the child's height and weight is important, and with the aid of previous

Table 4.1 Common gastrointestinal symptoms

Symptom	Cause	Age
Acute diarrhoea	Acute gastroenteritis	Any age
Chronic diarrhoea	Toddler's diarrhoea	6 months–5 years
	Food allergy	4 weeks–5 years
	Post gastroenteritis	Any age
	Coeliac disease	> 6 months
	Cystic fibrosis	Any age
Vomiting (effortless)	Gastro-oesophageal reflux	0–1 year (developmentally normal) Any age (developmentally abnormal)
Vomiting (short onset)	Infection	Any age
	Pyloric stenosis	1–4 months
	Poisoning	Any age
	Head injury	Any age
	Metabolic disease	Any age

Table 4.1 Continued

Symptom	Cause	Age
Abdominal pain	'Irritable bowel syndrome'	2 years–adulthood
	Constipation	Any age
	Food allergy	Any age
	Urine infection	Any age
	Peptic ulcer	5 years–adulthood
	Inflammatory bowel disease	5 years–adulthood
Constipation	Idiopathic	1–12 years
	Hirschsprung's disease	0–6 months
Jaundice (unconjugated)	Breast milk	0–6 months
	Hypothyroidism	0–6 months
Jaundice (conjugated)	Biliary atresia	0–1 years
	Hepatitis syndrome	0–2 years
	Infectious hepatitis	Any age

measurements (if available) a centile chart (*see* Figure 15.5, page 226) should be used to assess whether the child is growing appropriately for his or her sex, ethnic origin and parental size. The timing of growth failure may give important clues. For example, poor weight gain from birth may relate either to a feeding problem (with reduced intake) or to a disease such as cystic fibrosis. However, in coeliac disease, gastro-intestinal symptoms do not develop until after gluten has been introduced into the diet around the middle of the first year. A list of physical signs and their clinical significance is given in Table 4.2.

Table 4.2 Physical signs and clinical significance on abdominal examination

Physical sign	Clinical significance
Abdominal mass	Faecal mass in constipation
	Hydronephrosis
	Renal/suprarenal tumour
	Crohn's disease
Splenomegaly	Haemolytic disease
	Neoplastic disease
	Portal hypertension
Hepatomegaly	Chronic liver disease
	Neoplastic disease
	Storage disease
Anal fissure	Chronic constipation
	Crohn's disease
Ascites	Hepatic cirrhosis
	Nephrotic syndrome
Abdominal distension	Air swallowing
	Malabsorption

Nutritional requirements in childhood (*see also* Chapter 1)

The early stages of life are characterised by rapid growth and development and consequently, if the needs of the child are not met, failure to gain weight will occur very quickly and will be followed a few months later by failure of linear growth. The energy requirements of a newborn infant can exceed 120 kcal/kg/day (0.5 MJ/kg/day), compared with the adult, whose basal requirements are only about 40 kcal/kg/day (0.17 MJ/kg/day). Similarly, the protein requirements of the newborn infant are probably double those of the adult. Energy requirements are increased in children with cardiac or respiratory disease (where there is increased work of breathing), in children with malabsorption (where there is a loss of nutrients in the stool) and in children with major trauma and severe infection.

Box 4.1   Causes of gastroenteritis

Viruses
- Rotavirus
- Adenovirus
- Astrovirus
- Small round viruses

Bacteria
- *Campylobacter* sp.
- *Salmonella* sp.
- *Escherichia coli*
- *Shigella* sp.

Acute infective diarrhoea

Acute diarrhoea is a very common problem in young children. The causes are listed in Box 4.1. The most widespread pathogen is rotavirus (*see* Figure 4.2), and over 60% of cases are associated

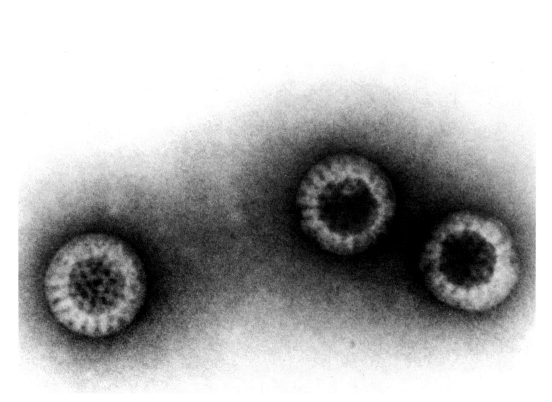

Figure 4.2   Electron micrograph of a rotavirus. (With thanks to Dr David A Gregory.)

with viral infections, although bacterial pathogens are more common in older children. Other features of acute gastroenteritis are the development of vomiting and fever, and other family members often have similar symptoms. In young children, symptoms may be more severe because the immature gut of the young child seems to be more susceptible to infection, particularly in children who have not been breastfed, and fluid loss from diarrhoea can quickly lead to dehydration. Pre-existing malnutrition greatly increases the risk of death from gastroenteritis.

Dehydration is assessed clinically by looking for a sunken anterior fontanelle and reduced skin turgor (see Table 4.3). The simplest treatment for mild to moderate dehydration, in the absence of persistent vomiting, is an oral rehydration fluid. The World Health Organization (WHO) rehydration solution contains sodium (75 mmol/l) and glucose (75 mmol/l), and through the action of a

Table 4.3   Clinical signs of dehydration

Dehydration level	Sign
2–3%	Thirst
5%	Increased thirst
	Reduced skin turgor
	Sunken fontanelle
	Sunken eyes
	Oliguria
10%	All above features *plus*
	Hypotension
	Tachycardia
	Peripheral shutdown
	Apathy
15%	All above features *plus*
	Coma
	Anuria

sodium/glucose co-transport protein on the brush border it greatly facilitates the absorption of water and electrolytes by the gut. As most enteric infections are self-limiting, this allows the child to be rehydrated and supported without the need for intravenous therapy. Commercial solutions for use in the UK are slightly more dilute than this, but the principle is the same (see Box 4.2).

Treatment with antibiotics is only very rarely indicated when the cause is bacterial, and anti-diarrhoeal drugs should never be used. Traditionally, it has always been taught that children with diarrhoea should be fasted and gradually re-graded back on to feeds. It is now known that this strategy prolongs their illness, and following rehydration there is no good reason for withholding solid or liquid food once a child feels like eating. Breastfed infants should continue to feed during the rehydration process.

In children with more severe dehydration, and in cases where vomiting prevents the use of oral rehydration solution, intravenous fluids are required. In the shocked child, a rapid infusion of isotonic saline may be needed. Most dehydrated children have a normal serum sodium concentration, but if the child has received overconcentrated feeds there is a risk of hypernatraemia, and great care is needed in the rehydration of these children, as rapid electrolyte shifts may lead to convulsions.

Most children make a complete recovery from acute gastroenteritis over a few days, although it is quite common for loose stools to persist for weeks after the acute illness. However, in some young children, damage to the gut may lead to the development of a transient lactose intolerance or sensitisation to cow's-milk protein. This also leads to prolonged diarrhoea accompanied by poor weight gain, and the use of a diet free of milk (i.e. hypoallergenic feed) may be indicated. In older children, dehydration develops less commonly, but diarrhoea may be complicated by blood in the stool, and with some strains of *E. coli* (e.g. *E. coli* type 157) the release of a toxin may cause haemolytic uraemic syndrome, which can progress to acute renal failure.

> **Box 4.2** Management of diarrhoea
>
> - Assess hydration.
>
> - Continue breastfeeding; stop milk feeds during rehydration (3–6 hours).
>
> - Continue solids if wished.
>
> - Give oral rehydration solution.
>
> - Do not give antibiotics unless a specific pathogen is identified.
>
> - Do not give antidiarrhoeal drugs.
>
> - Inform the parents of signs that would indicate dehydration.

Chronic diarrhoea

It is difficult to know exactly what bowel frequency is normal in young children, as there is great variation in stool consistency, frequency and sometimes also colour. Prior to toilet training, when the parents are able to observe the stool readily, a lot of anxiety can be generated if the stool does not conform to their perception of what is normal. One of the commonest causes of chronic diarrhoea in this age group is a benign condition called 'toddler diarrhoea'. The child is very well and growing entirely normally, does not appear ill, yet passes stools which are often very loose and watery, and which sometimes contain undigested food matter, in particular peas and carrots. The diagnosis can ususally be made from the history, but it is important that both past and present weights are accurately plotted on a growth chart so that normal growth can be confirmed. This may need a subsequent appointment to demonstrate normal weight gain. The family need explanation and reassurance that there is no serious underlying cause of the loose stools, that their child will almost certainly become toilet trained at the normal age, and that this condition does not delay the attainment of continence.

If the child is not thriving or atypical features are present, there is a need for a detailed dietary history and investigations as for growth faltering (*see* Boxes 4.10 and 4.11). Typical growth patterns for coeliac disease and cystic fibrosis are shown in Figure 4.3.

Inflammatory bowel disease

This term comprises the conditions Crohn's disease and ulcerative colitis, which present with diarrhoea, abdominal pain, weight loss and rectal bleeding. Crohn's disease normally affects the distal ileum and proximal colon, whereas ulcerative colitis can affect any part of the colon. Other features are shown in Box 4.5.

> **Box 4.3** Causes of chronic diarrhoea
>
> - 'Toddler diarrhoea'
>
> - Post-gastroenteritis lactose intolerance
>
> - Cow's-milk protein intolerance
>
> - Malabsorption:
>   - Cystic fibrosis (*see* page 78)
>   - Coeliac disease (*see* Box 4.4 and Figure 4.4)

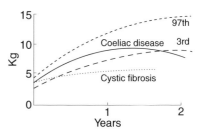

Figure 4.3 Comparison of the pattern of growth in coeliac disease and cystic fibrosis.

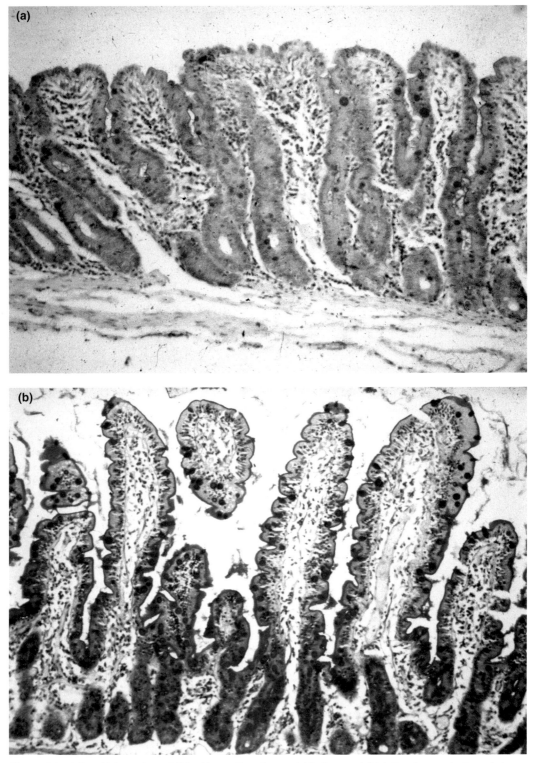

Figure 4.4 Jejunal biopsy in a child with coeliac disease (a) before and (b) following exclusion of gluten from the diet.

Box 4.4 Coeliac disease

- Sub-total villous atrophy develops following the ingestion of gluten in the diet (*see* Figure 4.4).
- It classically develops at about 9–12 months with weight loss and fatty stools.
- This presentation is now uncommon due to the general reduction in the gluten load in infants' diets.
- Children present as toddlers with more vague symptoms such as anaemia, poor weight gain or loose stools.
- Many patients are now diagnosed by screening at-risk groups (e.g. diabetes, Down syndrome).
- The condition can be cured by treating with a gluten-free diet.

Box 4.5 Features of inflammatory bowel disease

Crohn's disease
- Presents with abdominal pain, diarrhoea and weight loss, but this may be insidious.
- Non-gastrointestinal features are characteristic, including oral ulcers, intermittent fever, arthritis and uveitis.
- There may be finger clubbing.
- Diagnosed by barium follow-through, colonoscopy and biopsy.
- Treat with systemic steroids and sulphasalazine.
- Recurrence is common, and it may require surgery.

Ulcerative colitis
- Presents with bloody diarrhoea, usually in teenagers.
- Symptoms are mainly gastrointestinal.
- Rectum is always affected.
- Increased risk of malignancy in adult life.
- Diagnosis and treatment are as for Crohn's disease.

Vomiting in infancy

In a child who is otherwise well with a long history of regurgitation, the most likely diagnosis is gastro-oesophageal reflux. This condition arises due to the immaturity of the lower oesophageal sphincter, which allows the free regurgitation of milk in the young child. This is so common as to be normal in young children, but it may be a source of anxiety for the parents.

When the condition is more severe, the child may lose ingested calories and fail to gain weight, or the regurgitation may cause painful oesophagitis or lead to aspiration of gastric contents. Severe reflux is often seen in children with cerebral palsy, who may aspirate because of the lack of a cough reflex. In most cases, diagnosis is based on the history. The presence of reflux may be confirmed by a barium meal or more accurately by a 24-hour oesophageal pH study (*see* Figure 4.5).

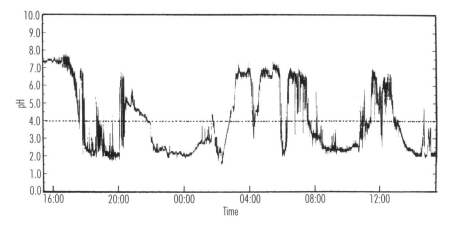

Figure 4.5 A segment of a 24-hour pH study showing prolonged episodes of reflux below a pH of 4.

Table 4.4   Treatment of gastro-oesophageal reflux

Symptom	Treatment
Mild reflux	Reassure parents *or* Feed-thickeners (Vitaquick or Carobel)
Moderate reflux	Feed-thickeners Alginates (Gaviscon) Prokinetic drugs (Domperidone)
Reflux with oesophagitis	H_2-blockers (ranitidine) added to the above
Failure of medical treatment with the development of complications	Surgery (wrap or fundoplication)

The presence of oesophagitis can be assessed at oesophagoscopy. Investigations are only needed in more severe cases or if complications are suspected.

The treatment of children with troublesome reflux is outlined in Table 4.4.

In an infant under 3 months old, with vomiting that develops acutely and leads to the development of dehydration and hypochloraemia, one should consider the possibility of pyloric stenosis (*see* Figure 4.6 and Box 4.6). This occurs most

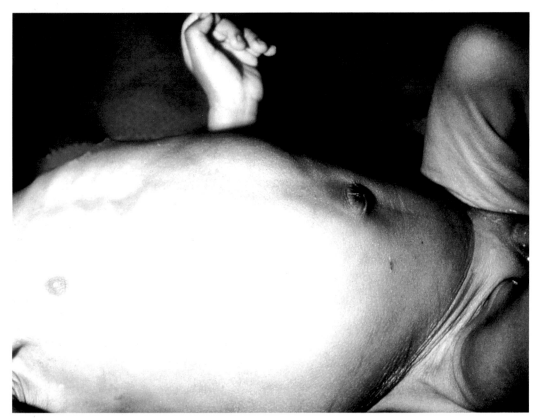

Figure 4.6   In pyloric stenosis, visible peristalsis is sometimes seen as 'golf balls' rolling across the upper abdomen from left to right. Note the visible peristalsis to the right of the midline and the obvious wasting in this infant.

commonly in males in the first month or two of life, and can be diagnosed clinically by a test feed which reveals a pyloric tumour on abdominal palpation. If the vomit contains bile, urgent assessment by a paediatric surgeon is needed. Vomiting may also be a symptom of any infection, and is a feature of metabolic disease, cardiac failure, poisoning and raised intracranial pressure.

Box 4.7 lists the differential diagnosis of vomiting in infancy.

Case study 1

Dawn, a 2-month-old infant, was breastfed for 2 weeks and was then transferred to the bottle because her mother had sore nipples. Her mother brought her to see the GP because of vomiting. She had a history of effortless regurgitation occurring almost immediately after feeds. Despite this she seemed to be a happy baby, and her regular weight checks showed normal growth. The vomit was at all times free of blood, and she did not have a cough or noisy breathing.

As Dawn was thriving well, her mother was advised to add a thickening agent to her milk feeds, and this resulted in some reduction in her regurgitation. Her mother was also reassured that Dawn's gastro-oesophageal reflux would probably get better as her diet became more solid and as she developed a more upright posture.

Box 4.6 Pyloric stenosis

- Projectile vomiting 2–3 weeks after birth
- No bile in vomit
- Associated weight loss and constipation
- Diagnosed by clinical examination
- Cured by surgery (pyloromyotomy)

Recurrent abdominal pain

Recurrent abdominal pain may affect up to 10% of children, and in many it is a manifestation of stress or distress. Where physical causes have

---

Box 4.7 Differential diagnosis of vomiting in infancy

- Overfeeding
- Oesophageal reflux – effortless vomiting from birth
- Pyloric stenosis – projectile vomiting from 2–3 weeks after birth (male predominance)
- Gastroenteritis (associated with diarrhoea)
- Bowel obstruction (e.g. intestinal atresia leads to bile-stained vomitus and abdominal distension)
- Metabolic disease (family history, acidosis)

---

been ruled out it is sometimes called 'periodic syndrome', and a full psychosocial evaluation will often reveal its origin. In some children the ingestion of particular foods may lead to abdominal pain, but in many no clear physical cause can be found. The periodic syndrome is essentially a diagnosis of exclusion, although the features are quite characteristic in the presence of emotional turmoil. If the child's abdominal examination, full blood count, erythrocyte sedimentation rate, urea and electrolytes, urine culture and abdominal ultrasound are all normal, and there is a normal pattern of growth, this will rule out most major pathologies.

If the pain is largely epigastric, associated with wakening at night or a positive family history of ulcer disease, the diagnosis of duodenal ulceration or *Helicobacter pylori* gastritis should be considered, and if the abdominal pain is associated with diarrhoea or the passage of blood in the stool, inflammatory bowel disease should be excluded. The common causes are listed in Box 4.8.

The basis for treatment of periodic syndrome is to recognise the factors that are causing and aggravating the abdominal pain and to try to eliminate them. In Case study 2 (overleaf) this involved alleviation of a stressful situation at school. In children with constipation, this condition should be treated with laxatives, or if it is suspected that certain foods are initiating the abdominal pain, a trial of dietary exclusions should be considered. Very often the uncertainty of not knowing what is causing the pain creates alarm in both the parent and the child, and reassurance may in itself help to alleviate the child's symptoms.

Box 4.8 Some important causes of recurrent abdominal pain

- 'Periodic syndrome'
- Stress (bullying, abuse)
- Depression
- Abdominal migraine
- Duodenal ulcer – pain before meals and at night, eased by food, often with a family history
- Inflammatory bowel disease
- Constipation
- Urinary tract infection
- Renal stone
- Gallstones (consider in obese adolescents)

Case study 2

Darren, aged 8 years, was brought to see his GP because of intermittent episodes of abdominal pain. This pain, which occurred two or three times a week, was central abdominal in location and generally colicky in nature. Darren's bowel habit was normal and he seemed to be growing well. On closer questioning, it was revealed that he was quite an anxious child, and his mother reported that his pain did seem to be worse on weekdays, particularly first thing in the morning, but that it was absent over the weekends and during the holidays.

The simple investigations outlined above were all negative, and it transpired that Darren was being bullied at school. Following a discussion with his teacher by Darren's parents, the problems were resolved and his pain slowly improved. He was encouraged to talk to his parents about problems he encountered at school, so as not to internalise them.

Persistent neonatal jaundice (see also Chapter 17, page 268)

Jaundice in early infancy should be taken seriously even if it is mild. The commonest cause is related to breastfeeding – the bilirubin is unconjugated and no specific treatment is required. If the bilirubin is conjugated, there is almost always serious pathology. Pale stools and dark urine suggest biliary obstruction, especially if the urine is positive for bilirubin on dipstick testing.

The most serious disease, which needs to be diagnosed within the first 8 weeks if treatment is to be successful, is biliary atresia. The diagnosis of biliary atresia is confirmed by a combination of liver biopsy, abdominal ultrasound and an isotope excretion scan. The treatment is a surgical porto-enterostomy (otherwise known as the Kasai procedure).

If surgery is unsuccessful, a progressive biliary cirrhosis leading to liver failure develops. Other pathologies which may present with conjugated jaundice, but which are not amenable to surgery, include metabolic disturbance (e.g. alpha-1-antitrypsin deficiency) and chronic viral infections. Often no specific cause can be found.

See Box 4.9 for a differential diagnosis of persistent jaundice.

Box 4.9 Differential diagnosis of persistent jaundice

First check whether the jaundice is due to conjugated (bilirubin in urine, pale stools and blood test) or unconjugated hyperbilirubinaemia.

Unconjugated
- Breast-milk jaundice
- Hypothyroidism
- ABO or rhesus incompatibility

Conjugated
- Biliary atresia
- Neonatal hepatitis
- Congenital infection
- Alpha-1-antitrypsin deficiency

Case study 3

At a 6-week check, Mary was noted by her GP to be jaundiced with yellow sclera. She was an otherwise healthy breastfed baby who had grown normally and fed well from birth. Her mother had noticed that she had dark urine and pale stools. The GP referred her urgently to hospital, where she was admitted for investigation when it was found that her bilirubin level was elevated at 120 micromol/l, and more than half of this was conjugated. The excretion scan showed delay, so Mary was referred to a centre with experience in paediatric hepatic surgery. A liver biopsy confirmed the diagnosis of biliary atresia. A Kasai operation was successful, and Mary's jaundice cleared within a few weeks as she made a good recovery.

Growth faltering

Failure to gain weight in infancy (formerly known as failure to thrive, and now termed growth faltering) is a common presentation, but can be complex to manage as it requires close attention to social, emotional, nutritional and medical factors. Assessment and management require a team approach. Most cases are not due to a 'medical' condition, and most often a combination of social, emotional and dietary factors is responsible, all resulting in deficient calorie intake (see Box 4.10). A multidisciplinary approach is needed, and it is essential that full attention is given to the support of the parents. In a small number of cases growth faltering may be a presentation of child abuse, and social services input should be sought.

Weight gain should be closely monitored in infants, especially those with feeding difficulty, and the weight should be charted on the centile chart kept in the personal child health record. Large babies may catch down in weight to their genetic centile, and the 6–8 week centile is a better predictor of weight at 1 year than the birth weight.

Investigation often requires an assessment by a paediatric dietitian as well as observation of feeding at home. It is taken for granted that bringing up a baby is something that comes naturally to most mothers. However, some mothers will have had negative experiences with their own parents, and in cases where the mother is young, single or unsupported, where there is evidence of parental mental illness or there are other major tensions within the family, good parenting can be impaired. The most important aspect of the history of a child who fails to gain weight is the dietary intake, and only when this has been confirmed to be normal should other causes be sought. The core medical investigations are listed in Box 4.11.

Box 4.10 Growth faltering

Definition

- A fall-off in weight across two centile lines on a 9 centile chart, related to the baseline at 6–8 weeks and lasting over a month.

Differential diagnosis

- Inadequate intake
  - Feeding mismanagement
  - Mechanical difficulty (e.g. cerebral palsy)

- Excessive losses
  - Vomiting
  - Diarrhoea
  - Malabsorption
  - Cow's-milk protein intolerance
  - Cystic fibrosis
  - Coeliac disease

- Increased requirements
  - Severe cardiac disease
  - Severe respiratory disease

- Failure of utilisation
  - Metabolic or liver disease

Box 4.11   Core investigations in growth faltering

- Urine microscopy for bacteriuria
- Blood pressure
- Urea, creatinine and electrolytes
- Full blood count
- Stool culture if there is chronic diarrhoea
- Sweat test for cystic fibrosis
- Endomesial antibodies for coeliac disease
- Immunoglobulins
- Chest X-ray if there are respiratory symptoms

Case study 4

Gemma, a 9-month-old infant, had been noted by her health visitor to be growing poorly, and had fallen from the 50th centile at 6 weeks of age to just below the 3rd centile. Her mother, Jill, aged 19 years, was a single parent living on her own in a council house with very little support. She had no relatives in the vicinity, did not now see the baby's father and was on income support. The health visitor had been concerned about the baby's feeding pattern. Gemma was prone to upper respiratory tract infections, and had had two episodes of diarrhoea, during which her mother was advised to stop feeding solids. Jill found her baby difficult to care for and frequently took her to the GP, who enlisted the help of the community paediatrician.

Gemma was assessed in the GP surgery by the community paediatrician and the health visitor together. The health visitor reported that Jill had a warm relationship with Gemma, but was short-tempered and did not have patience with her at mealtimes. Gemma was not an easy feeder, she was fussy about solids, and she cried a lot. Jill ate irregularly herself and Gemma followed this pattern. Jill had no one who could take Gemma for short periods to give her a break. Currently Gemma had no diarrhoea or vomiting, but she did have a mild upper respiratory tract infection. On examination she was found to be thin but well cared for. She did not appear pale, and there was no abdominal distension. The paediatrician decided to perform limited outpatient investigations.

An assessment by the community dietitian showed that Gemma's calorie intake was seriously low, as she had a limited intake of solid foods and could be difficult at mealtimes. Her milk intake was adequate but not her solid food intake, and as she had strong dislikes her mother mainly fed her low-calorie yoghurts and biscuits.

Jill agreed to try to alter her own eating pattern so as to have three regular meals a day, and to introduce a wider variety of high-calorie foods, using her own meals as a basis, with the addition of snacks such as full-cream yoghurt and bananas. She was encouraged to take Gemma to the mother and baby group at the local family centre, where she met other mothers and learned from their experience. A baby-sitting service was also organised through the centre so that she was able to have some evenings out and enjoy a break from baby care.

At follow-up 4 weeks later, Gemma was gaining weight and her mother looked much happier. She was able to develop her own interests through contact with other mothers at the family centre, and was also stimulating Gemma better. It was agreed that the health visitor would continue to monitor Gemma's weight in the baby clinic, and that the dietitian would review Gemma in 2 months' time.

Malnutrition

In the UK, malnutrition now presents mainly as obesity (*see* Chapter 2, page 30), which is increasingly common as well as difficult to treat. Other nutritional presentations seen in the UK include rickets (mainly in children of Indian and Pakistani origin) (*see* Box 4.12) and iron-deficiency anaemia (*see* Chapter 16).

Box 4.12 Nutritional rickets

- Deficient intake of vitamin D (dietary deficiency and lack of sunlight).
- Also occurs in metabolic disorders.
- Presents with misery, frontal bossing, rickety rosary (expansion of costochondral junction), bow legs and poor weight gain.
- Low calcium and phosphate and high alkaline phosphatase levels.
- Treated with oral supplements of vitamin D and with sunlight.

Internationally the commonest types of malnutrition are marasmus and kwashiorkor, conditions which would not occur if there was a fairer distribution of food between rich and poor countries and within poor countries. In both marasmus and kwashiorkor there is a deficiency of energy,

---

Box 4.13 Kwashiorkor and marasmus

Kwashiorkor
- Dependant oedema
- Skin changes
- Poor appetite
- Hypoglycaemia
- Hypothermia
- Diarrhoea

Marasmus
- Marked wasting without oedema
- No skin changes or metabolic derangement
- Child is usually hungry
- Characteristic picture in famine situations

---

although kwashiorkor tends to be more acute, with metabolic derangements and a high mortality rate (*see* Box 4.13).

Constipation and faecal soiling (encopresis) (*see also* Chapter 12)

Constipation

This is a surprisingly common presentation in infancy and early childhood, perhaps related to changing diets, with a higher proportion of more refined and convenience foods which have a low fibre content. However, there is also a considerable behavioural element in constipation. Children in the oppositional age range may use refusal to use the toilet as a way of getting their own way, while in some families the daily passage of a motion is seen as the key to good health, and therefore parental pressure to perform can be considerable. The relationship with diet is a close one, and increasing fibre and fluid content is the best way of relieving constipation.

It is important to take a good history to ensure that there is a common understanding of constipation by the doctor and the parent. Constipation is not present unless there is both infrequency of stool and difficulty in passage. The ideal frequency is not well known, but lies between daily and every 3–4 days.

Constipation is treated with diet, stool softeners and laxatives. However, the prolonged use of the latter is undesirable (*see* Box 4.14).

Box 4.14 Treatment of constipation

- Increase fluid intake (preferably water, not fizzy drinks).
- Aim for '5 a day' (five portions of fruit and/or vegetables daily).
- Increase fibre intake through wheat-based cereal (e.g. Weetabix) and wholemeal bread.
- Prune juice.
- Stool softener (e.g. lactulose).
- Laxative (e.g. senna) (this should be a last resort).

Soiling

This condition is stressful to the family and can be difficult to treat. Psychological factors are present in all cases, although they are not always causal. There is chronic constipation, and subsequently faeces impact in the rectum, with overflow incontinence. The initial constipation is compounded by the fact that defecation is painful, and this sometimes leads to the development of anal fissures with bleeding. The discomfort on passing stools often leads to the development of a toilet phobia, with further retention leading to continued constipation. With time, distension of the bowel leads to insensitivity of the rectum, and liquid stool from above bypasses the impacted rectum, leading to overflow and incontinence (see Figure 4.7).

Abdominal examination usually reveals palpable faeces in a loaded colon, and examination of the anus externally is often normal. With high doses of senna and lactulose the bowel will often empty, but if this does not work an admission may be necessary to disimpact the loaded bowel by the use of large volumes of fluid given through a nasogastric tube. The parents have to be helped to encourage more regular toileting, but if there is great fear of defecation, the expertise of a child psychologist may be needed. A 'star chart' and incentives can be used. In the long term, a high-roughage diet is helpful, and if further episodes of constipation develop they can be treated quickly with courses of oral laxatives.

Hirschsprung's disease

Most cases of simple constipation resolve quickly with treatment, but if the problem is allowed to continue for a prolonged period or if the child is not motivated to get better (as often occurs in children with developmental or psychological problems), the soiling may become chronic and relapse is likely. In addition, in a small number of children, abnormalities of the enteric nerves in the bowel may be found. The most severe form of this type of problem is known as Hirschsprung's disease, where there is aganglionosis which frequently leads to a presentation with constipation and intestinal obstruction in the first few weeks of life (see Box 4.15). However, Hirschsprung's disease usually presents in infancy and is rarely associated with faecal retention and overflow in mid-childhood. Occasionally, a rectal biopsy may be required to exclude aganglionosis in intractable cases.

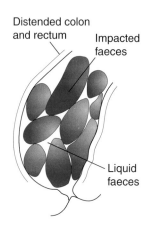

Distended colon and rectum

Impacted faeces

Liquid faeces

Figure 4.7 Faecal retention with overflow.

Box 4.15 Hirschsprung's disease

- Absence of ganglion cells from myenteric and sub-mucosal plexus of part of the large bowel.

- Presents in the neonatal period with intestinal obstruction.

- Associated with abdominal distension and bile-stained vomiting.

- Can present in later childhood with constipation, abdominal distension and growth failure, but no soiling.

- Investigation is by rectal biopsy.

- Requires surgery – colostomy followed by bypass.

Further reading

- Bisset WM (2003) Disorders of the alimentary tract and liver. In: N McIntosh, PJ Helms and SL Smyth (eds) *Textbook of Paediatrics* (6e). Churchill Livingstone, Edinburgh.

- Kelly DA (2003) *Disease of the Liver and Biliary System in Children*. Blackwell Publishing, Oxford.
- Walker-Smith JA and Murch S (1999) *Disease of the Small Intestine in Childhood*. Taylor and Francis, London.

Self-assessment questions

1 Pyloric stenosis:
(a) occurs in young infants   True/False
(b) may give rise to hypokalaemia   True/False
(c) has a characteristically palpable pyloric tumour   True/False
(d) has bile-stained vomiting   True/False
(e) causes rectal bleeding.   True/False

2 Diarrhoea:
(a) can be a completely benign symptom in toddlers   True/False
(b) when acute should be treated by stopping all oral intake   True/False
(c) may contain blood, if acute and caused by bacteria   True/False
(d) when acute is frequently caused by rotavirus   True/False
(e) is a major global cause of infant death.   True/False

3 In a child with abdominal pain:
(a) central pain is likely to be organic   True/False
(b) urine microscopy should be performed   True/False
(c) somatisation is commonly related to school difficulties   True/False
(d) threadworm is a common cause   True/False
(e) admission to hospital is necessary.   True/False

4 Growth faltering:
(a) requires a growth chart for diagnosis   True/False
(b) is suggestive of child abuse   True/False
(c) requires admission to hospital for treatment   True/False
(d) is usually due to calorie deficiency   True/False
(e) occurs most commonly in infancy.   True/False

5 Respiratory disorders

- Epidemiology of respiratory illness
- Normal and abnormal lung growth and development
- Chest signs
- Stridor and upper airway obstruction
- Asthma and wheezing illness
- Lower respiratory tract infections
- Cystic fibrosis
- Sudden infant death syndrome (SIDS)

Epidemiology of respiratory illness

Respiratory disease is the single commonest cause of admission to medical paediatric beds in industrialised countries and, alongside acute gastroenteritis (World Health Organization estimates), the commonest cause of death in the poorer countries of the world. In the under-5-year-old age group alone it has been estimated that more than 700 children die each day from acute respiratory infections (ARI) (*see* Figure 5.1).

Risk factors for serious morbidity and death are well known, and some are potentially remediable (*see* Box 5.1).

Although the agents responsible are somewhat different, with more bacterial infections causing problems in poorer countries, viral lower respiratory tract infections are common, particularly in infancy. Every year a predictable and remarkably constant winter epidemic of virally induced bronchiolitis, often caused by the respiratory syncytial virus, affects each new cohort of young infants (*see* Figure 5.2).

A remarkable feature in developed countries has been the rise in acute wheezing illness and asthma alongside an increase in atopic disease (*see* Figure 5.3).

This increase has yet to be explained, but possible culprits include indoor (house dust mite and gas cookers) and outdoor (car and industrial) air pollution, passive smoking and changes in the diet (low intake of vitamin C and other antioxidants and high intake of processed fats) and

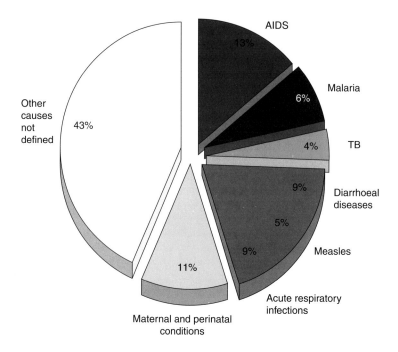

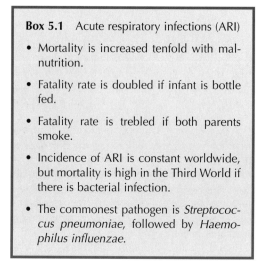

Figure 5.1   Child deaths (0–4 years) worldwide by main cause (data from the World Health Organization). Other causes not defined (43%) include accidents and unknown causes.

> **Box 5.1**   Acute respiratory infections (ARI)
>
> • Mortality is increased tenfold with malnutrition.
>
> • Fatality rate is doubled if infant is bottle fed.
>
> • Fatality rate is trebled if both parents smoke.
>
> • Incidence of ARI is constant worldwide, but mortality is high in the Third World if there is bacterial infection.
>
> • The commonest pathogen is *Streptococcus pneumoniae*, followed by *Haemophilus influenzae*.

reduced early exposure to infections, particularly gastrointestinal infections (the hygiene hypothesis). To a certain extent it may also be attributable to changes in diagnostic fashion, as what was once referred to as 'wheezy bronchitis' or 'lower respiratory tract infection' is now more likely to be labelled as asthma. However, this is unlikely to explain all of the observed increases, as allergic diseases, especially eczema and hay fever, have also increased.

Normal and abnormal lung growth and development

The lungs develop from the ventral part of the primitive foregut at approximately 8 weeks of gestational age, and airway development is complete by 16 weeks. Alveolar development commences at approximately 18–20 weeks, and it is this factor that is largely responsible for the limits of viability at approximately 22–24 weeks. Any disturbance to the ordered sequence of lung development can result in a range of congenital anatomical abnormalities, including pulmonary hypoplasia and a range of lung cysts and malformations.

The transition from liquid to air breathing is assisted by rapid lung liquid clearance via the lymphatic system and the vaginal thoracic squeeze during delivery. In some infants, lung liquid clearance is delayed, resulting in transient

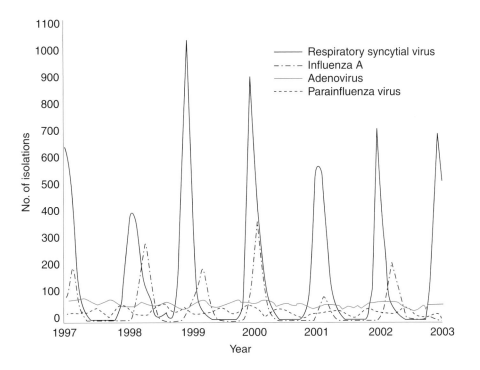

Figure 5.2 Epidemiology of respiratory syncytial virus, influenza A, adenovirus and parainfluenza virus in the Netherlands, 1997–2003. From van Woensel *et al.* (2003) *BMJ.* **327**: 36–40.

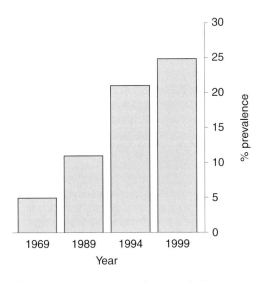

Figure 5.3 Changes in the population prevalence of asthma and atopic disease in Aberdeen schoolchildren between 1969 and 1999.

tachypnoea of the newborn (wet lung) (*see* Chapter 17). The pliable chest wall supports the lung relatively poorly in the first 1 to 2 years of life, and this results in poor peripheral airway function and an increased risk of airway obstruction.

In the premature infant, this feature is further complicated by poor production of surfactant and collapse of periperal lung units (*see* Chapter 17). Boys have functionally narrower airways than girls up to puberty, and this may in part explain the observed male preponderance of lower respiratory symptoms, including asthma, in pre-pubertal boys.

In addition to the important developmental considerations outlined above, significant infections and insults in early childhood may have lifelong consequences for adult respiratory health. These influences may even extend back to the intrauterine period. For example, smoking during pregnancy is associated with increased respiratory morbidity in early infancy.

Chest signs

The soft and flexible chest wall in the infant and very young child distorts when it is exposed to increased respiratory loads (e.g. in a wheezy baby). If the obstruction is mild, a groove adjacent to the lower rib-cage and anterolateral abdominal boundary appears with every inspiratory effort (*sub-costal recession*). As in the adult, suprasternal and intercostal recession may be seen, but in severely affected infants and young children under 2 years of age, *sternal recession* may also be evident. If the respiratory problem is prolonged, a more permanent deformation of the rib-cage is seen, with a groove or flattening of the lower chest wall – the so-called *Harrison's sulcus*, named after its first British observer. If the problem is associated with air trapping and hyperinflation, the forceful contraction of the diaphragm and associated increased anteroposterior thoracic dimension results in the so-called *pigeon chest* or pectus carinatum (*see* Figure 5.4).

Hyperinflation, as seen for example in acute asthma or bronchiolitis, also results in diaphragmatic depression and downward displacement of the liver, and is detected clinically as an increased anteroposterior dimension of the thorax, lack of cardiac dullness on percussion of the anterior chest, and an easily palpable liver edge. Care must be taken not to over-diagnose cardiac failure in the presence of respiratory disease, as fine crackles (crepitations) and an easily palpable liver edge are often found in acute infantile bronchiolitis, and crackles with or without wheeze are not infrequently found in pre-pubertal children with asthma. Cyanosis and nasal flaring are always signs of significant lower respiratory tract disease.

Noisy breathing

In acute upper airway obstruction associated with croup, for example, inspiratory stridor may be audible from the end of the bed, and in acute lower airway obstruction, expiratory wheeze will often be audible without the use of a stethoscope. It is always important to distinguish between upper and lower repiratory tract noises, as parents and untrained observers often find this difficult.

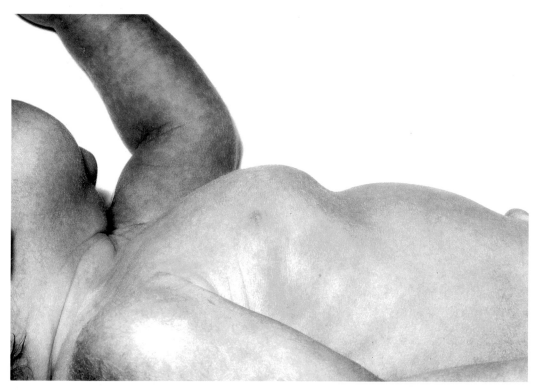

Figure 5.4   'Pigeon chest' (pectus carinatum) in an infant with severe lung disease of prematurity.

Table 5.1 Differentiation of upper airway obstruction

Croup (laryngotracheobronchitis)	Epiglottitis	Foreign body
Slow onset (2–3 days)	Rapid onset (< 24 hours)	No prodrome
Loud inspiratory stridor	Often quiet breath sounds	Sudden onset – often during unsupervised play
Well-looking child	Ill-looking child – pale	Coughing
Well-perfused	Poor perfusion	Unusual below 6 months
Low-grade fever	Toxic	
6 months–7 years	Drooling saliva	
	6 months–5 years	

Stridor and upper airway obstruction

Croup is the presenting symptom of upper airway obstruction and is always frightening to parents. The name 'croup' refers to the noise made by the child when breathing in, but also refers to the condition that most commonly causes this symptom, otherwise known as laryngotracheobronchitis, a viral infection.

Acute laryngotracheobronchitis can be difficult for parents and their family doctor to assess, and as a consequence many affected children are referred to hospital for a brief period of observation (see Table 5.1 and Box 5.2).

Box 5.2 Indications for admission for croup

- Possible foreign body or epiglottitis
- Severe chest wall recession
- Parents unable to cope

In any child with acute upper airway obstruction it is dangerous to examine the throat or to perform X-ray imaging, as the manipulation required may precipitate complete obstruction. A calm and confident approach is required, together with appropriate symptomatic therapy. Croup often worsens in the late afternoon and evening, and in severe cases it is wise to admit the child and observe them overnight. Traditionally treatment involves humidification of the inspired air using a bedside device. Systemic steroids hasten resolution (see Box 5.3). If obstruction is severe and epiglottitis or an inhaled foreign body is a possibility, an ENT surgeon and consultant anaesthetist should be alerted prior to the child's arrival. *Children with severe obstruction should be taken immediately to theatre and examined under anaesthetic and intubated.* As a temporising measure, nebulised adrenaline may give short-term relief, but with later rebound obstruction. Antibiotic therapy is mandatory for epiglottitis, and broad-spectrum cephalosporins are now commonly used, as many *Haemophilus influenzae* organisms are resistant to ampicillin. Although the number of cases has decreased since the introduction of *Haemophilus influenzae* type B (HIB) immunisation (see Chapter 22), recent evidence shows a resurgence that has resulted in recommendation for a pre-school booster programme.

Box 5.3 Management of croup

- Calm reassurance
- Humidification of inspired air
- In severe cases, consider nebulised adrenaline and systemic steroids

---

Case study 1

John, now aged 18 months, was born at term and was breastfed for the first 4 months. He has had an unremarkable development so far. He has had his triple (diphtheria, tetanus and polio) and HIB (*Haemophilus influenzae* type B) immunisations at 2, 3 and 4 months, and has recently received his measles, mumps and rubella immunisation. He has been in excellent health. Over the past 3–4 days he has developed upper respiratory signs of cough and runny nose, and over the past 12 hours his parents have noted a rasping cough which they describe as a 'bark like a sea-lion'. They have also noticed increased respiratory distress, and have observed that John's chest is now see-sawing up and down alarmingly. His parents have had a dreadful night and are extremely anxious. The GP deputising service was consulted in the early hours of the morning, and in view of the increasing respiratory distress of the child and the obvious anxiety of both parents, hospital assessment has been requested.

This is a common acute paediatric problem, and the history is very suggestive of croup or acute laryngotracheobronchitis. The differential diagnosis includes an inhaled foreign body and epiglottitis (*see* Table 5.1). Epiglottitis is *usually* associated with a more rapid onset, quiet respiration and a sick, pale-looking infant with or without drooling of saliva (a consequence of the acutely inflamed and swollen epiglottis). Although John is in the appropriate age group for an inhaled foreign body, this is unlikely as the onset was not sudden.

On observation, John is tired and irritable but can be diverted into play for at least a short period. He has marked subcostal and sternal recession and an easily audible high-pitched inspiratory stridor. A working diagnosis of croup is made. It is possible to manage mild croup at home, but as his parents are exhausted after their broken night, the symptoms are worsening, and John has features of respiratory distress, he is admitted to hospital.

Asthma and wheezing illness

Asthma is now the commonest chronic disease of childhood in developed countries. The reasons for its increased incidence along with related allergic conditions of eczema and rhinitis (hay fever) remain elusive (*see* page 289). Most children present with their first episode of wheezing before 3 years of age, and features that increase the risk of persistence of the disease through childhood into adulthood include coexistent allergy, severe episodes, female sex and taking up smoking. The diagnosis is based on the clinical features, among which documentation of wheezing heard on auscultation of the chest is key, together with typical symptoms of night cough and exacerbation of symptoms on exercise.

Management of acute episodes of asthma

Although acute hypoxaemia and death are unusual in children, with only about 20 child deaths each year in the UK, the prevalence of asthma has been rising (*see* Figure 5.3). These features may in part be explained by a lower diagnostic threshold and the use of effective prophylactic therapy, particularly inhaled corticosteroids (ICS).

The mainstay of acute asthma management remains bronchodilator therapy with beta-agonists either alone or in combination with ipratropium, and this may be required every 10–15 minutes until symptoms improve. Short courses (2–5 days) of systemic steroids are also indicated. Regular and frequent reassessment is needed in order to identify impending respiratory failure and the need for ventilatory support. The presence of hypoxaemia, inability to speak and pulsus paradoxus (defined as a fall in systolic blood pressure of > 10 mmHg during inspiration) are all important signs of severe disease and impending respiratory failure, and can be used in the assessment of severity (*see* Box 5.4).

Box 5.4 Signs of acute asthma

Acute severe asthma
- Too breathless to talk
- Too breathless to feed
- Respiration $\geqslant$ 50 breaths/minute
- Pulse $\geqslant$ 140 beats/minute
- Peak flow $\leqslant$ 50% of predicted or best value

Life-threatening features
- Peak flow < 33% of predicted or best value
- Cyanosis, silent chest or poor respiratory effort
- Fatigue or exhaustion
- Agitation or reduced levels of consciousness
- Pulsus paradoxus

Source: *British National Formulary (BNF) guidelines.*

Hypoxaemia must be dealt with as soon as possible, and nebulised drugs should always be driven with oxygen rather than with compressed air. In the presence of severe disease, rapid administration of appropriate drugs is required (*see* Table 5.2).

An objective assessment of severity can be made using arterial blood gas estimation, but this is reserved for children with severe disease in whom ventilation is being considered. As asthma improves it is common to find so-called 'early-morning dips' in peak expiratory flow rates, a feature that is also seen in poorly controlled asthma and that may require more intensive therapy, particularly in the evenings.

Management of chronic asthma

Most children, whatever their age, can be established on inhaled relievers (β_2-agonists) and preventers (inhaled steroids) by employing an age-appropriate delivery system. Infants and very young children can usually be established on aerosols and low-volume spacers, and older

Table 5.2 Treatment of acute asthma: summary

At home	*In hospital*
• Short-acting β_2-stimulant from metered-dose inhaler using large-volume spacer device may be as effective as use of nebuliser; dose is one puff every few seconds until improvement occurs (maximum 20 puffs), using face mask in very young children	• Short-acting β-agonist by nebuliser
	• Reassess every 10 minutes plus oral steroids
• Terbutaline may be given subcutaneously in severe episodes	• If child is too breathless, commence IV hydrocortisone
• Oxygen is of benefit	• Slow (10 minute) bolus of IV aminophylline, but halve dose if already taking oral xanthines
• A child who requires high-dose inhaled bronchodilators should also receive soluble tablets, prednisolone 1–2 mg/kg (maximum 40 mg) once daily for up to 5 days if necessary; child needs immediate referral to hospital if fails to respond	• Infusion of β-agonist may be used in addition for very severe cases
	• Oxygen is mandatory
• Aminophylline should no longer be used in children at home	

Source: *British National Formulary (BNF) guidelines.*

children on dry-powder devices or aerosols and standard spacers, although aerosols and spacers are the delivery systems of choice.

Long-term asthma management needs to be reconsidered in any child with increasing symptoms and with an acute life-threatening episode. Whereas intermittent bronchodilator therapy is adequate for very mild intermittent symptoms, once bronchodilator therapy is being used symptomatically more than twice a week, prophylactic therapy is indicated.

It is essential to check inhaler technique and use age-appropriate delivery devices (aerosol and spacers for the majority) (see Figure 5.5), adding a long-acting β-agonist and introducing other prophylactic medicines such as cysteinyl leukotriene antagonists or low-dose theophylline preparations if necessary. It must be remembered that many 'treatment failures' are due to poor adherence to recommended therapy.

The condition often remits in later childhood, particularly in boys. It is important to review children on prophylaxis at regular intervals so that attempts can be made to step down the treatment as the disease comes under control. High doses of inhaled steroids (see British Asthma guidelines at www.brit-thoracic.org.uk/sign/) should be avoided as systemic effects can occur, including adrenal suppression and subtle effects on growth and the skeletal system. However, in severe episodes systemic steroids are life-saving.

Many parents have concerns about possible side-effects of inhaled steroids on growth and bone metabolism, and they can be reassured that the doses used to control the vast majority of children (up to 400 μg of beclometasone or the equivalent per day) have no long-term effects.

Most asthma is managed by the primary care team, and specially trained 'asthma nurses' can significantly improve quality of life for affected individuals and their families. Community asthma clinics provide opportunities for patient education, including training in and monitoring of inhaler technique. Hospital clinics should be reserved for the 1–2% of severe or 'brittle' asthmatics, some of whom will require open access to hospital, and for the differential diagnosis of those with atypical features.

Exercise-induced symptoms are common, and can often be reduced by pre-treatment with a β-agonist. It is essential to allow the schoolchild with asthma to have access to their own inhaler, and to ensure that teachers feel supported.

The presence of atopic disease (asthma, hay fever and/or eczema) in first-degree relatives and its precipitation by a variety of circumstances, and not just by intercurrent viral upper respiratory tract infections, increases the likelihood of symptoms continuing into adult life. Measures to reduce household dust, particularly in the bedroom, may be of benefit in known atopic children.

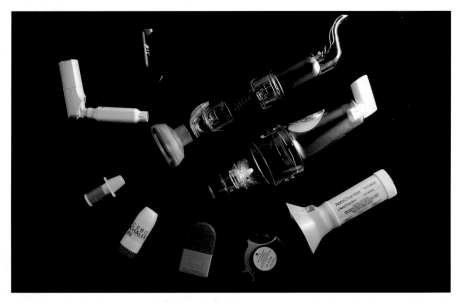

Figure 5.5 A range of devices and spacers for delivering aerosolised and dry powder anti-asthma medication.

Case study 2

Mhairi, aged 11 years, has a 5-year history of recurrent coughs and colds with breathlessness, and presents to the Accident and Emergency department distressed and too breathless to speak. She was first diagnosed as having asthma at the age of 8 years, and is currently using a dry-powder β-agonist inhaler for symptomatic relief. She has never been to hospital before, but both parents describe a gradual increase in the number of episodes so that she has been using her rescue (β-agonist) inhaler up to 2–3 times per week over the past 3 months. Her maternal uncle has asthma and her father has hay fever (he also had asthma as a child). Mhairi is a keen hockey player and her parents describe her distress at having to stop playing on occasion because of her episodes of wheezing.

On arrival, Mhairi is given nebulised salbutamol driven by oxygen rather than air because her oxygen saturation is 75% in air. An intravenous infusion is established and intravenous hydrocortisone is administered. A calm reassuring approach is adopted, and as soon as the nebulised salbutamol has finished, physical examination reveals a central trachea, chest hyperinflation, with an increased anteroposterior diameter (approximately equal to the transverse diameter), and a slightly peaked sternum. Mhairi has no nasal flaring but obvious intercostal recession and tracheal tug. On palpation of the radial pulse it appears to disappear on inspiration. Her oxygen saturation has risen to 90% in 100% oxygen, and she is now able to speak in short sentences. She is admitted to the ward.

Mhairi's treatment needs a full review before discharge, as her asthma is clearly not well controlled.

Lower respiratory tract infections

Pneumonia

Bacterial pneumonia is extremely common in developing countries but less so in developed countries. This is because of the association with poverty, overcrowding and passive smoking. The range of pathogens is remarkably similar across the globe, with *Streptococcus pneumoniae* being the commonest bacterial agent and respiratory syncytial virus (RSV) the commonest viral pathogen (*see* section on bronchiolitis below). Opportunistic pathogens (e.g. *Pneumocystis*) and tuberculosis are emerging in high-risk populations such as drug users and individuals with HIV infection.

Table 5.3   Pneumonia/lower respiratory tract infections

Infection type	At-risk groups
Bacterial	
Streptococcus pneumoniae	All ages
Haemophilus influenzae	Toddlers – becoming less common
Staphylococcus aureus	Uncommon – more in older children
Mycoplasma	School-age children
Tuberculosis	Rare in developed countries – risk increased in AIDS
Viral	
Respiratory syncytial virus	Mainly in infants
Parainfluenza virus types 1 and 3	Common at all ages
Influenza A and B	Common at all ages

Antibiotics are life-saving, and although widely used in the UK are rarely required, as the majority of lower respiratory tract infections are due to common respiratory viruses (*see* Table 5.3).

Clinical features

In addition to the classical features of cyanosis, chest and intercostal recession and nasal flaring, respiratory rate is a useful clinical feature, and in developing countries a respiratory rate of 50 breaths/minute or more is an indication for antibiotic use. The presence of wheezing can also be a useful sign, as this is rarely associated with bacterial pneumonia. As in many respiratory diseases in pre-pubertal children, male:female ratios are approximately 1.5:1, which may in part reflect differences in airway growth and development between the sexes. Other risk factors include passive exposure to cigarette smoke and in particular maternal smoking during pregnancy. It has been estimated that 10–15% of all paediatric hospital beds could be closed if parental smoking could be reduced to negligible levels.

Community-acquired pneumonia (CAP) typically presents after a brief prodromal pyrexial illness that progresses to an irritable unproductive cough with or without pleuritic chest pain. A high-grade pyrexia ($> 39°C$) is common unless the subject is immunosuppressed. Tachypnoea is usual, and the typical signs of lobar pneumonia may be evident, including localised bronchial breathing and crackles on auscultation.

CAP usually responds rapidly to first-line antibiotic therapy, penicillin or erythromycin, and resolves without long-term sequelae. Erythromycin is a good choice, although the gastric irritation often associated with its use occasionally makes it unpopular with patients. This problem can be avoided by using a second-generation macrolide such as clarithromycin. For children with more severe disease and who require admission to hospital, third-generation cephalosporins such as cefotaxime are indicated. A rare but well-recognised complication is empyema, which can be managed either conservatively with intrapleural urokinase (a fibrinolytic agent) or surgically (*see* Table 5.4).

After a single episode pneumonia is unlikely to recur unless there is an underlying problem such as gastro-oesphageal reflux, immune deficiency, a congenital lung anomaly (e.g. a lung cyst), ciliary dyskinesia or cystic fibrosis. Any child who has recurrent episodes or continuing symptoms (e.g. cough and sputum production) needs to have cystic fibrosis (CF) excluded, which at 1 in 2000 live births remains the single commonest recessively inherited disorder in Caucasian populations. Evidence of bronchiectasis with chronic radiological changes, particularly in the mid to upper zones, requires exclusion of CF (*see* page 78).

Associated failure to thrive and gastrointestinal symptoms would suggest undiagnosed CF. The finding of *Pseudomonas aeruginosa* in infected sputum is virtually pathognomonic of CF.

Table 5.4 Management of pneumonia

At home	In hospital
Antipyretics (most are viral)	Supplemental oxygen (if required)
Need for hospital referral based on clinical features (e.g. tachypnoea, cyanosis, poor feeding, pain)	Adequate hydration
Penicillin or macrolide (e.g. clarithromycin)	Cephalosporin (e.g. cefotaxime)
	Mobilisation of secretions (only if present)
	Consider atypical infections (e.g. *Mycoplasma*, *Chlamydia*)
	Consider drainage of empyema if present

Case study 3

John, aged 10 years, comes home from school early complaining of feeling hot and generally unwell. During the course of the evening he develops an irritable dry cough and pain in his left lower chest, which is more noticeable on breathing in. He is not cyanosed, but is tachypnoeic (25 breaths/minute) and has a central temperature of 39°C. Percussion note is slightly reduced at the left base. John is started on oral erythromycin with paracetamol 6-hourly as required, and his mother is instructed to re-contact the surgery if he fails to improve.

Next morning John is no better and his mother has noted that he is more breathless and that his left-sided chest pain is worse. She takes him to the surgery, where his doctor finds slight but definite tracheal descent and intercostal recession with quite definite dullness to percussion over the left posterior chest, with bronchial breath sounds and increased vocal resonance. He diagnoses lobar pneumonia and refers John to hospital, where a chest X-ray shows increased radiodensity in the left, mid and lower zone, consistent with the diagnosis. Blood cultures and a full blood count are taken, and an intravenous line is set up and a cephalosporin antibiotic commenced. Over the next 3 days, John's temperature slowly settles and his chest signs resolve, although at discharge on day 4 he still has dullness to percussion at the left base. Oral antibiotics are continued for a further 10 days.

Bronchiolitis

Bronchiolitis is a form of viral pneumonia that predominantly affects infants and which occurs in epidemics in the winter season (*see* Figure 5.2). Around 10–20% of affected infants and young children will have significant lower respiratory signs and symptoms, and 1% will require hospital admission. The peak incidence occurs in the third month of life, and although many adults and older children are affected, the symptoms are less severe.

The natural history of acute bronchiolitis typically exhibits a gradual worsening over a period of several days. A viral cause can often be established soon after admission (RSV immunofluorescence is usually available within a few hours of

Box 5.5 Features of bronchiolitis

- Winter epidemics
- Peak incidence at 2–4 months
- Respiratory syncytial virus (RSV) in 70% of cases
- Around 90% of all children acquire RSV before the age of 2 years
- High morbidity/low mortality (in developed countries)
- Bronchodilators are usually ineffective

pharyngeal aspirate being obtained). Antibiotics are not required, as secondary bacterial infection (particularly in developed countries) is rare. Other viral pathogens include parainfluenza viruses 1 and 3 and influenza A and B (*see* Figure 5.2 and Table 5.3).

Apart from exposure to environmental tobacco smoke, other risk factors include premature birth, immunodeficiency states and disrupted host defence.

Treatment of bronchiolitis

Bronchodilators are often given, usually by the nebulised route, with a variable response to β-agonists and ipratropium bromide. In infants under 6 months of age, bronchodilators are usually ineffective as most of the airflow obstruction is due to mucous plugging and mucosal oedema. Systemic steroids and high-dose inhaled steroids have also been shown to be of no benefit in the acute phase, but they may have a role in those infants who wheeze during the months following an acute episode. Despite the often severe airflow obstruction, very few infants require respiratory support. For a small number of high-risk infants the antiviral agent ribavirin may have a role in modifying the natural history of the disease by inhibiting viral replication. The roles of specific anti-RSV immunoglobulin and monoclonal RSV antibody in reducing disease risk and severity in high-risk infants, and when administered before each epidemic season, remain controversial (and they are extremely expensive).

Prognosis

Approximately 50% of affected infants continue with wheezing episodes over the next 6–12 months, often precipitated by intercurrent upper respiratory tract viral infections. In some of these infants this will be the first presentation of asthma, and this becomes more likely if there is a family history of atopic disease, particularly on the mother's part. The parents should be given an optimistic long-term prognosis for the child, as the majority of wheezing illness in infants and pre-school children resolves spontaneously later in childhood. Vaccination against RSV is not yet available.

Case study 4

Calum, aged 4 months, presents in mid-January with a history of increasing breathlessness over the past 24 hours. He has moderate chest wall recession and a wheezy cough, and is now unable to take bottle feeds.

Chest auscultation reveals high-pitched expiratory wheeze and showers of fine crepitations over all areas of his chest.

On examination, Calum is tachypnoeic at 60 breaths/minute, with subcostal recession and absence of cardiac dullness on percussion of the anterior chest wall. He also has a soft, easily palpable liver edge 5 cm below the costal margin. He has a dusky appearance, and pulse oximetry confirms hypoxaemia with an oxygen saturation in air of 85%, correcting to 95% in 40% oxygen. Calum is admitted to hospital, a chest X-ray reveals hyperinflation with areas of collapse/consolidation in the right upper and left lower zones, and nasopharyngeal aspirate is positive on immunofluorescence for RSV. Supplemental oxygen is required for the next 2 days together with nasogastric feeding. On day 3 Calum's respiratory rate has fallen to 30 breaths/minute and he begins to feed on his own. He is discharged home on day 5, although he still has a residual wheeze.

Tuberculosis

In a world context, tuberculosis is a major respiratory health problem that accounts for 20–30 million deaths per year. With the emergence of AIDS and multiple resistant organisms, the disease is becoming more prevalent in developed countries. Primary infection is usually pulmonary, and its early diagnosis requires a high level of suspicion. It should be considered in high-risk settings, in children at risk of AIDS (e.g. those with a drug-abusing mother), in children on immunosuppressive drugs for autoimmune disorders or cancer, and in children from mobile communities with a high risk of endemic disease.

Populations at increased risk include those from the Indian subcontinent, Central and East Africa and South-East Asia. Immunisation in the first week of life is recommended in high-risk communities, and affords up to 70% protection from the most damaging presentation of tuberculous meningitis (TBM). Routine immunisation of schoolchildren between 12 and 14 years of age remains the policy in the UK, but this may have to be revised if early disease becomes more widespread and more common.

Primary infection is by droplet spread, and may occur in the lung, skin or gut. This infection spreads to the local lymph nodes and forms the primary complex. Most of these complexes heal by fibrosis over the next 1 to 2 years, and some may calcify. The development of TBM is predominantly seen in infants. TBM has a poor prognosis and is a cogent reason for immunisation in the neonatal period in endemic areas and/or in high-risk populations.

Cystic fibrosis

Cystic fibrosis is a recessively inherited disorder for which the causative gene has been identified. The prevalence is approximately 1 in 2000 live births, with a carriage rate of 1:20 in the Caucasian population.

The primary defect is dehydrated and sticky mucus which affects both the lungs and the pancreas, leading to the presenting features of frequent infections and malabsorption (see Table 5.5).

A diagnosis of cystic fibrosis should be considered in any child with a history of chronic respiratory symptoms. However, with increasing awareness of this condition and the introduction of screening at birth by blood spot immuno-reactive trypsin (IRT), most new cases in those countries that undertake universal screening (including the UK) are now being diagnosed in infancy. Features that make cystic fibrosis more likely include failure to thrive and gastrointestinal symptoms, and in older children recurrent respiratory problems and nasal polyps (*see* Table 5.5). Male infertility due to blockage of the vas deferens may be a late presenting feature in mild cases; female fertility is unaffected. Effective management (*see* Table 5.6) requires a multi-disciplinary team.

Diagnosis

Cystic fibrosis is diagnosed by a 'sweat test', which involves driving pilocarpine into the skin with a small low-voltage electric current and detecting elevated levels of sodium and chloride. The underlying abnormality of the chloride channel is coded for on the long arm of chromosome 7.

Table 5.5   Features associated with cystic fibrosis

Respiratory system	Gastrointestinal system	Endocrine/reproductive systems
Bronchiectasis (progressive)	Neonatal meconium ileus	Diabetes mellitus
Haemoptysis	Rectal prolapse	Male infertilty (aspermia)
Nasal polyposis	Meconium ileus equivalent (distal intestinal obstruction syndrome)	
Chronic sinusitis	Pancreatic insufficiency	
Pneumothorax	Focal biliary cirrhosis/portal hypertension	

Table 5.6   Summary of cystic fibrosis management

Respiratory system	Gastrointestinal system	Endocrine/reproductive systems	Psychosocial support
Physiotherapy	Pancreatic enzymes	Insulin (maintain calorie-dense diet)	Family support
Antibiotics	Nutritional supplements	Fertility counselling	Individual support
Mucolytics	Injection of varices		Transition years (child/adolescent)
Palliative care			
Lung transplant?			

Sudden infant death syndrome (SIDS)

Sudden infant death syndrome (SIDS), sometimes termed cot death, refers to the devastating situation when parents find a previously well infant (commonly under 6 months old) dead in his or her cot. This condition is still not entirely understood.

A definition proposed at the 1994 Stavanger SIDS meeting underlined the importance of excluding explicable causes of death: 'the sudden death of an infant, which is unexplained after review of the clinical history, examination of the circumstances of death, and post-mortem examination'. Thankfully it is now less common than it was in the late twentieth century, and in the UK accounts for approximately 0.6 deaths per 1000 live births. The peak incidence is between 2 and 3 months of age, and it has a number of well-established risk factors, including maternal smoking (the strongest single risk factor), prone sleeping, preterm delivery, socio-economic deprivation, male sex and winter season. Although careful post-mortem examination is required to exclude organic disease, it has been estimated that up to 5% of cases may have an underlying metabolic cause, and up to 10% may be due to infanticide by what has been termed 'gentle smothering'. The latter suggestion is based on case histories and on the pathological findings, which almost invariably indicate an asphyxial end-stage event.

Although the 'Back to Sleep' campaign in which parents are advised to lie their infant on his or her back rather than on the front has been associated with a welcome fall in incidence, the cause or causes remain unknown. It is likely that causation is related to an interplay between the developmental changes in cardiorespiratory and/or temperature control and environmental factors such as environmental tobacco smoke exposure (ETS) and intercurrent viral infections. The sudden and unexpected death of an apparently normal and much loved infant is devastating for any family, and this is compounded by the required detailed enquiry by healthcare professionals and the police so that other causes of death can be excluded. Families may find the support offered by voluntary organisations helpful in coping with their loss.

Further reading

- Chernick V and Thomas F (eds) (1998) *Kendig's Disorders of the Respiratory Tract in Children* (6e). WB Saunders, Philadelphia.

- Dinwiddie R (1997) *The Diagnosis and Management of Paediatric Respiratory Disease* (2e). Churchill Livingstone, Edinburgh.

- Helms P and Henderson J (2003) Respiratory disorders. In: N McIntosh, P Helms and R Smyth (eds) *Textbook of Pediatrics* (6e). Churchill Livingstone, Edinburgh.

- Loughlin GM and Eigen H (eds) (1994) *Respiratory Disease in Children*. Williams & Wilkin, Baltimore.

- Phelan PP, Olinsky A and Robertson CF (eds) (1994) *Respiratory Illness in Children* (4e). Blackwell Science, Oxford.

Useful website

- British Asthma Guidelines 2003; www.brit-thoracic.org.uk/sign/

Self-assessment questions

1   Sudden infant death syndrome (cot death) is more common in:
(a) males   True/False
(b) upper social class infants   True/False
(c) infants over 6 months of age   True/False
(d) infants of low birth weight   True/False
(e) infants who sleep on their backs.   True/False

2   In acute lower respiratory tract infection and pneumonia in childhood:
(a) most cases have a viral origin   True/False
(b) crackles on chest auscultation indicate bacterial infection   True/False
(c) bacterial *Streptococcus pneumoniae* is the most likely organism   True/False
(d) broad-spectrum antibiotics are indicated in community-acquired pneumonia True/False
(e) maternal smoking is an established risk factor.   True/False

3   Alison, aged 6 years, has developed wheezing after a bad cold. Her peak
    expiratory flow rate (PEFR) is 70% of that predicted.
(a) She could be managed perfectly safely at home by her GP.   True/False
(b) She should be given a short course of penicillin.   True/False
(c) A β_2-agonist should be given by metered-dose inhaler and spacer. True/False
(d) She will need prophylactic treatment with inhaled corticosteroids once she
     has recovered from this episode.   True/False
(e) She needs to have an urgent chest X-ray.   True/False

4   Acute bronchiolitis:
(a) is usually caused by the respiratory syncytial virus   True/False
(b) is most common during the first year of life   True/False
(c) always requires hospital admission   True/False
(d) is often complicated by secondary bacterial infection   True/False
(e) has a peak incidence in late December/early January.   True/False

5   In cystic fibrosis:
(a) inheritance is by an autosomal recessive gene   True/False
(b) the gene is carried on the long arm of chromosome 16   True/False
(c) the stools often contain blood or mucus   True/False
(d) blood spot screening can detect asymptomatic cases in the neonatal period True/False
(e) females are infertile.   True/False

6 Ear, nose and throat problems

- Background
- Physiology and development
- Earache with fever: otitis media, glue ear
- Sore throat: tonsillitis, sleep apnoea, glandular fever
- Chronic nasal discharge

Background

Childhood ear, nose and throat problems are extremely common and make up a significant proportion of the workload of many GPs. Most of these problems are caused by the many upper respiratory infections to which young children are exposed. Existing as a recluse on a remote mountain top would protect against many of these ills, which can be seen as a consequence of normal social interaction, exacerbated by air-borne allergens in some, and probably also by passive smoking and environmental air pollution.

Most ear disease in children affects the middle ear, so that earache and deafness are the common symptoms. Otitis externa is also seen in children, and to the young child the external ear canal provides a tempting receptacle for a variety of foreign bodies. However, this temptation to insert objects into the ear canal is not limited to young children. The delicate nature of the deep meatal skin, eardrum and ossicles means that the

well-known advice to insert nothing smaller than one's elbow is generally sensible.

Sensorineural deafness is dealt with elsewhere in this book (*see* Chapter 10, page 144) and so will not be considered here.

A blocked and runny nose is a normal part of growing up, although in most children these symptoms are relatively infrequent and short-lived. A significant proportion have more persistent trouble and are often labelled 'catarrhal'. Most of this group have no serious pathology, and the symptoms reflect a transient tendency to upper respiratory infections (often associated with starting to attend playgroups, nursery or school), a degree of nasal allergy, or prominence of the naso-pharyngeal pad of lymphoid tissue (the adenoids).

Physiology and development

The tonsils and adenoids make up part of a collection of lymphoid tissue surrounding the

NB

Please see
erratum note
at front of
book.
(Refracted eardrum)
Turned through 180°

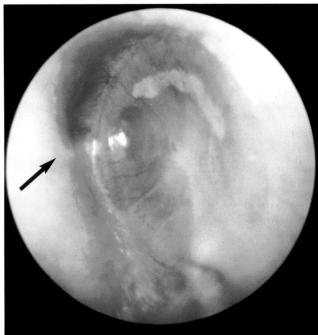

Figure 6.1 A normal eardrum. Note the light reflex.

upper aerodigestive tract. This arrangement is completed by lymphoid tissue in the base of the tongue (the lingual tonsils), and is known as Waldeyer's ring. The tonsils and adenoids are not usually apparent at birth, but enlarge through hyperplasia and multiplication of lymphoid follicles which in turn produce antibodies (immunoglobulins) – IgA locally and IgG and IgM systemically.

A pad of adenoids which is small in relation to the size of the nasopharynx usually causes no problems. The size of the adenoids increases after birth, usually reaching a maximum between the ages of 3 and 7 years. In the first few years of life the facial skeleton and the nasopharynx are relatively small compared with the cranium and the child as a whole, and enlargement of the adenoids can obstruct the nasopharyngeal airway, particularly in response to recent or recurrent infection. In addition, because of the situation of the adenoids close to the nasopharyngeal openings of the Eustachian tubes, enlargement or inflammation of the adenoids is thought to be a factor in the development of chronic otitis media in some children. Growth of the nasopharynx and regression of the adenoids with increasing

age ensure that problems due to the adenoids usually resolve before adolescence. The tonsils may also cause difficulties for the child because of their relative size. If the tonsils are particularly large (sometimes in a small child they may meet in the middle) then breathing may be impaired, particularly at night and when the adenoids are large, resulting in sleep apnoea.

Box 6.1 Causes of earache in children

- Acute otitis media
  - viral
  - bacterial

- Foreign body in ear canal (not necessarily painful)

- Trauma

- Impaired Eustachian tube function (e.g. during aircraft flight)

- Referred pain, usually from dental causes or tonsillitis

- Furuncle of external ear canal

Earache with fever: otitis media, glue ear

Earache is probably a universal symptom in childhood, although very young children have difficulty localising the pain and communicating the sensation to adults. Therefore in a sick child otoscopy is essential to assist in localising the illness. The severity of earache is not necessarily a good guide to the underlying pathology, as acute otitis media can be extremely painful yet resolve spontaneously, whereas the relatively uncommon form of chronic otitis media with destructive and potentially complicated cholesteatoma is usually painless. *See* Box 6.1 for the causes of earache.

A tendency to acute otitis media associated with upper respiratory infections is common in toddlers, possibly due to a sibling bringing home infections from playgroup or school. The history often begins after 6 months of age, when the effect of maternal immunity declines. The tendency to infection is often worse in the winter months, and may be linked to poor housing, poor nutrition and parental smoking. Acute otitis media often begins with a viral infection and resolves on symptomatic treatment alone, but bacterial infection may require antibiotics. A common complication of bacterial otitis media is rupture of the bulging tympanic membrane with resulting bloodstained discharge. The severe pain of the acute infection usually resolves with this rupture, and as the condition resolves the drum usually heals rapidly, although frequent infections may prevent healing and result in a chronic perforation. *See* Box 6.2 for a summary of the management of acute otitis media.

Acute mastoiditis, once a common emergency, is now relatively rare, the decrease in incidence

---

> **Box 6.2**   Management of acute otitis media
>
> - Analgesia
> - Antipyretics
> - Antibiotics
> - Advice to parents
>
> Many episodes of acute otitis media will resolve without antibiotics, which should be avoided if possible.

---

being due to antibiotics and also perhaps to a reduction in the virulence of the infecting organisms, so that an individual approach is necessary when attempting to quantify the problem (*see* Box 6.3).

Hearing loss in acute otitis media is usually transient and of little significance. In small children, particularly in the presence of recurrent upper respiratory tract infection, the middle ear fluid is slow to disappear and an effusion persists (glue ear), creating an environment in which a hearing impairment occurs. This may impair speech and language development, or in older children it may hinder school progress, and middle ear effusions are a frequent cause of failed hearing screening tests in young children. If the hearing loss or the tendency to chronic infection (*see* Figures 6.2 and 6.3 and Box 6.4) persists, a prolonged course (4–6 weeks) of a broad-spectrum antibiotic may bring about resolution. If this fails, surgical drainage of the middle ear with insertion of a ventilation tube in the eardrum (a grommet) may be indicated (*see* below).

Otitis media with effusion (OME, or glue ear) (*see* Box 6.5) also occurs in the absence of acute infections. The underlying pathology in this situation is thought to be poor Eustachian tube ventilation of the middle ear, which in certain children is associated with enlarged adenoids or nasal allergy. Medical treatment is disappointing. Surgical treatment of glue ear with grommets (and adenoidectomy in selected children) should be reserved for the minority of cases who suffer significant handicap from the condition.

The highly variable natural history of glue ear means that ideal management usually involves a period of 'watchful waiting' during which the child is monitored, with observation of their hearing, speech and language development, school progress, behaviour, and tendency to infection, before surgical intervention is contemplated.

Surgical intervention for glue ear consists of myringotomy (incision of the eardrum) with drainage of the middle ear fluid through this incision and insertion of a tiny plastic tube (a grommet) (*see* Figure 6.4 and Box 6.6) into the incision. The grommet therefore ensures ventilation of the middle ear, usually for between 6 and 12 months, before the tube is extruded from the eardrum.

Adenoidectomy is generally reserved for children whose adenoids are also causing troublesome nasopharyngeal obstruction or infection.

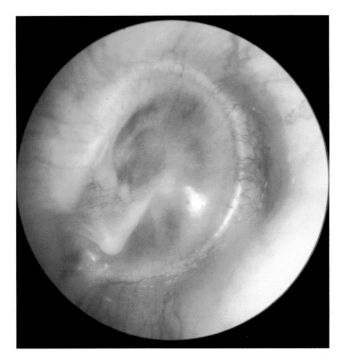

Figure 6.2 A retracted eardrum with amber-coloured fluid and tympanosclerotic scarring. This change is seen in chronic otitis media.

NB
See erratum
note at the
front of the
book.
(normal eardrum)
turned through 180°

Figure 6.3 Eardrum with dry central perforation and severe tympanosclerotic scarring.

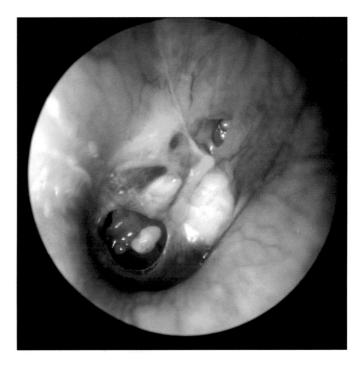

Box 6.3   Complications of acute otitis media

- *Acute mastoiditis*
  Now an uncommon complication. May resolve with antibiotics or require surgical drainage.

- *Perforation of tympanic membrane*
  Relatively common. Usually heals with minimal after-effects, but may become chronic.

- *Tympanosclerosis*
  Scarring of middle ear structures, including tympanic membrane. Usually minimal and of little significance.

- *Intracranial complications*
  These are rare, but can include meningitis and intracranial abscess.

Box 6.4   Chronic suppurative otitis media

1 *Persistent perforation of the tympanic membrane*
  This leads to hearing loss and a tendency to recurrent otorrhoea. Surgical repair is possible.

2 *Cholesteatoma*
  This is a collection of keratin from the skin of the eardrum and deep external meatus which accumulates in the middle ear and mastoid. Chronic infection causes local damage and complications. Surgical eradication is vital.

Box 6.5   Glue ear (chronic otitis media with effusion)

- Persistent viscous mucus in middle ear.

- Very common in pre-school children.

- May lead to hearing loss, poor concentration at school, and chronic middle ear damage.

- Initial management involves watchful waiting.

- Surgery (grommet insertion) is indicated for significant persistent deafness or recurrent infection.

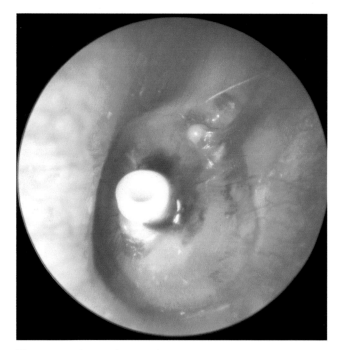

Figure 6.4   An eardrum with a grommet *in situ*.

Surgery for glue ear has become controversial, particularly as these operations are very frequently performed in Europe and the USA for a condition which is often self-limiting. It has been estimated that at least 75% of children in the UK experience glue ear at some time, but only 5% have persistent and bilateral middle ear effusions severe enough to warrant attention.

A small minority of children with ear disease have persistent structural abnormalities of the middle ear. A chronic perforation of the eardrum may be asymptomatic or may predispose to infection, especially if water enters the middle ear through the hole. Repair of the defect may then be indicated. A relatively rare but important form of chronic otitis media involves a perforation or retraction pocket in the attic or posterosuperior portion of the drum, through which the keratin of the squamous epithelium covering the outer surface of the drum and deep meatus can accumulate in the middle ear and mastoid air cells. This is known as cholesteatoma, and is associated with chronic, low-grade infection, often with offensive, smelly otorrhoea. Destruction of middle ear structures occurs, causing deafness, and the condition may slowly progress to cause facial nerve palsy, dizziness and occasionally intracranial complications. Surgery is usually required to eradicate the condition, and referral to an ear, nose and throat department is indicated.

Case study 1

Jamie, aged 18 months, the second of two children in the family, is brought to the GP's surgery irritable and hot, having had a poor night's sleep, and apparently crying with pain. The doctor sees from the records that he has a history of several episodes of acute otitis media over the past 10 months, each of which resolved on amoxicillin treatment.

Examination reveals Jamie to be pyrexial, and after a struggle the doctor can see that the right eardrum is red and bulging. Jamie's mother thinks that he hears well, although he often ignores her. His speech development seems to be slow. He failed the first health visitor distraction test of hearing at 8 months, passing the re-test 6 weeks later.

At Jamie's consultation, the GP prescribes amoxicillin in view of his general upset and the red, bulging drum. However, he is brought back to the surgery the following day, with no improvement. His mother reports that his right ear seems to be sticking out and very sore. Jamie appears drowsy and is again pyrexial, and the doctor sees that the right pinna is indeed more prominent than the left one. Closer inspection reveals a tender, boggy red swelling filling in the post-auricular sulcus and displacing the pinna forwards. The GP telephones the local ear, nose and throat department and arranges urgent admission to the paediatric ENT ward. On admission, Jamie is drowsy but rousable with no neck stiffness, and although he is uncooperative, there are no obvious cranial nerve abnormalities. A diagnosis of acute mastoiditis is made, and treatment with intravenous co-amoxiclav is started, along with intravenous fluids as Jamie is reluctant to drink. Over the next 24 hours there is a marked improvement in his general condition and the mastoiditis is settling. Jamie rapidly returns to health and is allowed home. Over the next 3 months there is a marked increase in his speech and language development.

Sore throat: tonsillitis, sleep apnoea, glandular fever

Sore throat is an extremely common presentation which is not easy to manage scientifically. Ideally, a bacteriological diagnosis should be made by taking a throat swab and sending it for culture to look for *Streptococcus haemolyticus* – type A is associated with serious complications in the form of scarlet fever, rheumatic fever (now rare) and acute glomerulonephritis. Most cases of tonsillitis are viral in origin and do not require antibiotics, and it is not certain whether an antibiotic will shorten the course even when a bacterium is the cause. However, throat swabbing is now rarely practised outside hospital, and it is conventional to treat with penicillin to cover a possible strepto-coccal origin. Can a bacterial tonsillitis be diag-nosed from the appearance? The answer is unfortunately not – even large red tonsils with white spots can be due to a virus such as Epstein–Barr virus (EBV) (*see* Chapter 3, page 42), the cause of glandular fever, well known for its association with a widespread rash if ampicillin is used in treatment (*see* Box 6.7).

If there are many large glands present in the submandibular and tonsillar regions, glandular fever should be suspected. This can be a severe illness with a prolonged course and subsequent fatigue lasting for several weeks, especially in older children and adolescents (*see* Box 6.8).

> **Box 6.8** Glandular fever (infectious mononucleosis)
>
> - *Cause*: Epstein–Barr virus.
>
> - *Transmission*: by intimate oral contact.
>
> - *Features*: fever, malaise, headache, anor-exia, petechiae over soft palate, lymph-adenopathy, splenomegaly, occasional rubelliform rash.
>
> - *Diagnosis*: excess of mononuclear cells, positive Paul-Bunnell test, positive mono-spot test.
>
> - *Treatment*: symptomatic.

Recurrent tonsillitis is common during the early school years, when children pick up infections from other children, and the autumn and winter months are usually the worst time of the year. Symptomatic treatment with oral fluids and paracetamol during acute attacks is indicated, and antibiotics are not always necessary, although they will shorten acute attacks and reduce the incidence of complications such as quinsy (peri-tonsillar abscess) (*see* Box 6.9).

The long-term management of recurrent tonsillitis largely depends on the frequency and severity of the individual episodes, the extent to which the child is disadvantaged by the condition

> **Box 6.7** Causes of sore throat in children
>
> - *Viral pharyngitis*
>   Associated with upper respiratory infec-tions. Mild, and does not usually impair eating and drinking.
>
> - *Acute tonsillitis*
>   Tonsils inflamed. Usually systemic upset. Impairs eating and drinking.
>
> - *Quinsy*
>   Peritonsillar abscess. In addition to symp-toms and signs of tonsillitis, drooling and trismus (inability to open the mouth widely) occur.
>
> - *Glandular fever*
>   Similar symptoms to acute tonsillitis, and also marked glandular enlargement.

> **Box 6.9** Management of recurrent tonsillitis
>
> - *Treatment of acute episodes*
>   Supportive measures: analgesics and antipyretics; antibiotics if resolution is slow or there is severe systemic upset.
>
> - *Management of recurrence*
>   Monitor progress, looking for spontan-eous improvement with age. Prolonged antibiotics may curtail frequent recur-rences.
>
> - *Tonsillectomy*
>   If there is a severe adverse effect on health or educational progress and no evidence of spontaneous improvement, this is an option.

(e.g. due to loss of time from school), and an estimate of the length of time the child will take to grow out of the condition.

Intervention usually means tonsillectomy, although a prolonged course of antibiotics, as in recurrent otitis media, may be effective in halting a cycle of frequent, recurrent tonsillitis, and thus avoid the need for surgery. A 'wait-and-see' policy, looking for signs of spontaneous improvement, is often the best approach (*see* Box 6.10).

Box 6.10   Indications for tonsillectomy

- Recurrent tonsillitis with significant adverse effects on health or educational progress and no sign of spontaneous improvement with increasing age.

- Quinsy, particularly if recurrent.

- Obstructive sleep apnoea.

Box 6.11   Sleep apnoea

- Episodes of cessation of respiration during sleep, which if significant lead to hypoxia. In children this is usually obstructive sleep apnoea due to enlarged tonsils and adenoids, and it is only rarely due to a central neurological cause.

- Diagnosis is made from the history from observers, usually the child's parents.

- Confirmed by monitoring during sleep, including pulse oximetry to assess severity and ECG to look for right heart strain.

Sleep apnoea

This condition is almost always due to enlarged tonsils and adenoids which obstruct the upper airway when the palatal and pharyngeal muscles relax in sleep, particularly in the supine position (*see* Figures 6.5 and 6.6). Typically, the child has

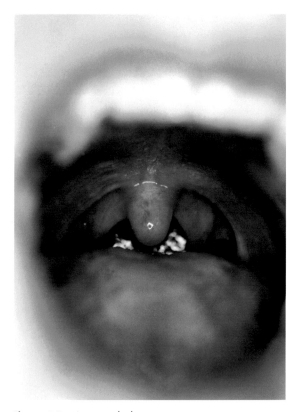

Figure 6.5   A normal pharynx.

Figure 6.6 Tonsillar hypertrophy in a child with obstructive sleep apnoea.

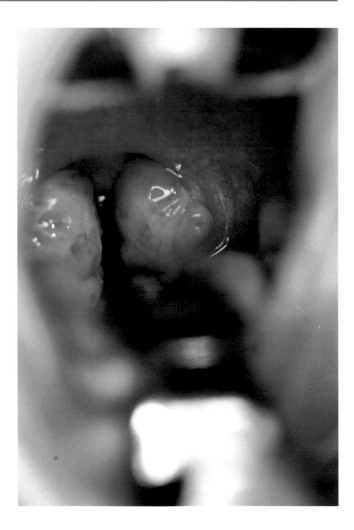

a restless sleep pattern that involves struggling to breathe. During periods of obstructive apnoea the arterial oxygen saturation falls, rousing the child, who will then usually change position and resume breathing until obstruction recurs. In severely affected individuals the quality of sleep is poor, resulting in daytime sleepiness, irritability and possibly poor intellectual performance. The condition can be documented in hospital, the most useful advance in this area in recent years being the pulse oximeter, a painless and accurate indicator of oxygen saturation. With this device it is possible to estimate the significance of the sleep apnoea as measured by the fall in oxygen saturation during apnoeic spells (*see* Box 6.11).

Rarely, sleep apnoea in children with extreme falls in oxygen saturation can lead to pulmonary hypertension and right heart strain.

Case study 2

Daniel, aged 5 years, is brought to the GP's surgery with a 2-day history of worsening sore throat and pain on swallowing. His mother reports that he is not his usual lively self, lacking energy and distressed. She also reports that his breath smells bad and he has swollen neck glands. The doctor examines Daniel, finding him hot and flushed with a rapid pulse. He has tender, enlarged glands below the angle of the lower jaw on both sides, and an open-mouth posture with a tendency to drool saliva. On opening his mouth, the boy's tonsils are seen to be enlarged, inflamed and with a white coating on the surface. The eardrums look slightly pink.

The doctor confirms the diagnosis of acute tonsillitis, and in view of the worsening clinical history over the past 48 hours, decides to prescribe antibiotics to add to the mother's management with paracetamol. The doctor notes from the child's record that Daniel previously developed a rash when on penicillin, so he writes out a prescription for erythromycin.

At this point the boy's mother complains that he always seems to be getting tonsillitis, she feels that he does not eat well and is not growing, and he has missed several weeks of school since he started last September. On further questioning from the GP, she reports that he snores extremely loudly at night and sleeps very poorly, especially when he has a sore throat. In addition to the snoring, Daniel struggles to breathe at times, and has spells when he stops breathing. The mother's own sleep is disturbed as a result, and she feels that something needs to be done to solve the problem. During the day Daniel always has his mouth open and seems unable to blow his nose.

Daniel has a clear history of upper airway obstruction at night, with snoring and sleep apnoea, and so is likely to have large adenoids in addition to his troublesome tonsils. If the tonsils are not large during the intervals between episodes of infection, yet the airway obstruction persists, then the adenoids can be assessed with a lateral X-ray of the nasopharynx. In view of his mother's concern and the history of sleep apnoea, Daniel's GP decides to refer him to an ENT surgeon. Although Daniel has no further tonsillitis over the next few weeks, his tonsils remain very large. His sleeping remains restless but the apnoea seems to be less noticeable. There is no history of nasal allergy, and the nasal mucosa appears normal. The ENT surgeon and Daniel's mother agree that there has been some overall improvement since the winter, and they opt for conservative management with a review in the autumn, although tonsillectomy and adenoidectomy remain a possibility.

Chronic nasal discharge

A chronically running nose may be due to chronic rhinitis, which may have an allergic cause (*see* Box 6.12). There is a tendency for small children to put items such as peas, beans, small toys and other objects up their noses. These normally give rise to a persistent foul-smelling discharge with total obstruction of the airway on that side, often with bleeding. The other common problem at this age is enlarged adenoids. These are easily demonstrated on a lateral soft-tissue X-ray of the nasopharynx.

Box 6.12 Nasal symptoms in children: pathology

- *Upper respiratory tract infections*
  - universal

- *Foreign body*
  - usually unilateral
  - foul discharge with or without bleeding

- *Chronic rhinitis*
  - allergic
  - vasomotor

- *Adenoidal hypertrophy*

Case study 3

Sarah is 3 years old and has been referred to her local ear, nose and throat department because of her persistently runny nose. Her mother reports that Sarah's nose is rarely dry, and that she tends to be a mouth breather with noisy breathing, especially at mealtimes and during sleep. There is no history of sleep apnoea. Sarah seems prone to upper respiratory tract infections, during which her nasal discharge turns thick and green, often persisting for weeks after the infection.

On examination, her nasal mucosa looks rather pale and purple rather than the usual pink colour, and there is excessive mucus in the nose, although it is clear and watery. Checking Sarah's nasal airway by holding a cold, shiny, metal spatula under her nose reveals a reasonable nasal airflow through both sides as shown by two mist patches on the spatula when she breathes out. Her throat and tonsils look healthy and unremarkable, and her ears look fine. Examination of her neck shows small, palpable and mobile glands on each side which are not tender.

In view of the history and the appearance of Sarah's nasal mucosa, the surgeon opts for treatment with topical steroids in the form of betametasone drops, one drop to be administered to each side of the nose twice a day. He advises the use of the drops for 2–4 weeks, as there may not be immediate benefit, and he suggests an X-ray of the adenoids only if there is no improvement. This is a condition that children usually grow out of.

Further reading

- Birrell JF, Cowan DL and Kerr AIG (1986) *Paediatric Otolaryngology.* Butterworth Heinemann, Oxford.
- Browning GG (1994) *Updated ENT* (3e). Butterworth Heinemann, Sevenoaks.
- Bull PD (2002) *Lecture Notes on Diseases of the Ear, Nose and Throat* (9e). Blackwell Science, Oxford.
- Kerr AG (ed.) (1997) *Scott-Brown's Otolaryngology. Volume 6. Paediatric otolaryngology* (6e). Butterworth Heinemann, Sevenoaks.

Self-assessment questions

1   In acute otitis media:
(a) the commonest causative organism is *Haemophilus influenzae*   True/False
(b) treatment should include an antibiotic   True/False
(c) rupture of the eardrum usually heals rapidly   True/False
(d) the diagnosis can be made with an auroscope.   True/False

2   A grommet is:
(a) an instrument for examining the adenoids   True/False
(b) indicated as treatment for glue ear   True/False
(c) only used by ENT surgeons   True/False
(d) likely to improve the child's hearing.   True/False

3 Acute tonsillitis:

(a) is associated with systemic upset   True/False

(b) may lead on to heart disease   True/False

(c) may be complicated by quinsy   True/False

(d) is worse in children of smoking parents.   True/False

4 Persistent nasal discharge:

(a) may be due to a foreign body   True/False

(b) is usually linked to significant pathology   True/False

(c) is suggestive of an anatomical defect   True/False

(d) may be allergic in origin.   True/False

7 Eye disorders

- Clinical assessment
- Squint
- Cataract
- Retinopathy of prematurity

Visual maturity is reached at about 8 years of age, but the most critical period of visual development is up to 2 to 3 years of age. Any block to clear vision during this time has a profound effect on vision in later life – the earlier the visual block occurs, the greater the eventual deficit will be. Therefore early diagnosis of all childhood visual problems is essential. Early detection of treatable disease may be best achieved by screening either the whole population or certain at-risk groups.

Severe bilateral visual disability is rare in childhood (2–3 per 10 000 population), but early and accurate diagnosis is important to allow parental support, assessment of special educational needs and appropriate genetic counselling.

Most visually impaired children now attend normal local school, but their visual impairment service teacher acts within the child's home and in conjunction with the class teacher. The visual impairment teacher advises and helps with stimulation of the impaired sight of the affected child, and can help to arrange for enlargement of printed matter, use of ideal lighting and low-vision aids at home and/or at school. The visually impaired child is always encouraged to be as independent as is safely possible, and to join in the same sports and pastimes as their normally sighted peers and siblings.

Clinical assessment

Parental concerns regarding vision should always be taken seriously. Important points in the history are a relevant family history (e.g. refractive error, squint or cataract in childhood). Visual problems are also common in children with a variety of medical conditions (see Box 7.1).

Vision in infants is measured by preferential looking and/or visually evoked cortical potential

---

Box 7.1   Groups at high risk for visual problems

- Family history of squint, refractive error or childhood cataract
- Premature infants (< 32 weeks' gestation or < 1500 g birth weight)
- Children with neurological or metabolic disease
- Children with other disabilities, including cerebral palsy
- Long-standing insulin-dependent diabetes (regular screening for retinopathy)
- Pauciarticular juvenile rheumatoid arthritis (regular screening for uveitis)

(VECP). Preferential looking relies on the fact that an infant will look to a striped black-and-white pattern in preference to an even grey target of the same overall luminosity. The spatial frequency of the stripes is increased until the infant shows no preference for the striped over the grey target. The VECP consists of electrical responses measured from occipital skin electrodes while the child sees an alternating or 'on/off' black-and-white checkerboard pattern on a television screen.

The examination of a baby requires a visual target. A face is better than a torch. The examiner notes visual attention and the ability of the eyes to follow a moving target. However, even a blind baby can appear to follow a face when they hear the examiner's voice. The examiner may need to use speech or a noisy toy to engage the baby's visual attention, but then visual fixation should be central, steady, and maintained in the absence of sounds. The examiner looks for smooth pursuit movements in response to a moving target.

Unilateral visual impairment due to refractive error can only be detected when the child's vision is assessed monocularly. A hand or a sticky patch is used to occlude one eye while measuring acuity in the other. Abnormal eye movements (nystagmus) are looked for. Pupillary constriction to light should be present when using a pen torch in a dim room. Vision testing in the non-verbal child is difficult, and if there is concern about vision, an ophthalmologist should assess the child.

At around 3 years of age a child will match letters or pictures of reducing size held at a distance of 3 or 6 metres by the examiner. The child holds a key card and picks out the letter or picture by pointing with a finger. The right and left eye are tested separately using a sticky patch to occlude the other eye (*see* Figure 7.1). At 4–5 years of age a child will read the letters on the Snellen test type held at a distance of 6 metres (*see* Figure 7.2). Some normal children do not achieve adult visual acuity (6/6) using the Snellen test until 6–7 years of age.

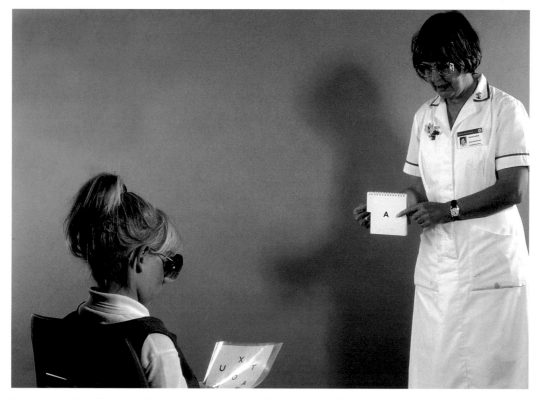

Figure 7.1 The Sheridan Gardiner test. The visual acuity of each eye is measured with the other eye occluded with a patch. Jodie identifies the letters, held at 3 metres or 6 metres, by pointing to the same letter on her key card.

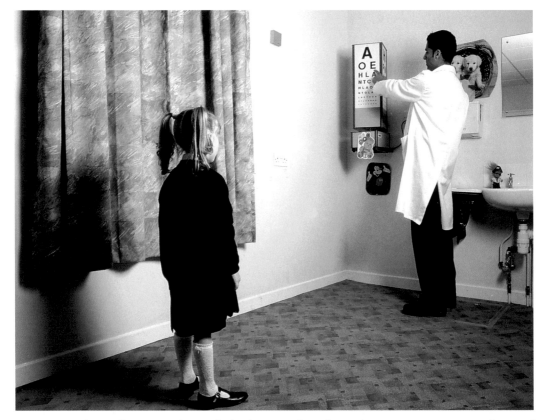

Figure 7.2   The Snellen test. Jodie reads the letters with each eye from 6 metres. A minor degree of unilateral amblyopia may be detected by a reduced acuity in one eye with the Snellen test when the visual acuity is the same in both eyes with a single-letter test (Sheridan Gardiner test). The adult with normal vision is able to read the reference-sized letter on the Snellen chart at 6 metres (i.e. 6/6).

Squint

Squint is a misalignment of the visual axis of one eye, or it may alternate between both eyes. It is a common problem, occurring in approximately 4% of all children. Parents usually recognise a squint, and any parental report of squint should always be taken seriously. The condition is often familial. Squint is detected by the corneal reflection test or by the cover test. The latter requires the child to fixate on an object while first one eye

and then the other is covered. Any movement of the uncovered eye is noted (*see* Figure 7.3).

The young squinting child does not have double vision because the image of the squinting eye is suppressed. If the squint is constant, amblyopia (*see* Box 7.2) rapidly ensues, resulting in reduced vision in the squinting eye. Surgery has a role in maintaining binocularity in an intermittent squint, but is usually only cosmetic for a constant squint of long duration.

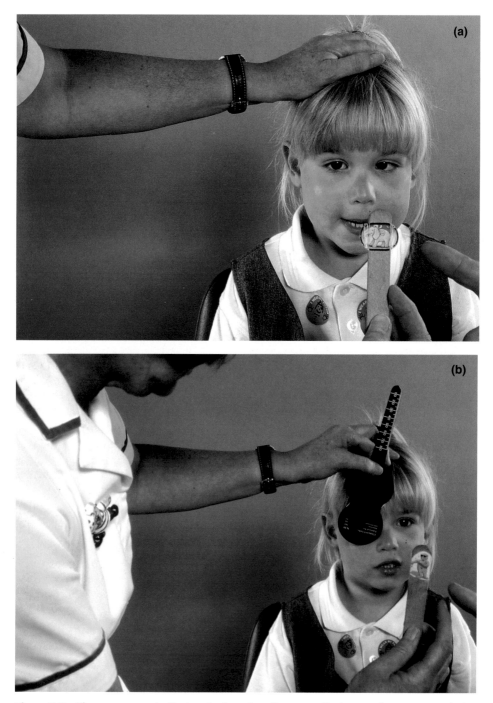

Figure 7.3   The cover test. Jodie is asked to describe a small picture, the accommodative target, held about 0.3 metres in front of her. Any misalignment of the visual axes is noted. (a) She has a left convergent squint, which is obvious when she fixates to a near object. When the squinting eye is covered the fixing eye does not move. (b) When the fixing eye is covered the squinting eye moves to take up fixation. The test is repeated with a larger target at 6 metres.

Box 7.2 Amblyopia

- *Definition*: reduced vision due to disuse of one or both eyes in infancy or childhood.

- *Causes*:
  - squint
  - refractive error
  - cataract
  - ptosis
  - corneal scar.

Case study 1

Scott was 2 years old when his mother first noticed his right eye turning in towards his nose. This squint was intermittent at first, but had become constant in recent weeks, which prompted his mother to take him to see the family practitioner. The GP confirmed that there was definite asymmetry of the light reflection on the cornea, especially when she spoke to Scott and moved her head from side to side. This clearly showed the convergent right eye from the lateral position of the reflection of her pen torch on Scott's right cornea as opposed to the central position of the reflection on his left cornea.

Scott was referred to an ophthalmologist. At 2½ years of age his binocular visual acuity was 3/6 with the Kay picture test. He did not cooperate with monocular vision tests. He had a constant right convergent squint and objected strongly to occlusion of his left eye. He fixed a small picture held at 1–2 metres with his left eye, but did not fix well with his right eye when his left eye was covered with an occluder. Cyclopentolate (1%) eyedrops were instilled into both of his eyes, and after 30 minutes retinoscopy was performed.

Scott was found to be long-sighted. His right eye had 4 dioptres of long sight and his left eye had 2 dioptres of long sight. (The power of a lens in dioptres is the reciprocal of its focal length measured in metres.) Ophthalmoscopy was normal in both of Scott's eyes. He was given spectacles to be worn constantly to correct his long sight, and his mother was instructed to patch his good left eye for 4 hours each day, ideally when he was looking at books and pictures or watching television. When he returned to the eye clinic after 6 weeks he was tolerating his left eye patch for the full 4-hour period each day. When he was wearing his spectacles, his right convergent squint was noticeably less than without them. The patching regime was supervised by the orthoptist. At 3 years of age his visual acuity was 6/6 in his right and left eye with the Kay picture test, and his daily occlusion treatment was no longer required.

Cataract

It is most important that every newborn is screened at birth for congenital cataract using the ophthalmoscope (*see* Figures 7.4 and 7.5). Congenital cataract is the commonest cause of treatable visual impairment or blindness occurring in infancy. The pupillary red reflex is seen through the ophthalmoscope held at about 30 cm from either eye of the baby after first focusing the examiner's free thumb held at a similar distance in front of the instrument. The ophthalmoscope is held close to the examiner's eye. Any congenital cataract will show up as a black area within the pupillary red reflex (*see* Figure 7.6). If diagnosis is delayed until the child's mother notices that her child does not see fully or his or her eyes develop irregular movement, or nystagmus, a normal adult level of vision will not be achieved. Causes of congenital and infantile cataract are listed in Box 7.3.

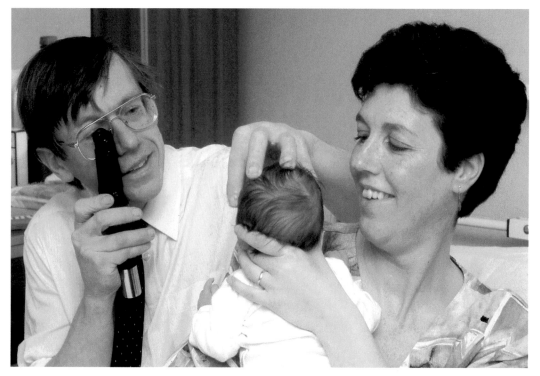

Figure 7.4   Examination of newborn for congenital cataract. Normally a clear even red reflex is seen in each pupil when viewed through the ophthalmoscope. Cataract will show up as a black area in the red reflexes. Dim room lighting and a new battery in the ophthalmoscope are required!

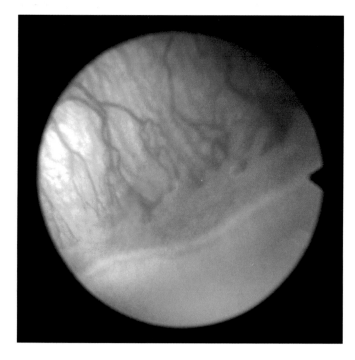

Figure 7.5   Retinopathy of prematurity (*see* page 102). At 8 weeks of age this premature infant (birth weight 800 g) has a ridge of neovascular tissue at the advancing edge of the retinal vessels, with white avascular retina seen beyond the ridge. The ridge extends for 12 clock hours around the retinal fundus.

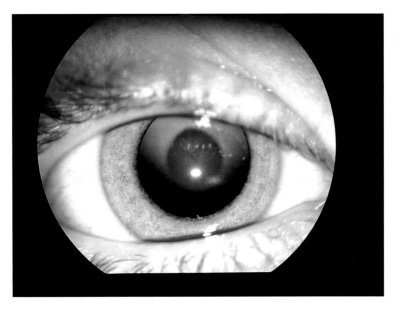

Figure 7.6 A congenital cataract is seen as a black object blocking the pupillary red reflex.

An important but rare cause of absence of the pupillary red reflex is retinoblastoma (*see* Box 7.4). This is a malignant ocular tumour of childhood that occurs in approximately 1 in 20 000 live births. Around 40% of cases are hereditary, and of these 10–15% have a microdeletion on chromosome 13.

Case study 2

Kay was born as a home delivery as this was her parents' preference. Her mother had been immunised against rubella in childhood, and this was her second pregnancy. There was no family history of any problem with vision. Kay's pupillary red reflexes were not examined with the ophthalmoscope at birth. At 3 weeks her mother became worried when she noticed that Kay did not look at her and that her eyes moved about aimlessly. Her family practitioner found that Kay did not fix a face with her eyes. She did follow a light at 1.5 metres with both eyes open. She had a constant coarse roving bilateral nystagmus. When both eyes were examined with the ophthalmoscope, a red reflex could be seen but no retinal details were visible. There appeared to be a central black area within the red reflex. The GP immediately telephoned the local ophthalmologist, who saw Kay the same day.

Kay was admitted for a full neurological assessment, which was normal apart from the cataracts. Electroretinograms were performed with both eyes tested together, as was a visually evoked cortical potential (VECP) in response to a flash stimulus to both eyes. Both tests were normal. VECP to a pattern stimulus would have been reduced by the light-diffusing effect of the cataract. Three days after her initial consultation, Kay underwent left lensectomy and anterior vitrectomy under general anaesthesia. Her left eye was padded until right lensectomy was performed 6 days later. Next day she was later given 30-dioptre extended-wear contact lenses for both eyes, focusing her eyes at about 1 metre.

At 4½ years of age her visual acuity was right 6/9 and left 6/36 with distance spectacle correction. Her right eye was patched for 5 hours a day. At 5 years of age her visual acuity was right 6/9 and left 6/12 with spectacles. She still has a slight fine irregular jerking of both eyes (nystagmus) and a small variable left squint. She attends a normal school.

Retinopathy of prematurity

The developing retina first receives oxygen and nutrition from the choroidal vessels. As the retina develops in complexity, its metabolic requirement increases and blood vessels grow across the retina from the optic disc. This vascularisation is not complete until full term. Extreme prematurity may interfere with normal vascularisation of the retina, resulting in retinopathy of prematurity (ROP) and sometimes severe visual impairment.

To detect ROP, all premature infants less than 32 weeks' gestation or 1.5 kg birth weight are screened using binocular indirect ophthalmoscopy through dilated pupils from about 7 weeks of age. At this time retinal vascularisation has proceeded two-thirds of the distance from the optic discs to the ora serrata in each eye. In retinopathy, retinal vascular growth stops and a ridge of pink-coloured neovascular tissue projecting slightly forward into the vitreous forms at the front edge of the advancing retinal vessels for 360° around each eye (see Figure 7.5). The ocular media are clear and posterior pole retinal vessels are usually normal. Many premature babies develop mild or moderate retinopathy, but this mostly regresses without treatment.

A few babies with progressive disease need treatment. This involves anaesthetising the baby and ablating the avascular retina between the neovascular ridge and the ora serrata of each eye with a diode laser through a binocular indirect ophthalmoscope. This reduces further neovascular proliferation and decreases the incidence of traction retinal detachment by 50% compared with untreated eyes. A later complication of ROP is myopia that requires spectacle correction.

Further reading

- Forrester J, Dick A, McMenamin P and Lee W (1996) *The Eye: basic sciences in practice*. WB Saunders, London.
- Khaw PT and Elkington AR (1999) *ABC of Eyes* (3e). BMJ Publishing Group, London.
- Taylor D (1997) *Paediatric Ophthalmology* (2e). Blackwell Science, Oxford.
- Taylor D and Hoyt C (1997) *Practical Paediatric Ophthalmology*. Blackwell Science, Oxford.

Self-assessment questions

1   Amblyopia in children may be due to:
(a) congenital cataract   True/False
(b) torticollis   True/False
(c) age-related macular degeneration   True/False
(d) squint   True/False
(e) corneal scar.   True/False

2   Assessment of vision:
(a) is impossible in infants   True/False
(b) needs to be differentiated from responses to voice   True/False
(c) can be undertaken using visually evoked cortical potentials   True/False
(d) acuity is measured using the cover test   True/False
(e) squint is assessed using a Snellen chart.   True/False

3   Squint:
(a) is not serious if it is noticed under 1 year of age   True/False
(b) normally requires corrective surgery   True/False
(c) is diagnosed by the cover test   True/False
(d) may lead to loss of vision in one eye   True/False
(e) is treated by patching one eye.   True/False

4   Visual impairment:
(a) is not diagnosable in the first 6 months of life   True/False
(b) requires the child to be in a special school   True/False
(c) can be detected by screening   True/False
(d) requires referral to an ophthalmologist   True/False
(e) is associated with Down syndrome.   True/False

8 Neurological disorders

- Epilepsy
- Febrile convulsions
- Headache and migraine
- Coma, encephalopathy and encephalitis

At least 20% of children who are admitted to hospital have a neurological problem as either the sole or an associated complaint. Many childhood neurological disorders have a genetic (and sometimes metabolic) basis. Congenital malformations such as myelomeningocele (spina bifida, *see* Chapter 10) arise during embryogenesis. Fetal cerebrovascular accidents, intrauterine infections and inborn errors of metabolism may all produce a legacy of neurological impairment in infancy and childhood.

Paediatric neurology has a large network of interconnections – the neurosurgeon, neuroradiologist, neurophysiologist, child psychiatrist and child psychologist, ophthalmologist, geneticist, orthopaedic surgeon and ear, nose and throat surgeon are all close professional colleagues of the discipline. Treating the child with a neurological disorder is often best seen as a multidisciplinary exercise that transcends the artificial barriers of hospital and community services, and of course we must not forget that it is the parental role which is usually pivotal to success (*see* Chapter 10 for cerebral palsy and Chapter 3 for meningitis).

Epilepsy

Epilepsy is the tendency to have recurrent seizures. Both the complexity and the fascination of childhood epilepsy lie in its heterogeneity. At one end of the spectrum we find the child who attends normal school and is achieving, and at the other is the child with multiple disabilities, the seizure disorder being only one of these. Somewhere along the spectrum is the child who shows unblemished neurodevelopment until 18 months of age and then develops infantile spasms, almost guaranteed to blight his or her future potential, or the child who develops absences (*petit mal*) at 6 years of age, only to outgrow the condition at 10 years. Epilepsy is a disease that was well known to Hippocrates and which across the centuries has been mystified and stigmatised, and even modern-day parents consider the diagnosis with dread. The explosion of new antiepileptic drugs, new developments in surgical approaches to treatment and new discoveries in genetics have brought a welcome optimism to the management of the child with epilepsy.

The most important aid in the diagnosis of an episode that may be a convulsion is a clear witnessed account of the 'funny turn' in question. Often the parents have been too frightened by the event to observe the details, or sometimes the event has occurred at school. The history is of utmost importance, and in case study 1 (*see* page 108) we are given the description of an initial simple partial seizure (consciousness retained, left-sided facial twitching) which becomes secondarily generalised (consciousness lost and tonic-clonic seizures of the whole body following). This is typical of the condition known as benign Rolandic epilepsy, and is found in up to 20% of children with epilepsy. The electroencephalogram (EEG) shows the typical features of this condition. The purpose of performing an EEG is not to make the diagnosis of seizures, because the diagnosis is based on the clinical history. Rather the EEG is used to define the type of epilepsy and the location of abnormal discharges.

We must always be certain about the diagnosis of epilepsy before labelling a child with this disorder, as it has profound implications for both the child and their family (*see* Box 8.1). About 5 in every 1000 schoolchildren have epilepsy. Most of these will have primary or idiopathic epilepsy

---

Box 8.1 Conditions that can be confused with seizures

- Breath-holding attacks
- Simple faints
- Acute confusional migraine
- Cardiac dysrhythmias
- Narcolepsy
- Night terrors
- Reflex anoxic seizures
- Benign paroxysmal vertigo
- Neonatal jitters
- Sleep myoclonus
- Benign infantile myoclonus
- Tics
- Benign paroxysmal ataxia
- 'Pseudo-seizures'

(i.e. no underlying cause will be evident), but some will have secondary epilepsy due to a cause such as head injury, meningitis, birth asphyxia or tuberose sclerosis (*see* Box 8.2).

Box 8.2 Secondary epilepsy

- Head injury
- Meningitis
- Encephalitis
- Birth asphyxia
- Tuberose sclerosis
- Inborn errors of metabolism

There are many ways of considering the diagnosis of epilepsy. There may be a specific cause, but we also need to consider a seizure-type diagnosis. The most recent classification of the epilepsies is shown in Table 8.1. It divides the epilepsies into those that are generalised (i.e. the whole of the brain is involved) and the partial (or focal) epilepsies (i.e. where the aberrant activity involves only a part of the brain). Another useful concept is to consider the epilepsies as age-related phenomena, and Table 8.2 shows an example of this approach.

Prognosis in the childhood epilepsies is very variable. There are some clearly benign conditions, such as *petit mal* (childhood absence epilepsy), Rolandic epilepsy and juvenile myoclonic epilepsy, which if managed properly have an excellent prognosis. Most of the refractory epilepsies are found in children who have multiple disabilities, or children who have acquired one of the malignant epilepsies (e.g. West's syndrome or the Lennox–Gastaut syndrome), which are associated with an inexorable decline in intellectual ability. Prolonged seizures ('status epilepticus') are most often seen in this group. The less common and less well-recognised 'nonconvulsive status', where the child seems perpetually 'far away' and may have lost communication skills, also requires urgent attention.

Treating epilepsy is about far more than controlling fits. A full explanation must be given, especially when, apart from an EEG, no further investigation is required. The child needs an explanation of what is happening to him and why he needs to take medicine. The school nurse and

Table 8.1   International classification of epileptic seizures

I   Partial seizures (seizures beginning locally)

   A   Simple partial seizures (consciousness not impaired)
     (1)   with motor symptoms
     (2)   with somatosensory or special sensory symptoms
     (3)   with autonomic symptoms
     (4)   with psychic symptoms

   B   Complex partial seizures (with impairment of consciousness)
     (1)   beginning as simple partial seizure and progressing to impairment of consciousness
     (2)   with impairment of consciousness at onset

   C   Partial seizures becoming secondarily generalised

II   Generalised seizures (bilaterally symmetrical and without localised onset)
   A   (1)   absence seizures
      (2)   atypical absence seizures
   B   Myoclonic seizures
   C   Clonic seizures
   D   Tonic seizures
   E   Tonic-clonic seizures
   F   Atonic seizures

III   Unclassified epileptic seizures

Source: adapted from *Commission on Classification and Terminology*, 1989.

Table 8.2   Epilepsy as an age-related phenomenon

- A neonatal period which extends to 3 months of age, during which seizures are related to a structural pathology and the prognosis is poor

- 3 months–4 years, during which period the seizure threshold of the central nervous system is low and reactive seizures, especially with fever, are common. Serious epileptic syndromes such as infantile spasms (West's syndrome) and the Lennox–Gastaut syndrome (severe myoclonic epilepsy of early childhood) occur in this epoch

- 4–9 years, during which period there is a predominance of primary or idiopathic generalised and partial epilepsies (e.g. childhood absence epilepsy and benign Rolandic epilepsy). Complex partial seizures secondary to structural brain abnormality also become better defined in this epoch

- 9 years onwards, when primary generalised epilepsies such as well-defined juvenile myoclonic epilepsy occur, while complex partial seizures are also more frequently encountered

Source: from Aicardi (1998) and O'Donohoe (1995).

Box 8.3   Prolonged seizures ('status epilepticus')

- Medical emergency
- First aid – place in recovery position
- May be treated with buccal/rectal benzodiazepines (by parents or GP)
- May need intravenous barbiturate in hospital

schoolteacher (with the child's parents' permission) should be informed, just in case he has a seizure in class. Children with epilepsy occasionally become the butt of teasing or are bullied by their peers, and it is important to be mindful of this so that the problem can be tackled. Children must be encouraged to have a full, normal childhood, with a few restrictions in activities. Both the child with epilepsy and his parents must be left feeling that the world is his oyster (just as it was for Agatha Christie and Julius Caesar, both of whom had epilepsy).

The need for further investigations (see Box 8.4) is determined by the seizure type (e.g. focal seizure) and the presence of positive findings on examination. Most parents wish to start medication, although benign Rolandic epilepsy resolves spontaneously in the second decade of life, whether treated or not. It is important to acknowledge the trauma that the parents suffered on witnessing their child's first fit (most parents in this situation think that their child might die). Giving them basic first-aid instructions on how to deal with possible future episodes increases their confidence. It is also important to discourage them from developing overprotectiveness, which is always counter-productive. In addition, side-effects of the chosen anticonvulsant need to be discussed. Providing the parents with literature and showing them the videos supplied by the Epilepsy Association and pharmaceutical firms is extremely helpful.

Box 8.4   Further investigations of seizures

- Neuroimaging – CT, MRI, ultrasound in infants
- Biochemical investigations
- 24-hour EEG
- Videotelemetry

Box 8.5   Restrictions in activities

- Swimming only with supervision
- Not riding a bicycle in traffic
- Not climbing heights

Case study 1

Dougal, who was 6 years old, was sent up to the outpatients with a history of a 'funny turn' at night. He shared a bedroom with his 10-year-old brother Angus, who had been awakened at night by a noise. Angus found Dougal thrashing around in the bed, and he hurriedly woke his parents. At this point, all the parents could describe was that Dougal could not be wakened, he appeared rather stiff, and both his arms and legs were jerking. By the time the GP arrived it was all over and Dougal just wanted to go back to sleep.

The GP spent most of his time allaying the parents' anxieties. While awaiting a hospital appointment, it was decided that Dougal's father, who was a very light sleeper, should share Dougal's room in case there was a recurrence. Three weeks later there were further attacks, and his father was able to provide a good description of these. He was woken by Dougal making a grunting noise (laryngeal spasm), there was an odd movement of Dougal's face with his mouth pulled to the left, and he was drooling. He was trying to say something but could not get the words out. Shortly after this he seemed to lose consciousness, he went stiff, and then there was jerking of all four limbs. The whole episode lasted for 3–4 minutes. When Dougal recovered he could talk, and he said that his face had felt funny at the beginning, but now he was very sleepy. He went back to sleep and the next morning he was entirely normal.

This story would fit well for a seizure, but it is important not to jump to this conclusion too quickly, as there are various other conditions that can be confused with seizures. Most children with suspected seizures are referred to hospital for further evaluation, so Dougal was seen in the outpatient clinic.

Dougal was a previously well child whose perinatal history was normal, and who had had no head injuries or serious illnesses. He had been perfectly well and normal on the nights before these attacks occurred. There was no relevant family history, and Dougal was entirely normal on both general and neurological examination. A diagnosis was made of benign Rolandic epilepsy, and an EEG was requested which confirmed this.

Dougal's parents were anxious to know what further investigations might be needed, whether to restrict his activities, and whether he should be given treatment. They wanted to know what to do if he had another fit, and whether he needed to be followed up at the hospital.

Febrile convulsions

The tendency to febrile convulsions often runs in families, sometimes in an autosomal-dominant pattern, and this may emerge when grandparents can contribute a family history. A first febrile convulsion may be the precursor to others, but prophylactic treatment with anticonvulsants is ineffective in the short term, and does not modify the outcome in the long term. The natural history of simple febrile convulsions is benign – children grow out of them by school age, and there is no long-term risk of epilepsy.

> **Box 8.6** Simple febrile convulsions
>
> - Neurologically normal child
> - No previous history of fits (except simple febrile convulsion)
> - Fever
> - Age 6 months–6 years
> - Duration less than 30 minutes
> - Generalised fit

Febrile convulsions have a specific definition (see Box 8.6). Management and prevention include:

- the use of antipyretics (paracetamol or ibuprofen, but not aspirin because of its rare association with Reye's syndrome – encephalopathy with fatty degeneration of the viscera)
- the avoidance of over-heating
- resisting the temptation to strip all clothing off and expose the child in a cold room or give them a cold bath – because cutaneous vasoconstriction results, and the core temperature can actually rise further

- explaining that the tendency to have febrile convulsions is often familial
- advising on basic first aid (recovery position, and calling an ambulance after 5 minutes if the fit does not stop by itself).

Children usually make a rapid recovery, generally because the cause has just been an acute viral infection, but they need to be observed for a while to make sure that the fit is not associated with a serious illness such as meningitis or septicaemia.

> **Case study 2**
>
> Andrew, aged 2 years, developed a running nose and a cough on a Saturday night, and became progressively more feverish on the Sunday. His parents called the GP, and a member of the deputising service saw him, at which point his temperature was 37.9°C and he was quite well. On the maternal grandmother's advice he was given a drink and put to bed, well wrapped in blankets, close to a radiator. An hour later the parents heard a strange noise, and going to him they found him stiff and blue. They attempted mouth-to-mouth resuscitation and called an ambulance, which brought him to the Accident and Emergency department. On arrival there he was pink, not responding to his parents, and there were jerking movements of all his limbs. He was clearly having a seizure. From the account of the ambulance crew and the parents it appeared that the fit had lasted for nearly 10 minutes.
>
> The background was that Andrew had been a completely normal child neurologically, with no previous history of convulsions. The seizure was seen to be generalised (although

the onset was not witnessed). It transpired that Andrew's mother had had two short seizures with a fever when she was about the same age. Examination of Andrew revealed no other physical sign apart from his temperature (now 38.9°C) and his evident coryza.

As with any other first fit, the parents were terrified, and consequently they needed a great deal of understanding and support. They were given written information which they could read at leisure and discuss later with their own GP. An hour later Andrew was playing happily in the waiting area, dressed only in a nappy and a T-shirt. His parents could see that there was nothing to be gained by admitting him to hospital, and they took him home.

Headache and migraine

Headaches worry children, their parents and their GP. There are usually two parallel problems – the first is the headaches and the second is the tremendous unvoiced family anxiety that the headaches may have a sinister underlying cause (e.g. cerebral tumour).

Migraine is strongly suggested when the story is characteristic – the headaches are often described as 'being all over, or sometimes over one eye', starting at any time of day and usually persisting for several hours. Children find it difficult to describe the nature of the pain, but it sometimes makes them cry. They often have abdominal pain, feel sick and may vomit. Visual experiences, such as spots before the eyes or blurred vision, are unusual in younger children but are sometimes reported by adolescents. Lying down in a quiet, darkened room usually helps. Sleep usually resolves the headaches.

Even when the history is strongly suggestive of migraine, it is important to ascertain a number of other key points. Are there any relevant psychological stressors (e.g. marital conflict or financial worries in the family)? Is there a family history of bad headaches or migraine? Is there any evidence of clumsiness, wobbliness, slurring of speech, change in personality or loss of skills?

Thorough examination includes measuring the head circumference and auscultating the skull

(for an arteriovenous malformation, which often has a bruit). The cranial nerves must be examined and, of course, the fundi. When the neurological examination has been completed, the skin must be inspected for evidence of neurocutaneous syndromes and the blood pressure should be measured (see Box 8.7).

Box 8.7 Examination for headache

- Examine the fundi and the cranial nerves.
- Measure the head circumference.
- Measure the blood pressure.
- Percuss and auscultate the skull (for an arteriovenous malformation, which often has a bruit).
- Ataxia suggests a space-occupying lesion, or hydrocephalus.
- Inspect the skin for evidence of neurocutaneous syndromes.

If there are no abnormal physical findings on full neurological examination, we can be very reassuring to the parents, indicating that by far the most likely diagnosis here is migraine. When the parents have witnessed a thorough examination of their child, they almost always accept this (with great relief), and it is rare for even the most anxious to demand some form of neuroimaging.

We then need to offer an appropriate explanation for the child's symptoms, sympathising with his headaches but acknowledging that although they may be very severe, they are not serious and are not associated in any way with a problem like a brain tumour. (Nine-year-olds are more sophisticated in their superficial medical knowledge since the advent of television soap operas!)

The severe throbbing headache of migraine is associated with dilatation of the cerebral vasculature (see Box 8.8). In cases of 'classical' migraine, this is preceded by an aura, which is thought to be associated with cerebral vasoconstriction. Migraine attacks may be provoked by stress, exercise, head trauma, dietary factors, menstruation, etc. In childhood, and especially in young children, migraine commonly has features such as cyclical vomiting, recurrent abdominal pain, and other periodic phenomena such as recurrent fever and paroxysmal limb pain that have been described as the 'periodic syndrome' (*see* Chapter 4). Often, it is only when such episodes are replaced by migraine that the earlier episodes are appreciated as migraine equivalents. Some rarer forms of migraine may also present in childhood, and these can present a considerable diagnostic challenge.

Box 8.8 Defining migraine

The headache is paroxysmal and has three of the following features:

- throbbing nature
- unilateral location (less common in children)
- relieved after sleep
- presence of an aura
- associated abdominal pain, nausea or vomiting
- family history of a similar condition.

Having explained the various precipitants or triggers of migraine headaches, it is useful to ask the child and his parents to keep a diary of his headaches over the next 8 weeks, and to record his dietary intake for 4–8 hours prior to each headache. When he returns to the outpatient clinic in 2 months' time, he may have identified a particular food (e.g. cheese, cola or chocolate) which has consistently precipitated his headaches. Removing the culprit from the diet is the best form of treatment, but obsessional elimination dieting must be avoided. It is more likely that no particular food can be incriminated. If a stressful situation at school has been identified as a trigger, it can be helpful to enlist the help of the community paediatrician in order to try to relieve this. Regular meals and sufficient sleep should be recommended, and a lifestyle of 'moderation in all things'. In the long term, childhood migraine

has a good prognosis. Long remissions occur and many children outgrow their attacks. Commonly the child and his parents report that the headaches are still happening but that 'they just don't bother him any more' (*see* Box 8.9).

Box 8.9 Managing migraine

- Identify triggers, such as food or stress (e.g. school anxiety).
- Promote regular lifestyle.
- Discuss drug treatment for attacks.
- Consider prophylaxis if attacks are frequent, or if the child is having significant time off school.

Box 8.10 Medication for migraine

- *Treating the attack*:
  - paracetamol
  - ergotamine tartrate (orally or rectally)
  - chlorpromazine (rectally if vomiting)
  - buclizine (e.g. Migraleve)
  - sumatriptan or zolmitriptan.

- *Regular prophylaxis*:
  - pizotifen
  - clonidine
  - propranolol
  - calcium-channel blockers.

If the headaches are still troublesome, as they will be in about 10% of children, and further examination reveals no abnormal signs or any other problems, medication will need to be discussed (*see* Box 8.10). Many children do not respond to antimigraine treatment, and it should be further explained that a lack of improvement when treated with various medications is entirely compatible with the diagnosis.

Table 8.3 Some causes of headache other than migraine

Brain tumour: intermittent, often nocturnal; vomiting, neurological signs

Vascular malformation

Fixed location headache: neurological signs, seizures

Malignant hypertension: throbbing pain, seizures, transient visual disturbance

Hydrocephalus (and congenital malformations): no characteristic quality, large head

Paranasal sinusitis: fullness, pressure, tenderness over sinus

Intracranial abscess/chronic meningitis: neurological or meningeal signs

Benign intracranial hypertension ('pseudo-tumour cerebri'): non-distinctive, papilloedema, diplopia

Cluster headaches: periodic, facial pain, lacrimation, Horner's syndrome

Psychogenic headache: pressure, aching, tightness, anxiety and/or depression

Post-concussion syndrome: history of head injury, dull aching headache, anxiety and/or depression

Ophthalmological problems: can cause headache (rare)

Source: from Aicardi (1998).

Other headaches

Headache is an important symptom in childhood because it is extremely common. Around 4–5% of children suffer from migraine. The challenge of the clinical problem lies in separating the rare headache of severe organic cause (e.g. brain tumour, cerebral abscess) from the mass of benign ones (*see* Table 8.3).

'Psychogenic' or 'tension' headache is often described as a feeling of pressure or tightness which increases as the day wears on. This continuing low-intensity headache has no associated symptoms or signs. It is usually caused by stress (which the child is unlikely to recognise), and the appropriate treatment is to clarify the underlying psychological cause and attempt to relieve it.

At all ages (except infancy) headache is an important symptom of brain tumour, especially those in the posterior fossa, where the majority of childhood brain tumours arise. Sometimes the headache is paroxysmal with intervals of remission, mimicking migraine, but it is exacerbated by factors that influence intracranial pressure, such as coughing, exercise and sleep. Sometimes the headache of brain tumour may precede any other signs or symptoms, but certainly by 4 months after its onset almost all children will have neurological signs, a change in personality, a slowing of growth, or other features (*see* Box 8.11).

Box 8.11 Symptoms of brain tumour

- Headache:
  - all ages except infancy
  - sometimes paroxysmal, mimicking migraine
  - worse with coughing, straining, exercise and sleep
- Change in personality
- Clumsiness or loss of motor skills
- Nausea, vomiting
- Slowing of growth

Coma, encephalopathy and encephalitis

Any state which involves a change in the level of consciousness is termed an 'encephalopathy'.

A large number of disorders may lead to encephalopathy, and the primary pathology may arise within or outside the central nervous system. The commonest cause of acute non-traumatic childhood encephalopathy is intra-cranial infection, but this is closely followed by hypoxic ischaemic insult (*see* Box 8.12).

Box 8.12 Some important causes of childhood encephalopathy

- Trauma
- Poisoning
- Hypoxia/ischaemia (near-miss sudden infant death syndrome, near drowning)
- Meningitis, encephalitis
- Mass lesions (haematoma, abscess, tumour)
- Fluid and electrolyte disorders (severe dehydration)
- Blocked CSF shunt
- Status epilepticus
- Hypertensive encephalopathy
- Hemiplegic or basilar migraine
- Endocrine dysfunction (hypoglycaemia, diabetic ketoacidosis)
- Renal failure
- Hepatic failure (Reye's syndrome)
- Inborn errors of metabolism
- Haemorrhagic shock/encephalopathy
- Iatrogenic causes (over-rapid correction of dehydration, drug overdosage)

The hospital management of a child with a depressed level of consciousness is a team effort. It is important to make a rapid general assessment of the patient immediately to ensure that no cardio-respiratory support is necessary at this stage. Provided that there is no evidence of shock and that respiration appears to be adequate, one member of the team can set about inserting an intravenous line and drawing blood for baseline biochemical investigations, while a nurse inserts a nasogastric tube and empties the stomach.

A careful history often provides clues to the diagnosis (*see* Table 8.4). Acute deterioration suggests a metabolic disturbance, poisoning or cerebrovascular accidents. Deterioration over a period of days or weeks is consistent with infections, chronic ingestions or raised intracranial pressure.

Table 8.4 Encephalopathy: clues from the history

Immediate: recent viral infection (encephalitis); found lifeless in cot (near-miss sudden infant death syndrome); empty drug bottle nearby (drug/substance abuse)

History of pre-existing disorder: diabetes, epilepsy, migraine, sickle-cell disease, CSF shunt

Family history: tuberculosis, epilepsy, previous unexplained deaths in infancy

Social history: always consider the possibility of non-accidental injury in young children

---

Should an urgent lumbar puncture (LP) be performed? It is well recognised that some deaths in cases of bacterial meningitis are associated with 'coning' (herniation of the brainstem through the foramen magnum) following LP. Most children with acute meningeal signs come to no harm from LP. However, in the seriously ill child whose consciousness is impaired, and where there are fundoscopic signs of raised intracranial pressure, focal signs or other signs of incipient coning, it is wise to treat with antibiotics first and defer the LP for 24 hours.

When dealing with a sick child, close contact must be maintained with the parents to keep them informed of events. It is important to spend plenty of time with the parents, encouraging them to talk and to express their thoughts and concerns.

Box 8.13 Herpes encephalitis

- Is caused by herpes simplex virus.
- Presents with encephalopathy, and occasionally with seizures.
- Has characteristic but not consistent EEG changes.
- Is diagnosed by detecting viral DNA in cerebrospinal fluid.
- Is treated with acyclovir.
- Children often require intensive care and respiratory support.
- With early aggressive treatment, it usually has a good outcome.

Case study 3

On her return from school, 13-year-old Kirsty complained of headache and refused her tea. The following morning her mother found her very drowsy in bed and called the GP. Kirsty had been a previously well child, there was nothing relevant in the family history, and her mother felt that the possibility of substance abuse was remote. The GP found that Kirsty's level of consciousness was diminishing at an alarming rate, and arranged an emergency admission.

There were no clues on examination (*see* Table 8.5). Kirsty opened her eyes to pain, made grunts but not words when spoken to, and was able to localise pain, giving her a score of 9 on the Adelaide Paediatric Coma Scale (*see* Table 8.6). Although she was encephalopathic, she was not deeply unconscious, there was no meningism, brainstem function was intact (corneal, pupillary and oculocephalic reflexes were normal, and respiratory pattern and heart rate were normal), there were no focal signs and the presence of severely raised intracranial pressure was unlikely (*see* Table 8.7).

Although the level of suspicion of bacterial meningitis was not high (no high-grade fever and no meningism), Kirsty was immediately treated with antibiotics and acyclovir (an antiviral agent). An urgent CT scan revealed a 2 cm dense lesion in the left temporal lobe which was surrounded by some oedema (*see* Figure 8.1). There was no midline shift and there were no signs of raised intracranial pressure. An urgent EEG demonstrated high-voltage, slow-wave activity seen over the posterior left hemisphere. These investigations suggested a diagnosis of herpes encephalitis (*see* Box 8.13).

A lumbar puncture was performed. The cerebrospinal fluid showed a mild lymphocytosis with normal glucose levels, and the protein concentration was moderately elevated. It was positive for herpes simplex nucleic acid by polymerase chain reaction (PCR), confirming the diagnosis.

Kirsty was treated with acyclovir administered intravenously for 7 days. She developed no seizures and made steady, slow progress. Throughout the admission her parents required a great deal of support.

At discharge, Kirsty was well and had no neurological impairment. Herpes simplex encephalitis can have devastating effects on cerebral function, and commonly did so before the advent of acyclovir, but Kirsty was diagnosed early and she was treated promptly and adequately (*see* Box 8.13). Psychometric assessment carried out several months later revealed an average IQ, and long-term follow-up did not reveal any delayed sequelae such as epilepsy.

Table 8.5   Encephalopathy: clues from the examination

Breath odours: diabetic ketoacidosis, glue sniffing, aminoacidopathies

Bruises, abrasions, burns, torn frenula, bruised genitalia: non-accidental injury

Skin abnormalities: neurocutaneous disorder, minor abrasion (toxic shock), cold sore (herpes), petechial rash (meningococcaemia), bleeding into skin/orifices (haemorrhagic shock/encephalopathy), parotid swelling (mumps, meningo-encephalitis)

Head: large circumference, splayed sutures, crackpot sound on percussion (hydrocephalus), bulging fontanelle (raised intracranial pressure), bruits (arteriovenous malformation), shunt present (blockage)

Meningism: bacterial meningitis, intracranial bleed

Midline pit over spine: CNS infection due to dysraphism

Eyes: proptosis, unilateral exophthalmia

Papilloedema: raised intracranial pressure from any cause

Table 8.6   Comparison of Adelaide Paediatric Scale (APS) and Glasgow Coma Scale (GCS – appropriate for older children)

Paediatric scale (APS)		*Adult scale (GCS)*
Eyes open		
Spontaneously	4	
To speech	3	As in paediatric scale (APS)
To pain	2	
None	1	
Best verbal response		
Orientated	5	Orientated
Words	4	Confused
Vocal sounds	3	Inappropriate words
Cries	2	Incomprehensible sounds
None	1	None
Best motor response		
Obeys commands	5	
Localises pain	4	
Flexion to pain	3	As in paediatric scale (APS)
Extension to pain	2	
None	1	

Table 8.7 Symptoms and signs of acutely raised intracranial pressure

All age groups	Infants	Toddlers and older children
Decreased conscious level	Reluctance to feed	Anorexia
Lethargy	Irritability	Headache
Vomiting	Full fontanelle	Nausea
Convulsions	Spreading of sutures	Diplopia
Decorticate/decerebrate posturing	'Sunsetting' eyes	Papilloedema
Respiratory arrest	Crackpot sign	False localising signs
	Rapid increase in head size	

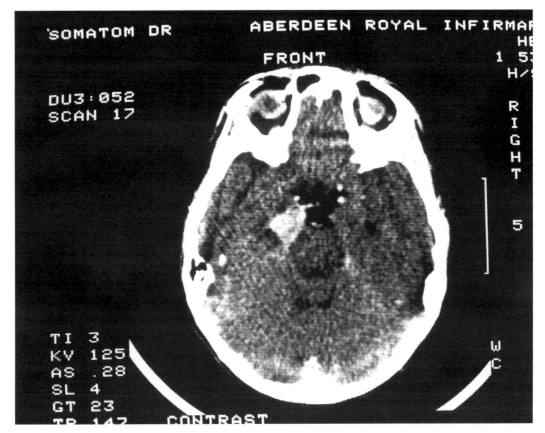

Figure 8.1 Transverse computerised tomography (CT) scan showing an enhancing dense lesion approximately 2 cm in diameter in the left uncus with 1 cm of surrounding oedema. This is characteristic of herpes encephalitis.

Further reading

- Aicardi J (1998) *Diseases of the Nervous System in Childhood*. MacKeith Press, London.
- Brett EM (ed.) (1997) *Paediatric Neurology*. Churchill Livingstone, Edinburgh.
- O'Donohoe NV (1995) *Epilepsies in Childhood*. Butterworth Heinemann, Sevenoaks.

Self-assessment questions

1 The purpose of an EEG is to:

(a) diagnose epilepsy   True/False

(b) define the type of epilepsy   True/False

(c) exclude cardiac dysrhythmias   True/False

(d) diagnose brain tumours   True/False

(e) reassure the parents.   True/False

2 Simple febrile convulsions:

(a) can be prevented by treating with aspirin   True/False

(b) always start focally   True/False

(c) often run in families   True/False

(d) occur up to 10 years of age   True/False

(e) last for less than 10 minutes.   True/False

3 Migraine in childhood:

(a) is commonly associated with abdominal pain   True/False

(b) can have a dietary trigger   True/False

(c) should always be intensively investigated, including brain imaging   True/False

(d) if unilateral, suggests an underlying tumour   True/False

(e) is caused by cerebral vasoconstriction.   True/False

4 Epilepsy:

(a) is still a stigmatising condition   True/False

(b) requires attendance at a special school   True/False

(c) should be treated with a single drug   True/False

(d) requires a child to avoid sport   True/False

(e) is associated with behaviour problems.   True/False

9 Orthopaedic disorders

- Limping in a toddler
- Limping in a young child
- Limping in an adolescent
- Painful limp
- Miscellaneous conditions:
  - growing pains
  - bow legs
  - knock-knees
  - intoeing
  - foot deformity (talipes)
  - flat feet (infantile pes planus)

Orthopaedic disorders represent 10–15% of children's health problems. Eliciting an accurate history may be difficult; examining a screaming child is impossible. The approach must always be slow and gentle. Use of the unaffected limb for comparison of movement is useful – joint movement varies with the age of the child. In this chapter some of the common problems will be discussed, together with their presentation and treatment. With many conditions early diagnosis and treatment are essential to prevent permanent bone damage leading to long-term disability.

Limping in a toddler

A limp is an abnormal gait pattern which varies with the causative agent. There are several common causes of limping.

Box 9.1 Causes of limp

- Pain: trauma, infection
- Instability: developmental dysplasia of the hip
- Shortening of one limb
- Spasticity of the muscles
- Weakness of the muscles
- Ataxia

Relevant factors include the age and sex of the child, their general health, the onset of the limp and the presence of pain. The commonest cause of a painful limp is trauma, but the history may not be forthcoming – the younger child forgets, and the older child may prefer to forget! (*See* Boxes 9.1 and 9.2.)

(See Boxes 9.1 and 9.2.)

Box 9.2 Differential diagnosis of the toddler with a limp

- Developmental dysplasia of the hip

- Trauma

- Infantile coxa vara (a small angle between the femoral shaft and the femoral neck)

- Infection

- Talipes

- Cerebral palsy

Developmental dysplasia of the hip (DDH) (formerly known as congenital dislocation of the hip)

Developmental dysplasia of the hip is the term now used for a spectrum of conditions in which the head of the femur is displaced from the acetabulum. It includes dislocation, subluxation and instability. The condition is screened for by examination at birth and at 6 weeks of age. It is more common in girls and is more frequent after breech delivery. DDH should always be considered in a toddler who limps. It is normally diagnosed in the newborn period, but it may be missed (*see* Box 9.3).

The Ortolani test for DDH is routine in the newborn (*see* Chapter 17, page 267). The hip ligaments are lax, and a positive test, producing a clunk, indicates a dislocatable hip. If positive, this would be followed by the application of an abduction splint to stabilise the hip until the

---

Box 9.3 Developmental dysplasia of the hip (DDH)

- Occurs in 1–2 in 1000 live births.

- Is more common in girls.

- Around 50% of cases are bilateral.

- Most common in breech presentations.

---

capsule tightens. Unfortunately, a significant number of cases are missed, so untreated DDH remains a problem. Any limp in a toddler requires urgent referral and an X-ray.

The prognosis for developmental dysplasia of the hip at this age, if treated by gentle closed reduction, is that 80% of cases will have a successful outcome. If treated at birth, the hip should become completely normal – hence early diagnosis is extremely important.

Case study 1

Emma, aged 16 months, has limped since she walked on her own at 14 months. Her parents initially thought that she was unsteady, and only became concerned when the limp persisted, when they decided to take her to see their GP. The limp did not distress Emma. Her parents were uncertain whether she had had a hip test at birth, as she was a premature baby.

Emma walked in quite happily but with an obvious dipping gait – the Trendelenburg gait (when the weight is transferred on to the unstable hip, the pelvis dips on to the opposite side). Examination of the hips confirmed shortening of the right leg with tightness of the right adductor muscles. The telescoping test for instability of the right hip was positive. The X-ray showed that the left femoral head was outside and above the acetabulum, confirming the diagnosis of developmental dysplasia. Emma was admitted for treatment with her mother. She was nursed in a cot, head down at a 45° tilt, with fixed traction on the left leg and weighted traction on the right leg. This gradually stretched out the tight soft tissues and the hip came down opposite the acetabulum. At this stage, the hip could be gently reduced under general anaesthetic, dividing the tight adductor muscles subcutaneously first. Plaster was then applied with both hips flexed, abducted and externally rotated.

Emma will spend several months in plaster, until X-rays confirm that the femoral head and acetabulum are developing normally. The longer the hip is out of joint, the longer the treatment will be.

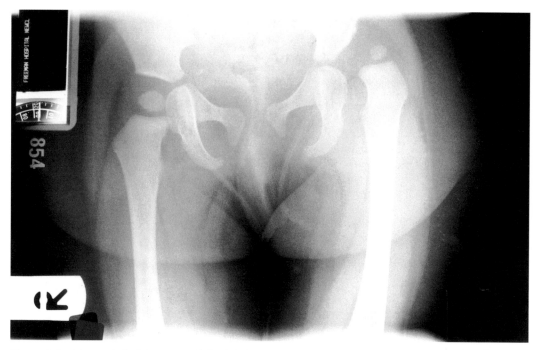

Figure 9.1   Congenital dislocation of the left hip. Note the upward and outward displacement of the femoral head. The left femoral head is smaller than the right, and the left acetabulum is shallower and more open or sloping.

Limping in a young child

The causes of limping in an early school age child are different from a toddler and are listed in Box 9.4. Perthes' disease is a serious chronic condition affecting this age group.

Perthes' disease

Perthes' disease (pseudo-coxalgia) (*see* Box 9.5) is an avascular necrosis of the upper femoral epiphysis. Its aetiology is unknown, but possibly involves a combination of genetic factors and trauma to the hip causing an intra-articular effusion. This increases the intra-articular pressure and compromises the circulation to the epiphysis, leading to necrosis of the latter. The dead bone is then gradually removed, and new bone is laid down, producing a fragmented appearance on X-ray (*see* Figure 9.2). During this stage, the femoral head is rather plastic and can be moulded by outside pressure. The final phase is that of bone healing, and any residual deformity will be permanent.

Box 9.4   Differential diagnosis of a limp in a young child

- *Hip*
  Perthes' disease (pseudo-coxalgia)
  Trauma
  Infection
  Irritable hip syndrome
  Juvenile arthritis
  Missed coxa vara

- *Knee*
  Discoid meniscus
  Baker's cyst

- *Feet*
  Talipes

- *General*
  Shortening of the limb
  Cerebral palsy
  Early manifestation of a dystrophy

In a young child, revascularisation is relatively rapid (*see* Figure 9.3), and minimum treatment is necessary.

In the 7- to 8-year-old group, revascularisation takes much longer and some protection for the femoral head may be necessary. This is achieved by taking the weight off the affected hip or by allowing weight bearing with the hip abducted.

Above the age of 8 years the prognosis is not as good, because of the length of time that the femoral head will take to heal. Surgery to improve the 'containment' of the femoral head may be appropriate here.

Box 9.5   Perthes' disease (pseudo-coxalgia)

• Perthes' disease occurs between the ages of 3 and 11 years.

• It is four times more common in boys.

• Around 15% of cases are bilateral, but not necessarily simultaneously.

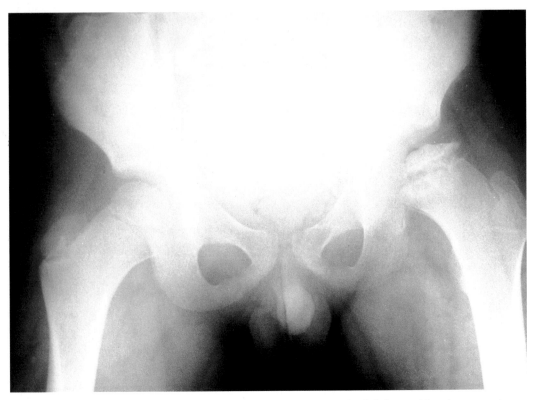

Figure 9.2   Perthes' disease. Early phase of necrosis, age 6 years. The left femoral head appears denser relative to the decreased density of the metaphysis. The ossific nucleus is smaller, but the cartilage space is thicker.

Figure 9.3 *see pages 123 & 124*   Perthes' disease. (a) Phase of revascularisation, age 6.75 years. The central dense area (arrowed) is where new bone is being laid down on the dead trabeculae in the nucleus. (b) The head is now looking 'fragmented' as new bone is laid down and dead bone is resorbed, age 6.75 years. (c) The healing phase. The head is 'filling in'. Note how the metaphysis has broadened a little, and the femoral head has broadened and become partially subluxed, age 7.75 years. (d) Healing complete, age 12 years. Note the residual deformity (broadening and flattening of the femoral head). The articular cartilage is normal.

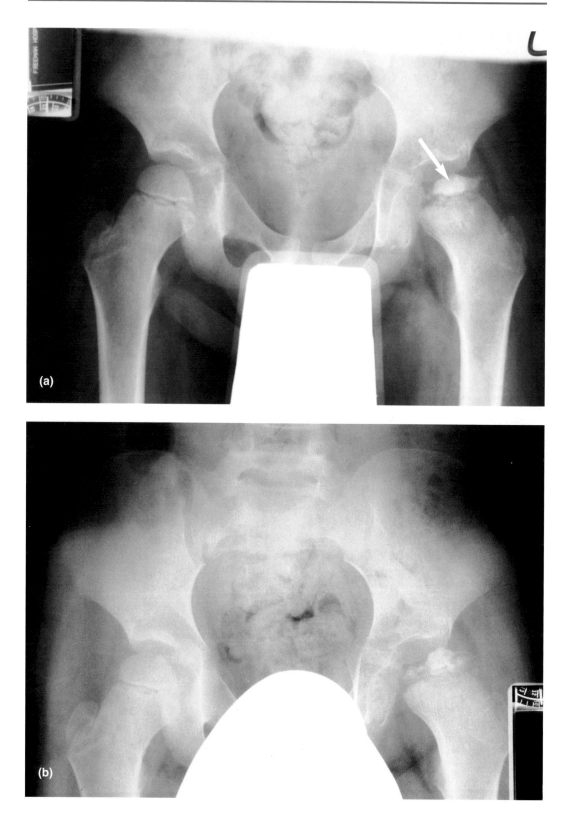

(a)

(b)

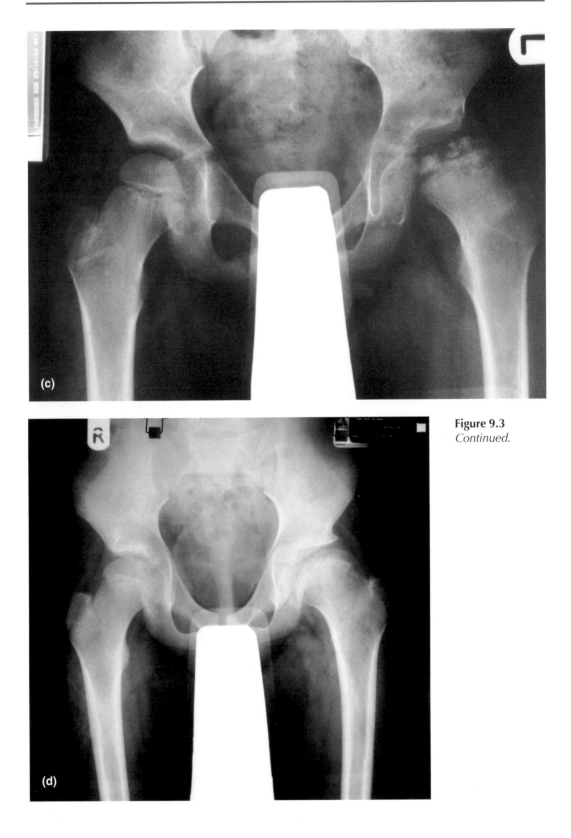

Figure 9.3
Continued.

Case study 2

Peter, aged 6 years, is a fit child who walked at 1 year. Two months ago he started to limp. Occasionally he said that his left knee was sore, but he continued to play happily. His parents could remember no injury. Initially, Peter's limp was hardly detectable, but after walking up and down it became more obvious.

Lying on the couch, he held the left hip semi-flexed and externally rotated. The knees were normal. He had marked restriction of abduction and internal rotation in the left hip – the classical signs of Perthes' disease, which were confirmed on X-ray.

Peter was admitted the following day. He was put on traction, gradually increasing the abduction and internal rotation of the hip. After 3 weeks this was almost normal, so he was allowed up gradually. No further limp developed, and after 1 week he went home. He has to sleep with a pillow between his legs to abduct his hips, and he cannot jump or play games, but he can go to school. This regimen will continue until his X-rays show that the left hip has healed. This may take up to 1 year.

Limping in an adolescent

Slipped upper femoral epiphysis (SUFE)

This condition occurs in the 10–15 years age group and is more common in boys, particularly the overweight (*see* Box 9.6). Around 30% of cases are bilateral.

Box 9.6 Slipped upper femoral epiphysis (SUFE)

- Most common in boys.
- Age group affected: 10–15 years.
- Around 30% of cases will be bilateral.
- Affected girls: often tall and thin.
- Affected boys: often overweight.

All cases of SUFE will require surgery. This may involve simple pinning of the epiphysis where the slip is minimal, or correcting the alignment of the femoral neck by osteotomy and then pinning. Any attempt to manipulate the head back on to the femoral neck would have dire consequences for the blood supply and would lead to avascular necrosis.

The aetiology is thought to be related to an imbalance between the growth hormone (too much) and the sex hormone (too little), which weakens the epiphyseal plates, predisposing to the slipping.

Case study 3

John, aged 13 years, has been 'walking badly' for several months. A keen fan of cowboy films, he was thought to be emulating his heroes – walking with his feet turned out, rolling from side to side. His parents had not been concerned, and John had never complained. It was a friend, who was a nurse, who suggested that John might have a problem. He was somewhat overweight, with a tendency to female distribution of fat. General examination revealed under-development of his genitalia.

Examination of the hips revealed loss of internal rotation, limitation of abduction, and as the hips were flexed the legs rotated outwards, suggesting slipping of both upper femoral epiphyses (SUFE). This was confirmed by X-ray, particularly the 'frog view' – with the hips abducted and externally rotated (*see* Figures 9.4 and 9.5). Both upper femoral epiphyses had slipped downwards and backwards in relation to the femoral neck. This was a chronic bilateral SUFE and it required surgery.

After operations on both hips (*see* Figure 9.6 for placement of nail) and 3 months in bed, John is now mobilising well. The end result is still in the balance.

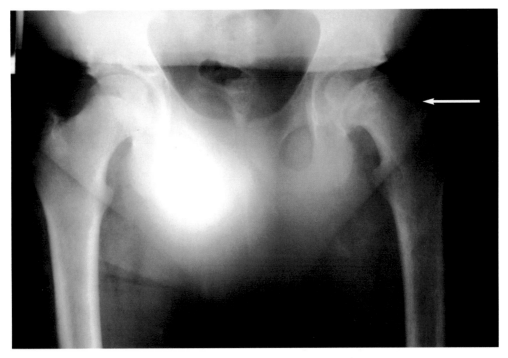

Figure 9.4 Slipped upper left femoral epiphysis (SUFE). Note the more prominent appearance of the femoral head, a consequence of its downward 'slip'. Bone 'build-up' around the epiphysis indicates that this is a chronic slip.

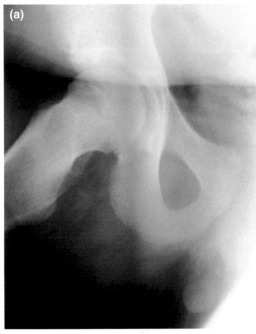

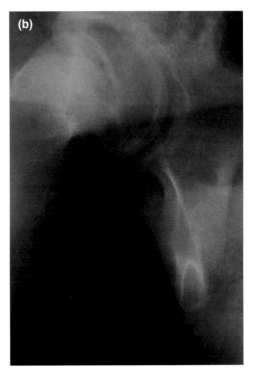

Figure 9.5 (a) SUFE normal hip in lateral view. (b) SUFE showing slipping of femoral head.

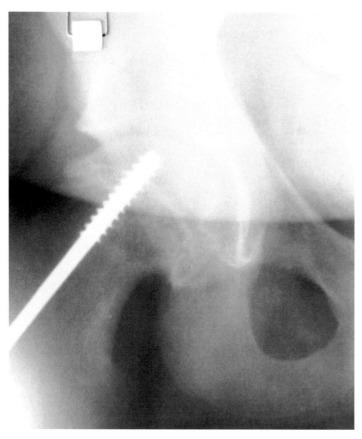

Figure 9.6 SUFE – healing with nail *in situ.*

Painful limp

A child who limps with pain is in urgent need of investigation, as an infectious cause is highly likely. Trauma is also possible. The differential diagnosis is shown in Box 9.7.

Box 9.7 Differential diagnosis of painful limp

- Osteitis
- Trauma
- Septic arthritis
- Cellulitis
- Rheumatoid arthritis
- Rheumatic fever

Osteitis

Osteitis is a disease of growing bone (*see* Box 9.8), and in 90% of cases the causative organism is

---

Box 9.8 Symptoms of osteitis

- Pain
- Pyrexia
- Local skin tenderness
- Local skin warming
- Bone extremely tender to percussion
- Associated restriction of joint movement
- Minimal local swelling in the early stages
- X-rays initially normal, but become abnormal after 7–10 days

---

Staphylococcus aureus. The portal of entry may be mild skin trauma or sepsis of the upper respiratory tract, particularly infection in the ear.

Case study 4

Philip is 5 years old. Three days ago he fell and grazed his right knee. Two days later he became unwell, developed a temperature and refused to walk, so his parents took him to the surgery. Philip was obviously ill and pyrexic. He pointed to the pain on the inner side of his knee. There was some local swelling just below the knee and the overlying skin was warm. He would not allow anyone to touch his knee.

He was admitted to hospital and put to bed. His left leg was splinted and elevated, blood was taken for cell counts and culture, and the leg was X-rayed (to exclude a fracture in a febrile child). The diagnosis of osteitis was made, and intravenous flucloxacillin was started with intravenous fluids.

Blood tests confirmed a raised white cell count and a raised erythrocyte sedimentation rate. X-rays were normal. After 12 hours there was very little improvement. As it was suspected that Philip was developing a subperiosteal abscess, he was taken to theatre and the abcess was drained. His blood cultures were negative, but fortunately he had responded to the flucloxacillin. Culture of the pus from the small abscess grew *Staphylococcus aureus.* The antibiotic was continued for 3 weeks.

Philip eventually made a full recovery.

Septic arthritis

This presents with a similar clinical picture to osteitis, and it can complicate osteitis. In the older child the disease is acute and rapidly progressive. Pyrexia associated with severe joint pain, muscle spasm, and virtually no movement at the joint because of pain are the presenting signs. There may be a visible joint effusion. Immediate antibiotic treatment must be given and diagnostic aspiration performed. If pus is obtained, the joint must be opened, cleaned out and then immobilised. Failure to remove the pus from an infected joint leads to destruction of the articular cartilage and irreversible joint damage.

In the infant the presentation is less acute – possibly an irritable infant with restriction of movement in the joint. Fever may be mild and the blood counts may be only slightly raised. An X-ray may show distension of the joint and some displacement of the femoral head in the case of the hip. As with the older child, treatment involves aspiration to confirm the diagnosis, followed by arthrotomy and cleansing of the joint, antibiotics and immobilisation.

Transient synovitis

This condition is benign, but it is the commonest cause of limping in young children. There are similar features to septic arthritis, but there is no systemic illness, the white cell count is not raised, and the X-ray is normal.

Juvenile chronic (rheumatoid) arthritis

This chronic illness can be very debilitating in children. It presents in three forms, namely systemic arthritis (in which the child is generally ill), polyarticular arthritis (characterised by painful swelling and restricted movement of both large and small joints) and pauciarticular arthritis (occurs in girls under 4 years of age and involves few joints – usually knees, ankles and elbows). The latter is associated with iridocyclitis, which may lead to loss of vision (*see* Box 9.9).

Box 9.9   Rheumatoid arthritis (juvenile chronic arthritis)

- 9% systemic (Still's disease) with acute illness and high fever, anorexia, rash, splenomegaly and anaemia
- 16% polyarticular seronegative
- 3% polyarticular seropositive adult type
- 49% pauciarticular (usually knees)
- multidisciplinary team required for management

Management of juvenile chronic arthritis is by the use of anti-inflammatory drugs and physical and occupational therapy.

Miscellaneous conditions

Growing pains

This strange condition presents with leg pain although not with limp. The diagnosis requires the exclusion of other more sinister conditions. It may be caused by oedema of the fascial sheaths. The pain occurs at night and may wake the child. Treatment is symptomatic and should also include reassurance.

Bow legs

This condition is a common developmental anomaly in toddlers. In a child aged between 1 and 3 years it is normal, although the parents may become quite anxious about the appearance of the child. They may be reassured that by 5 or 6 years of age the legs will have straightened out. The main differential diagnosis is rickets, and an appropriate history should be obtained and, if necessary, X-ray and bone biochemistry performed.

Knock-knees

Knock-knees are part of normal child development, and most cases improve spontaneously. Most children are born with some varus of the knees, which usually corrects by 2 years of age. Some then overcompensate to produce the valgus or knock-knee. Knock-knees are a manifestation of general ligamentous laxity (in this case the medial collateral knee ligaments), and therefore tend to look worse when standing.

Most cases are physiological and resolve spontaneously by the age of 7 years. They are more common in overweight children, and improve if the weight is reduced.

Some rarer causes are shown in Box 9.10.

Assessment

The standard measurement is the intermalleolar separation measured while standing and sitting,

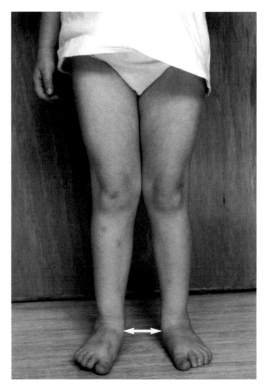

Figure 9.7   Knock-knees. Arrow indicates intermalleolar separation.

with the knees just touching. The intermalleolar separation is the gap between the medial malleoli (*see* Box 9.11 and Figure 9.7).

Box 9.10   Rarer causes of knock-knees

- *Metabolic*: e.g. rickets (vitamin D deficiency or renal).
- *Congenital*: arachnodactyly.
- *Traumatic*: previous epiphyseal or high tibial fractures.

Box 9.11   Intermalleolar separation in knock-knees

Standing measurement:

- 1–2 cm: mild
- 2–4 cm: moderate
- > 4 cm: severe.

See also Box 9.12 for definitions of valgus and varus.

Treatment of knock-knees

In physiological cases, the aim is to prevent deterioration and overstretching of the medial ligaments. Mild cases do not require treatment. Moderate cases probably do not require treatment under the age of 7 years, unless they are deteriorating or have associated valgus heels (around 50% of cases). In these children, there is a place for valgus wedges in the shoes. Night splints are usually reserved for severe cases, especially in older children.

In pathological cases, any metabolic causes would need to be treated. This group may require surgical correction when growth ceases. Apart

---

Case study 5 (young child)

Peter, aged 5 years, attends the clinic because his parents are concerned about his knock-knees and the way he wears his shoes. The knock-knees were noticed about a year ago and seem to be getting worse. He is a fit child, although he is rather overweight, as is his mother.

He walks with obvious knock-knees and is wearing his shoes down on the inner side of the heels. When he is standing, the gap between the malleoli is 3 cm, and when he is sitting it improves to 2 cm. Also when Peter is standing it is noticeable that his heels roll in – over into valgus.

He has a physiological knock-knee and at his age will probably grow out of it. However, he has the problem of valgoid heels, often associated with knock-knees. It will therefore be worth putting valgus wedges under the heels of his shoes on the inner side to control this. His mother will also be given appropriate dietary advice for him.

This regimen should correct the problem within 2–3 years, but if there is no improvement in 2 years' time, or he deteriorates, simple night splints to correct the deformity may be considered.

---

from knock-knees being an unattractive condition, in adult life it does increase the risk of degenerative joint disease in the knee.

There is still a great divergence of orthopaedic opinion as to whether knock-knees should be treated.

Box 9.12   Knock-knees: definitions

Valgus: the line of the joint angles away from the midline.

Varus: the line of the joint angles towards the midline.

Case study 6 (adolescent)

Mary, aged 13 years, came to the clinic with her mother. She has been knock-kneed for years and has 'not grown out of it' and wants her legs straightened. She is not overweight, and she is an attractive girl with a very obvious knock-knee. The intermalleolar gap is 5 cm when standing and 3 cm when sitting. Her feet are normal. Mary's growth years are limited. She is very cooperative and is an ideal case for night splints, which should correct the deformity, as there is no pathological cause of her knock-knee.

Intoeing

Intoeing is a common developmental anomaly.

At birth, the femoral neck is anteverted 50° on the femoral shaft. This gradually decreases towards the adult range of 15–20°. Only very rarely is corrective osteotomy necessary. In some children a compensatory external rotation of the tibia develops, where the knees remain turned in but the feet are straight – the so-called 'squint knees'. No treatment is necessary.

Case study 7 (school-age child)

Michael, aged 6 years, has always intoed. He is very fond of watching television and always sits on the floor with his hips and knees internally rotated and his feet out to the side – the TV or W position (*see* Figure 9.8). When walking, his knees, ankles and feet are turned in (i.e. the problem is with the hips – persistent femoral neck anteversion).

Michael's mother has been reassured that the condition will improve spontaneously, but she must stop him sitting with his legs turned in. If possible she must get him to sit with his legs crossed 'tailor' fashion.

Talipes

Of the congenital foot abnormalities, talipes equinovarus (club foot) is the most common,

occurring in 2 in 1000 live births (*see* Figure 9.9). It is more common in boys than in girls, and 50% of cases are bilateral. The severity of the condition is assessed by the rigidity of the deformity, not by the appearance. The deformity cannot be corrected manually. This differentiates the condition from postural equinovarus.

The deformity arises during early embryonic development. The muscles of the posterior and medial compartments of the calf are short, and the affected joint capsules become fibrosed and contracted on the concave side. This produces secondary changes in the developing bones and joints (*see also* Box 9.13).

Box 9.13   Features of club foot (talipes equinovarus)

- Equinus at the ankle – foot points down.
- Varus at the subtalar joint – heel turns in.
- Adduction and supination of the forefoot.
- Internal torsion of the tibia.

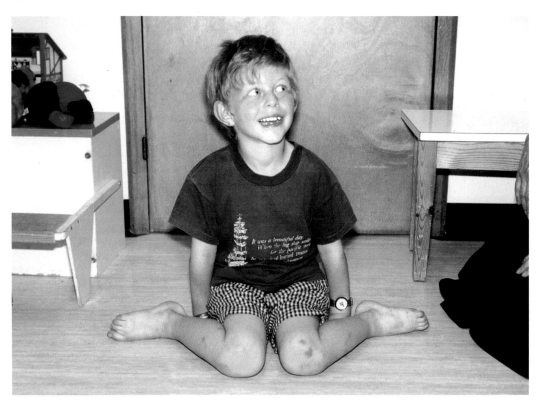

Figure 9.8   'TV' position.

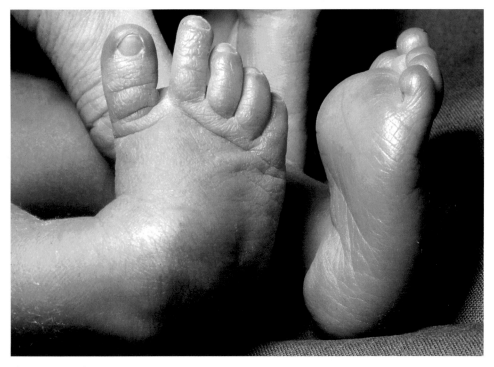

Figure 9.9 Talipes equinovarus.

Treatment begins at birth and requires a regimen of stretching, strapping and splinting carried out by specially trained physiotherapists. If the foot has not corrected by 3 months of age, surgical intervention will be necessary to release contracted soft tissues and joint capsules and lengthen shortened tendons. In the older child, corrective bone surgery may be necessary. Even when the foot is well corrected the child may be left with a shorter foot and also some shortening of the tibia (usually 1–2 cm).

Case study 8

After a normal delivery it was obvious that baby Sean's feet were not normal. The feet were pointing down, the heels were turned in, and the forefeet were rotated in (supinated) so that the little toes were almost touching.

The paediatric orthopaedic surgeon found that the right foot was very rigid and resisted passive correction. The left foot, although it looked the same, was more mobile and corrected moderately well when passively manipulated.

Baby Sean had a severe right talipes and a moderate left talipes. Treatment was started immediately.

Talipes calcaneo-valgus

This deformity is mainly postural and is due to intrauterine pressure, with the foot folded up to the tibia. Most cases respond to passive stretching and possible bandaging. The condition is often ignored, and in more severe cases may cause delay in walking due to the over-stretching of the Achilles tendon. When the child stands, the feet roll markedly into valgus (to be differentiated from infantile pes planus). The use of supportive boots with heel lifts and valgus wedges will encourage walking as the lax tissues tighten.

Infantile pes planus

The majority of children will look 'flat-footed' when they begin walking. This is due to the presence of a fat pad under the arch of the foot. This normally disappears by the age of 3–4 years.

Flat foot (dropping of the longitudinal arch) must be differentiated from the valgus foot (pes valgus, where the heel rolls inwards), in which there is the appearance of a flattened arch. Persistent flattening of the arch is helped by exercises and arch supports. Pes valgus requires the insertion of valgus (medial) wedges in the heels of the shoes to correct the heel deformity. *See* Figure 9.10.

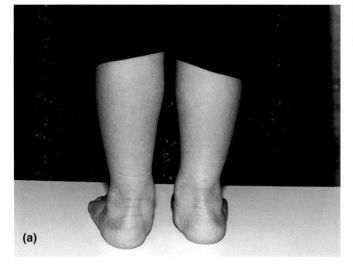

(a)

Figure 9.10 (a) Infantile pes planus. Heels are neutral. (b) Valgus ankles, showing 'roll-in' effect of ankles.

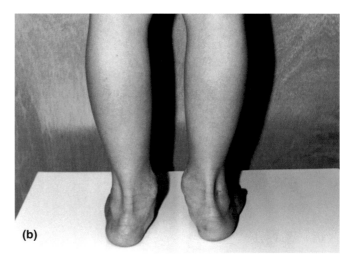

(b)

Further reading

- Benson KDM, Fixsen JA, Macnicol MF and Parsch K (2001) *Children's Orthopaedics and Fractures.* Churchill Livingstone, London.

- Sharrard WJW (1992) *Paediatric Orthopaedics and Fractures.* Blackwell Science, Oxford.

Self-assessment questions

1   Developmental dysplasia of the hip is:

(a) a hereditary condition   True/False

(b) curable if treated within the first month of life   True/False

(c) reliably diagnosed by physical examination   True/False

(d) associated with shortening of the affected limb.   True/False

2   In septic arthritis:

(a) the commonest agent is *Staphylococcus aureus*   True/False

(b) the commonest joint is the hip   True/False

(c) osteitis is normally associated   True/False

(d) immunodeficiency is likely to be associated.   True/False

3   Bow legs in a toddler:

(a) is an early sign of rickets   True/False

(b) occurs in normal children   True/False

(c) requires surgical treatment   True/False

(d) is a sign of early obesity.   True/False

4   The following orthopaedic conditions may be screened for:

(a) developmental dysplasia of the hip   True/False

(b) talipes equinovarus   True/False

(c) flat feet   True/False

(d) Perthes' disease.   True/False

10 Disability

Feeling beastly – nasty,
Many discuss me so –
Can he hear? Can he see?
Can fools fly? Evidently no!
  (Christopher Nolan (1980) *Damburst of Day
  Dreams.* Weidenfeld & Nicholson, London)

Writing became Joseph Meehan's
Word-World. Brain-damaged, he had for
years clustered his words, certain that some
cyclops-visioned earthling would stumble on
a scheme by which he could express
Hollyberried imaginings.

  (Christopher Nolan (1987) *Under the Eye of
  the Clock.* Weidenfeld & Nicholson, London)

These two quotations from the writings of
an exceptionally talented person with spastic
quadriparesis poignantly contrast the exterior
image with the interior illumination. His definition
is his writing, not his cerebral palsy. Such talent is
rare, and it illustrates the importance of potential.
The aim of those who work with children with
disability is to help each child to reach his or
her potential, whatever that may be. Achieving
that potential depends on early identification of
handicap, careful assessment, teamwork in treatment, and support and commitment from parents
and carers.

Definitions

The words *impairment*, *disability* and *handicap*
have different meanings. The dictionary definition
is quoted in Box 10.1, followed by a definition
in the context of this chapter. Box 10.2 illustrates

135

Box 10.1 Definitions

Impairment: an injurious weakening – any loss or abnormality of physiological or anatomical structure.

Disability: a want of ability – any restriction or loss of ability due to an impairment in performing an activity in a manner or range considered normal for a human being of that developmental stage.

Handicap: a disability that makes success more difficult – a disadvantage for an individual arising from a disability that limits or prevents the achievement of desired goals (an uncompensated disability).

Box 10.2 Summary of the differences between WHO terms and the equivalent terms used in other medical conditions

WHO model	Medical model
Impairment	Aetiology
Disability	Pathology
Handicap	Manifestations

---

the differences between the World Health Organization (WHO) terms and the equivalent terms used in other medical conditions.

For example, a long eyeball (*impairment*) results in myopia (*disability*), but spectacles prevent *handicap*.

Disabled people themselves do not always agree with this definition, which equates a disability with a pathology. They prefer to use a social model of disability which places the onus on society to normalise the world for the disabled person (*see* Box 10.3 and Figures 10.1 and 10.2).

A *special need* used in the terms of the Education Act (1981) is an educational need of a child which is not usually met by the normal provision for a child of that age.

Special provision is what an education authority provides to meet special needs.

Early identification of special needs gives the most time to alleviate handicap and to reach potential. It also gives parents the best opportunity to come to terms with their child's disability. Early

---

Box 10.3 Medical and social models of disability

Medical model: locates the problem within the individual to be treated or cured. A disabled person is seen as being outwith the normal.

Social model: locates the problem in society. Individual limitations are acknowledged but are seen as less important than society's failure to ensure that the needs of disabled people are taken into account in its organisation and facilities.

---

identification is based on sound knowledge of the normal development of the child, set out in Chapter 1. Assessment of development is based on the appreciation of the 'normal' and its variations.

Development does not progress in a linear fashion, but in a stepwise manner with 'treads' and 'risers'. The staircase is uneven, and some stages of development constitute a quantum leap, the achievement of which opens up new possibilities. For example, erect locomotion (a gross motor skill) frees the hands for the myriad of fine motor tasks that are subsequently learned.

The different developmental 'streams' (gross and fine motor, hearing and speech and social development) are interlinked but run at different rates, and experience is needed to determine when dissociation between them becomes pathological. Cultural and rearing practices influence developmental patterns. A baby who is stimulated will always do better than a baby of the same endowment who is deprived of stimulation.

The general health of an infant plays its part, too. A baby who is seen during or after an acute illness may well have decreased tone and apparent delay, but will often catch up. Chronic illness will also slow down development, as will frequent hospitalisation. Socio-economic factors are of great importance, as parents living in poverty and under stress may stimulate their child less, with delayed speech or motor development being the sequel.

The case studies that follow illustrate the principles of management of the disabled child.

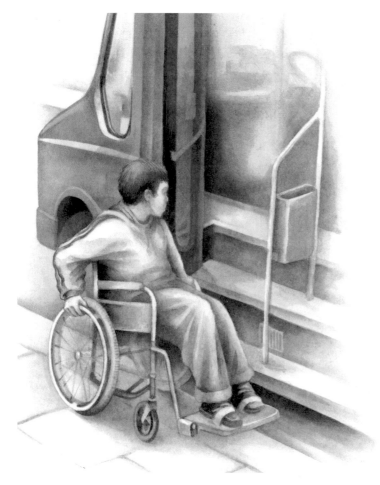

Figure 10.1   Child with disability unable to get on bus.

Figure 10.2   Disabled teenager using a Maltron keyboard.

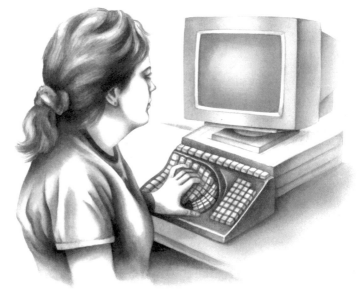

Down syndrome

Down syndrome was first recognised as an entity in 1866 by Dr John Langdon Down in England. In 1959, Lejeune and his colleagues demonstrated that this syndrome was associated with an extra chromosome 21. It is one of the commonest causes of mental disability.

Down syndrome is normally recognisable at birth. The key features of the syndrome are shown in Boxes 10.4 and 10.5. Every baby is an individual, but there are many common features both in the facial appearance (*see* Figure 10.3) and in the moderate to severe learning difficulty which occurs. There is also a high incidence of heart and intestinal defects. Children with Down syndrome have many positive features, and at the time of diagnosis there should not be too much emphasis on defects as opposed to assets.

It is very important that the diagnosis is presented to the parents sensitively. This is outlined in Case study 1 opposite and summarised in Box 10.6.

Box 10.4   Key features of Down syndrome

- Mongoloid slant of eyes
- Single palmar creases and other characteristic dermatoglyphics
- Small head size with brachycephaly
- Hypotonic features
- Developmental delay and learning difficulties
- Tendency to develop heart and intestinal disease and leukaemia
- Dry skin and associated hypothyroidism
- Trisomy 21

Box 10.5   Down syndrome

Cause: trisomy, translocation or mosaicism of chromosome 21.

Overall incidence: 1 in 600; incidence increases at both extremes of maternal age (i.e. at maternal age of 45 years, 1 in 30 risk).

Clinical features: round face, flat profile, flat occiput, epicanthus, 'mongoloid' slant to eyes, Brushfield's spots on iris, protuberant tongue, broad short-fingered hands, clinodactyly (curving of the little finger), single palmar crease, wide-spaced big toe, short stature, hypotonia and general learning difficulties.

Associated problems: congenital anomalies, including heart disease, duodenal atresia, Hirschsprung's disease, hypothyroidism and increased risk of leukaemia.

Associated minor problems: dry skin, feeding difficulties, recurrent upper respiratory tract infections, glue ear, feeding difficulties, hypermetropia and myopia.

Prognosis: normal life span, increased incidence of Alzheimer's disease in later life and increased risk of myeloid leukaemia.

Box 10.6   Telling parents about a disability

- Tell the parents together.
- Tell them as soon as possible.
- Tell them in a quiet place without interruptions.
- Tell them without an audience of staff.
- Tell them honestly and directly, with warmth and understanding.
- Allow them privacy after the initial interview.
- Meet them again to allow them to ask questions.
- Give them time and space to consider their feelings.

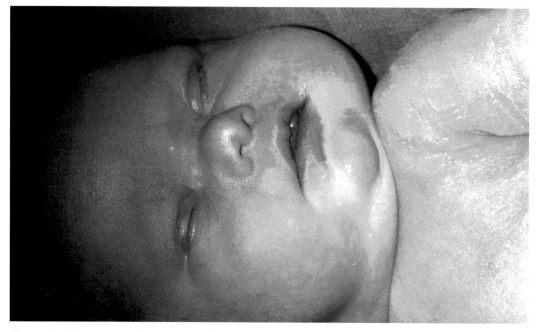

Figure 10.3   Newborn with Down syndrome.

Breaking bad news

One of the most important tests for a paediatrician, and one which requires great skill, is informing parents that their child has a disability.

The reaction of a parent is summarised in Box 10.7, and Case study 1 describes the process.

Box 10.7   Different stages of reacting to bad news

1 Shock

2 Anger

3 Disbelief, denial

4 Acceptance

Case study 1

John was born at term after a normal delivery, and is the first child of Jim and Brenda, who are in their mid-twenties. The Senior House Officer (SHO) is called to see the baby, as the nurses think he may have Down syndrome.

Elaine, the SHO, examines the baby and agrees with the diagnosis. Brenda is aware that something is not right, and she asks what is wrong with the baby. Breaking the news is a consultant task and both parents should be present, but if Elaine is sure then she should not conceal the information. If she is uncertain then she should say that there may be something not quite right and that the consultant is coming to see them.

Parents prefer to be told this kind of news as soon as possible, and when they are together. The baby should be present, as this will help the consultant to explain the situation. This is a private matter, not one for the open ward, and disturbances must be minimised. It is helpful to have someone known to the mother (perhaps a midwife or sister) present, and providing that numbers do not get too great, the social worker or liaison health visitor of the child development team may find it useful for future management to hear what has been said.

There are different ways of breaking the news. One effective approach is to examine the baby with the parents, gently indicating the features of the syndrome and explaining that although individually they can occur in normal people, the overall features indicate Down syndrome, and that this will be confirmed by a blood test. This approach avoids raising a false hope that the test will be normal and that all of this will have been a bad dream.

Once the words 'Down syndrome' have been said, parents have told us that they cannot take in any more information.

All questions should be answered, but this information will have to be reiterated on a follow-up visit when further questions can be answered. The inability to take in information after bad news is part of a well-described reaction to tragedy which parents take a variable time to work through. Parents say that they welcome practical information about the day-to-day management of their child as well as details of the problems that are likely to occur.

A karyotype is necessary both for accurate genetic diagnosis and to assess the likelihood of recurrence of Down syndrome. Around 95% of all Down syndrome cases are due to non-disjunction trisomy 21 (see Table 10.1 and Chapter 11, page 154).

Blood should be sent for a karyotype for assessment of the genetic risk, and cardiac ultrasound should be arranged because of the possibility of a congenital heart defect. The child's hearing should also be tested.

John could be placed in a 'mainstream school' with extra support or in a 'special school' or a special unit attached to a mainstream school. He will need regular follow-up of his vision, hearing, height and weight, and his thyroid function tests will need to be checked. Down syndrome children are prone to recurrent upper respiratory tract infections, which can lead to conductive deafness. Some develop hypothyroidism, weight problems, or long or short sight.

Table 10.1 Recurrence risk in Down syndrome

Type of syndrome	Parents' chromosomes	Likelihood of recurrence
Trisomy 21	Normal	1 in 100 if mother is under 40 years. If mother is over 40 years, twice usual probability for her age
Translocation with chromosome 13, 14, 15 or 22	Normal Mother a carrier Father a carrier	Usual probability for mother's age 1 in 8 1 in 40
Mosaicism	Normal	Unknown, probably the usual probability for mother's age

Source: Selikowitz (1997).

Cerebral palsy

The conditions known as 'cerebral palsy' were first described by William John Little in 1863, but it was William Osler who coined the term in 1886. Cerebral palsy is the commonest cause of physical disability in the UK. It is usually but not always associated with prematurity or birth asphyxia. It is non-progressive but remains for life, and it mainly affects the use of the muscles, the characteristic feature being spasticity. All or part of the body may be affected, and there is wide variation in severity. Learning difficulties are common but by no means always present, and careful testing is needed to find the cognitive development potential (*see* Box 10.8).

Box 10.8   Cerebral palsy

Definition
Cerebral palsy (CP) is a disorder of movement and tone caused by a non-progressive brain lesion.

Incidence/types
2 in 1000 live births
Spastic (hypertonic) 70%
Athetoid ⎫
Ataxic   ⎬ 20–25%
Mixed   ⎭

Pattern
Hemiplegic: one side of the body involved
Diplegic: lower half of the body involved
Quadriplegic: all of the body involved

Associated problems
CP alone: *c.* 30%
CP + epilepsy: *c.* 30%
CP + learning difficulties: *c.* 30%

Therapy for cerebral palsy should be coordinated by a paediatrician. Therapy services (physiotherapy, occupational therapy and speech therapy) are central, and drug therapy is commonly used to reduce the spasticity. Surgery is occasionally required if there are severe contractures. Seizures are common and require treatment, and support will be needed in the educational setting. The parents are the key therapists for the child, and they need to be empowered to take on this role while at the same time recognising their own need for information and support.

Case study 2

Beth is 9 months old. She is just beginning to sit up and is still wobbly. Her mother, who is a single parent, has observed that she is left-handed, and draws your attention to this when she presents with a respiratory infection. She had a preterm birth but there were no complications.

Examination shows increased tone on the right, the hand is clenched, the thumb is adducted, there is weakness in that arm and the reflexes are brisk on that side. Hand preference at this age suggests that there is a neurological problem, in this case cerebral palsy. The picture is one of a right-sided weakness with hypertonia and upper motor neuron signs.

Investigations such as computerised tomography (CT) or magnetic resonance imaging (MRI) scan and a genetic opinion may be useful. Physiotherapy will be arranged, directed at reducing spasticity, maintaining the range of movement and improving strength. The local child development team should be involved. Orthotics may provide a light-weight splint to prevent shortening of the Achilles tendon (ankle foot orthosis, AFO), and a muscle relaxant, baclofen, can be used to reduce tone. The social worker on the team can discuss benefits and allowances.

When Beth is 3 years old, she is able to walk independently with an ankle foot orthosis on the right leg. She has regular physiotherapy and occupational therapy. Her mother wonders whether she will cope in school.

Preparing for school will require a Statement of Special Educational Needs (in England and Wales) or a Record of Needs (in Scotland) in line with the Education Act (1981). Beth's parents have a statutory right to be involved in the record/statement process and to receive a copy of the record or statement. An educational psychologist will take the lead role in this process. The record or statement describes Beth's strengths and weaknesses and sets out her needs. Beth's IQ is in the normal range and her needs are centred around her physical problems. She will be reviewed regularly. She should attend mainstream school with extra help.

Delayed walking

This is an important presentation which can signify a number of different conditions (*see* Box 10.9 for differential diagnosis). The mean age for learning to walk is 15 months but there is a wide range, and delay should be considered at over 18 months. As walking is such an important milestone, parents become quite anxious if their child is a late walker. One of the commoner reasons is the familial 'bottom-shuffler' (*see* Box 10.10), but do not assume that this is the cause without considering other more serious conditions which may require specific treatment. In all late-walking boys the creatine kinase level should be checked in order to exclude muscular dystrophy (*see* Box 10.11 and Case study 3).

Box 10.9 Differential diagnosis of late walking

- Extended normal range
- Familial late walker
- Bottom-shuffler
- Isolated motor delay
- Global delay
- Cerebral palsy
- Rarities, including muscular dystrophy

Box 10.10 Features of bottom-shuffling

- An alternative developmental pathway
- Sit–shuffle–walk, normally but late
- Occurs in 2% of children
- Often has a positive family history
- Dislike of prone position
- Relative lower limb hypotonia
- Absent/decreased caudal parachute response
- Does not crawl

Case study 3

Benjamin is 18 months old and has not yet started to walk. His elder brother, William, walked at 12 months. His mother Gwen initially felt that Ben was 'just lazy', but is now concerned about him.

Ben sits and crawls. He does not cruise, but pulls himself up to the furniture. All other development is reported as normal. He has had no serious illnesses, and he was a full-term, normal delivery. All of the family members except Gwen walked at about 12 months. She bottom-shuffled and walked at 17 months.

Ben is well. There are no abnormalities on examination. Neurological examination shows normal power, tone and reflexes. He appears well-muscled. Developmental examination shows normal fine motor development, normal speech, language and hearing development, and normal social and adaptive skills. Ben's gross motor development is as his mother described. He also demonstrates Gower's sign in that he 'climbs up his legs' when getting up from a prone or seated position on the floor.

It was felt that he might be a 'shuffler' like his mother, but that it was important to check his creatine kinase (CK) level.

Ben's CK level was 10 000 units per litre (normal < 160 IU/l), which is a grossly elevated value and points to a diagnosis of muscular dystrophy. The definitive diagnosis is made by muscle biopsy.

The muscle biopsy was positive, showing an increased variation in fibre size and an increase in rounded fibres staining with eosin. This confirmed the diagnosis.

Ben's prognosis is progressive muscular weakness, with loss of walking between the ages of 7 and 13 years and death in the late teens or early twenties. Physiotherapy aims to maintain a plantar grade foot to help Ben to walk for as long as possible. Ankle foot orthosis (AFO) can also assist, and an Achilles tenotomy may be required. These measures require teamwork. Ben will eventually need a wheelchair.

Genetic counselling is necessary for the family with an affected male, for although the condition can arise *de novo* it is usually transmitted down the female line. The DMD gene has now been localised on the short arm of the X-chromosome and its product, dystrophin, has been identified (*see* Chapter 11).

Box 10.11   Duchenne muscular dystrophy (DMD)

Incidence
1 in 3000

Aetiology
X-linked recessive gene, carried by asymptomatic females, 50% of whose daughters will be carriers and 50% of whose sons will be affected. The affected boys lack the protein dystrophin in muscle. Antenatal diagnosis is now possible

Diagnosis
Creatine kinase and muscle biopsy

Prognosis
Loss of walking at 7–13 years
Death in the late teens or early twenties

Associated problems
Lower than average IQ
Muscle contractures
Scoliosis
Progressive weakness
Respiratory problems

Speech delay

This is an increasing problem in the UK, and it is one of the commonest reasons for referral to a developmental paediatrician. According to their teachers, up to 10% of 7-year-olds are difficult to understand. There is a strong social class distribution due to the higher prevalence of ear infections in lower socio-economic groups, and also less language stimulation. Speech delay has a major impact on educational and social achievement and should therefore be investigated and managed actively with an emphasis on early detection (*see* Box 10.12).

Behavioural difficulties are common in children with communication difficulties. Most children with speech delay should be referred to a speech and language therapist.

Case study 4

Richard is 2 years old, the second of a professional couple's two children. He has no words, and is prone to temper tantrums. His sister Elizabeth, aged 4 years, is a chatterbox. His mother is concerned about him and asks what can be done.

Richard babbled but got stuck at the 'da da da' stage after a bad cold. He does not seem to understand instructions, particularly the word 'No'! He is never the first to the front door when the bell rings. Richard's mother felt that Elizabeth was 'doing all the talking for him and he would come on'. Examination shows glue behind both eardrums.

The audiometrician performs a hearing test which shows a 60-decibel hearing loss across all of the frequencies in both ears.

Further tests, including evoked-response audiometry, establish that Richard's hearing loss is conductive, and that he has glue ear (*see* Chapter 6, page 85). Grommets are inserted (*see* page 88), and later Richard's parents note that he is taking more notice, is less loud and does not study faces so intently, and that he is uttering an increasing number of single words.

Richard starts to progress, and within a few months he is starting to put words together.

Box 10.12   Speech delay

Incidence
2.4% of children are totally unintelligible at age 7 years, according to teachers (National Child Development Survey)
4 male:1 female

Associated problems
Non-reading
Poor number work
Motor learning difficulties
Impaired visual acuity

Differential diagnosis
Global delay
Hearing loss
Lack of stimulation
Specific language disorder
The autistic continuum
Elective muteness

---

conductive loss and approximately 3 in 1000 will have a sensorineural loss. There are many genetically determined causes of deafness. Although universal screening of neonates by oto-acoustic emissions is soon to be introduced throughout the UK, parents may also be effective screening agents. If a parent thinks that their child has a hearing problem, the child must have their hearing assessed and proved normal or otherwise.

Box 10.13   Causes of deafness

Conductive	*Sensorineural*
Foreign body	Drug-induced
Wax	Meningitis
Serous otitis	Encephalitis
(glue ear)	Asphyxia
	Hyperbilirubinaemia
	Congenital infection
	Genetic

The deaf child

Deafness can have many causes (*see* Box 10.13). Around 5–10% of children will have a significant

Certain acquired medical conditions carry a high risk of deafness, and all children who have had a meningitic or encephalitic illness should have their hearing tested on recovery. If a hearing child becomes deaf as a result of such an illness, a cochlear implant is a possible option, but this

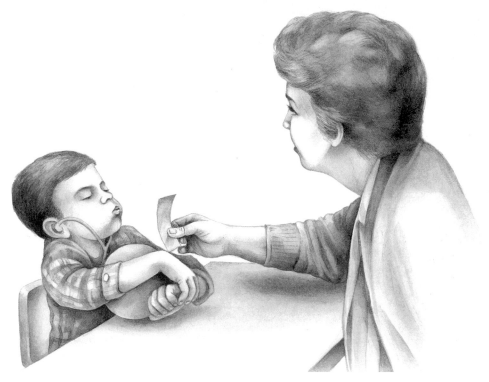

Figure 10.4   Specialist provision is needed for the deaf child.

is not appropriate for the majority of deaf children.

A team approach to the management of a hearing-impaired child is important. Awareness of a child's problem and the correct classroom positioning will help. Deaf children do not just have a problem with hearing and speaking. They can also find it difficult to learn written language, which is a system of symbols representing speech, which is in turn a system of sound symbols representing both abstract and concrete thoughts. Thus there is a need for specialist provision, whether this is integrated into a mainstream school or provided in a special school (*see* Figure 10.4).

Stigma still exists with regard to deafness – hearing-impaired individuals face discrimination and bullying in society. Parents should always be put in contact with a support group, which is one of the ways of countering this problem.

Visual impairment

In this section we shall be considering problems that are severe enough to affect daily life and education (*see also* Chapter 7). Visual impairment can be very mild (squint, or short or long sight) or very severe, and if severe is often associated with other defects. The learning capacity of visually impaired children can be considerable, and with the use of aids of various kinds there are few pursuits which are not open to them. The causes are listed in Box 10.14.

Beware of the word 'blind' – parents do not like it. Pause a moment and think, what would a blind person see? Blind is not 'blackness', or only very rarely is it so.

Parents tend to think that the word 'blind' does mean blackness and that it also means for ever. Instead, try to convey to them the concept of functional vision. If a child has a visually directed reach then he or she is not blind. 'Blind' is an administrative category or level of visual acuity below which certain benefits are payable.

Box 10.14   Visual impairment

Definition in UK
Visual acuity 3/60 or less in better eye with correction

Incidence of blindness
32 in 100 000 children

Causes in the developed world
- Delayed visual maturation
- Genetic disease: congenital cataract, albinism, retinal dystrophies
- Perinatal disease: retinopathy of prematurity, birth hypoxia
- Non-genetic congenital malformation: microphthalmos, congenital glaucoma
- Congenital infection: rubella

Associated problems
In the UK, many cases of blindness are associated with other severe handicaps, including cerebral palsy, epilepsy and learning disability

---

Case study 5

James, aged 8 weeks, was brought to the clinic. At a 6-week check, his mother reported that he was not 'looking at her'.

James was full-term, with no adverse history. He did not have cataracts or an abnormal retinal reflex. His pupil reactions were present, but there was no 'threat blink'* and no fixation. In other respects his development seemed to be normal. Further investigations, including fundoscopy under anaesthesia, electroretinograms (ERGs) and visual evoked responses (VERs), were carried out. Examination and ERGs were normal, but VERs showed reduced amplitude and delayed pattern.

With visual stimulation James started to respond, vocalising to light and then to face, and by the time he was 1 year old his visual skills were normal for his age.

This presentation could represent delayed visual maturation (DVM). Just as there can be delay in gross or fine motor skills, there can also be delay in visual maturation. If there is no associated mental retardation, a child with isolated DVM is likely to have useful vision by 6 months of age. If there is associated mental retardation, useful vision will also be delayed. A visual stimulation programme can be helpful.

*A 'threat blink' is elicited by bringing a closed hand to the outer canthus of each eye in turn and then suddenly opening the fingers, avoiding the face. By doing this you avoid a draught, which could elicit a corneal reflex blink.

Learning disability

The terms *mental handicap, mental retardation* and *general learning disability* are all synonyms. The existence of such synonyms is an indication of a lack of acceptance of mental handicap within society and the progressive adaptation of technical terms as terms of abuse by the public ('retard' in the USA and 'mental' in the UK).

Learning disability is different from the other problems discussed which cause special need. It is not a disease, a disorder, a syndrome or a specific disability. It is a blanket or administrative term for a wide variety of different genetic, social, educational and specific medical conditions with the common feature that 'affected' individuals repeatedly score below 70 on specific IQ tests. Learning disability is sometimes an indication of brain dysfunction, just as epilepsy or cerebral palsy are, but often it is not.

IQ scores are not used as the sole delineator of learning disability. A comprehensive assessment by an educational psychologist acting as part of a team is required. When conducting epidemiological studies, IQ testing is relevant.

Behaviour problems are common in children with learning difficulties. There is a temptation for carers to 'make allowances' and over-protect the child. Consistent, firm management is advisable, not allowing any undesirable behaviour to become entrenched. The child should be encouraged and taught to be as independent as possible within his or her level of ability.

Case study 6

Mary is just over 3 years old. Her birth and early history were quite normal, but she was a slow walker at 18 months, and a slow talker, saying her first words at 18 months, and linking words at 2 years 6 months. At her 3-year developmental surveillance she is functioning at about the 2-year level. Otherwise she is well. Her mother needed some remedial help in school herself and so is not particularly worried about Mary. There is nothing obvious on examination.

On paediatric review, the history is confirmed. Physical examination is normal, with no specific clues. The Denver Screening Test confirms functioning at around the 2-year level at a chronological age of 3 years 3 months. Mary's birthday falls at such a time that her school target date is in September, 13 months away. Thyroid function tests, urine amino acids, chromosomes and DNA studies for fragile X syndrome (*see* Chapter 11, page 160) are all normal. Vision and hearing tests are also normal.

Mary's IQ is found to be 60. Her speech delay is commensurate with her general delay, her fine motor skills are at the same level, and there is no significant gross motor impairment.

Mary's needs are mainly educational. She requires a coordinated assessment directed towards establishing a Record/Statement of Needs within the next year. This process requires input from her parents, the educational psychologist, teacher, a speech therapist and the community paediatrician.

Mary's special needs are identified as a requirement for a highly structured developmental curriculum, small group teaching, one-to-one teaching with extra classroom support, a speaking environment with regular professional speech therapy and occupational therapy review with advice as necessary. These needs could be met either in special school or in her local primary school with additional support. Her mother chooses special school (*see* Box 10.15).

Mary does well at special school, but at the age of 9 years her mother mentions that she is having difficulties with her behaviour at home, although no similar report is received from school.

Box 10.15   Special school vs. mainstream

Special school	*Mainstream school*
May be far from home	Near to home
May be stigma to child	Good for mixing, but there may be bullying
Specialised teachers	Specialised support may be lacking
Good for parental support	Enables child to be with siblings

Dyslexia (specific reading difficulty)

A specific difficulty with reading and spelling that is not associated with any general impairment is present in approximately 5% of school-age children.

Case study 7

David is 8 years old. He is having problems at school with reading, spelling and written work. Numbers are not too problematic, and he likes drawing and physical education. He has been receiving help from a remedial teacher. His father had some difficulties at first in school, but there is no other relevant history. David's mother wonders whether 'anything more can be done'.

This problem is different from the others discussed in this chapter. David is older than the other children, his problem is not a disease, and its remedy lies outside the medical arena. There are several things that can be done, the most important being to get the correct diagnosis. Review the history, look at examples of David's schoolwork, examine him, paying attention to the neurological system, look for evidence of motor learning difficulty, ascertain hand, foot and eye laterality, ask him to draw and write, and check for squint and visual acuity.

The only 'abnormality' you have uncovered is that David seems to lack a fixed reference eye and that there is prima facie evidence of a specific learning difficulty with reading. Two steps are appropriate, namely referral to an orthoptist and referral to an educational psychologist.

Reading difficulty is commonly seen in practice because reading is fundamental to most education. Dyslexia tends to be a socially 'acceptable' special need. It is necessary to distinguish specific learning difficulty from a more general learning difficulty.

Spina bifida

The term 'spina dorsi bifida' was coined by Professor Nicolai Tulp in Amsterdam in 1652. It is a central nervous system malformation in which the spinal cord fails to close during fetal development, and in the severest forms is exposed to the surface when the baby is born. There is a greater or lesser degree of lower limb paralysis and often associated hydrocephalus due to the Arnold–Chiari malformation (a downward displacement of the cerebellum and medulla oblongata through the foramen magnum).

The prevalence in the UK is currently about 1 in 1000, and it is falling because of antenatal diagnosis and the prevention of recurrence by the use of folic acid supplementation.

The policy of early surgery for all spina bifida babies led to the survival of large numbers of children with a subsequent poor quality of life. Certain adverse factors were recognised as being associated with a bad outcome, and these are now regarded as relative contraindications to surgery (*see* Box 10.16).

Once there has been an affected child in the family there is an increased risk of neural-tube defects in that family. The inheritance of neural-tube defects is multifactorial. Genetic counselling is possible, as is antenatal diagnosis.

Case study 8

Michael is a full-term, normal delivery baby and is noted to have a spina bifida. He will require careful evaluation by a paediatrician or paediatric neurologist and a paediatric surgeon. It is important to allow the parents to participate in an informed debate about what should be done.

Michael's mother asks you to let her see his back. It is best to allow this, as it will assist explanation later, and often what is imagined is worse than the reality.

Michael's defect is a lumbar sacral myelomeningocele covering L4, L5, S1, confirmed on X-ray. There is no hydrocephalus, spinal deformity or other major defect.

Early surgery is performed, involving closure of the back and insertion of a Spitz–Holter ventriculo-peritoneal shunt to allow drainage of cerebrospinal fluid into the peritoneal cavity.

With a lesion at the level of Michael's, walking with short calipers is possible. There may be orthopaedic problems associated with muscle imbalance. Kyphosis and scoliosis may occur, and will need to be watched for. There may be problems with urinary continence and infection, and there may also be bowel problems. Learning difficulties are not uncommon, and there may be sexual problems in adult life.

Box 10.16   Adverse factors in spina bifida

- Thorax-lumbar lesions, motor level L3 and upwards
- Spinal deformity, severe kyphosis or scoliosis
- Gross hydrocephalus, occipital frontal circumference (OFC) > 2 cm above 90% percentile
- Other motor defects

Hydrocephalus

This condition, known to the lay person as 'water on the brain', is commonly associated with spina bifida, but may be caused by other conditions such as intracranial haemorrhage in a preterm infant, meningitis or other infection, neoplasm or congenital abnormality. There is a blockage of the flow or reabsorption of cerebrospinal fluid in the ventricles.

Hydrocephalus would be suspected on finding a rapidly enlarging head circumference in an infant together with a wide fontanelle, frontal bossing (swelling in the frontal region) and the 'sunsetting sign' (sclera visible above the pupil) (*see* Box 10.17).

Treatment involves the insertion of a shunt between the ventricle and the peritoneum or right atrium of the heart (usually the former).

Box 10.17   Signs of hydrocephalus

- Rapidly enlarging head circumference
- Wide and bulging fontanelle
- Frontal bossing
- Sunsetting sign
- Raised intracranial pressure

Support for parents

Parents are a very important part of the team. Most parents are a great asset to a disabled child. Sadly, however, occasionally a parent can contribute to handicap. Support for carers is an important role of the team. Breaking the bad news and the stages of grieving have been discussed in the section on Down syndrome, but the principles apply to all disabilities.

When a baby is born, it is expected to be perfect. If it is not, many parental dreams and hopes are shattered. Some parents will adjust, but not all of them. The quotations at the beginning of this chapter could not have been written if Christopher Nolan had not been read to and had not been fully involved in his family's love of literature.

Parents with limited education and from a poorer socio-economic background may find it harder to deal with the complex issues and also the multiple contacts with various service providers, and will require additional support and advocacy on their behalf.

Parents need information about causation, the current situation, future prospects and genetic implications. They need practical help in alleviating their child's handicap, including aids to easier living, access to appropriate appliances, and environmental adaptations.

They need the essential break – respite from care – but they may not know this at first. Such respite may be short- or long-term or crisis relief, and can take a variety of forms including hospital provision in cases where there are very special needs. These parents need financial assistance and help to gain access to the statutory benefits that are available (*see* Box 10.18).

Parents need information about the services that are available, which may come from specialist social workers, liaison health visitors, books or support agencies.

They frequently benefit from the mutual support of other parents who have children with similar problems. There are many different syndrome support groups in existence. The organisation 'Contact a Family' acts as a coordinating network and can be used to put families in contact with self-help groups for a wide variety of different conditions.

Box 10.18   Allowances and financial support

Disability living allowances

Care component

Lower level: small amount of care at specific times

Medium level: attention or help needed by day or by night

Higher level: constant attention or help needed by day and by night

Mobility component

Lower level: can walk, but needs more supervision than a child of the same age

Higher level: virtually unable to walk

Family Fund, PO Box 50, York YO1 2ZX Funded by the Government, administered independently by the Joseph Rowntree Trust. Provides help for the families of severely handicapped people in areas that are not the responsibility of other agencies

---

Teamworking

The problems mentioned in this chapter all require a team approach if the children involved are to reach their full potential. The team consists of a core group of professionals who work together regularly, both helping individual children and planning and developing services for children with special needs as a group.

Teams need to meet regularly, and most evolve their own pattern – weekly meetings about clinical problems and monthly meetings about broader issues are usual. Child development teams also require a clear lead, and this will often be provided by a consultant paediatrician.

Further reading

- Baron-Cohen S and Bolton P (1993) *Autism: the facts*. Oxford University Press, Oxford.
- Cunningham C, Morgan P and McGucken RB (1984) Down's syndrome: is dissatisfaction with disclosure of diagnosis inevitable? *Dev Med Child Neurol*. **26**: 33–9.
- Emery AEH (1994) *Muscular Dystrophy: the facts*. Oxford University Press, Oxford.
- Griffiths M and Clegg M (1988) *Cerebral Palsy: problems and practice*. Souvenir Press, London.
- Hall DMB and Hill P (1996) *The Child With a Disability* (2e). Blackwell Science, Oxford.
- Selikowitz M (1997) *Down Syndrome: the facts* (2e). Oxford University Press, Oxford.
- Shaw C (1993) *Talking and Your Child*. Hodder and Stoughton, London.
- World Health Organization (1980) *International Classification of Impairments, Disabilities and Handicaps*. World Health Organization, Geneva.

Useful organisation

- Contact a Family; www.cafamily.co.uk

Self-assessment questions

1 Down syndrome is:
(a) caused by trisomy of chromosome 23   True/False
(b) present only in boys   True/False
(c) associated with intestinal obstruction   True/False
(d) able to be diagnosed antenatally.   True/False

2 A disability is:
(a) a limitation of achievement   True/False
(b) due to an impairment   True/False
(c) treated by physiotherapy   True/False
(d) an abnormality of physiological or anatomical structure.   True/False

3 The following are disabilities:
(a) visual impairment due to squint   True/False
(b) myelomeningocele   True/False
(c) glue ear   True/False
(d) hemiplegia in cerebral palsy.   True/False

4 Management of learning disability requires:
(a) physiotherapy   True/False
(b) assessment of special educational need   True/False
(c) placement in a special school   True/False
(d) chromosome testing.   True/False

11 Genetics

- Role of the clinical geneticist
- Modes of inheritance
- Marfan's syndrome
- Cystic fibrosis (autosomal recessive)
- X-linked disorders

Role of the clinical geneticist

Although a genetic disorder may affect an individual child, it is important to remember that the diagnosis of a genetic disorder has implications both for the immediate family and often for the wider family. It is this family-orientated approach which characterises clinical genetic practice. The human genome contains around 20 000–25 000 genes, mutations in which may cause specific genetic diseases. The range of possible genetic disorders is vast, and although genetic disorders as a group are relatively common (about 1 in 20 individuals under the age of 25 years have a genetic disorder), each individual disease may be rare. They also represent a substantial paediatric workload. For example, congenital malformations, many of which are genetic, account for 2% of all live births but for 30% of bed-days occupied in a children's hospital.

The clinical geneticist fulfils three main roles in the care of children and families with genetic disorders. First, they are involved in the clinical assessment and diagnosis of children with possible genetic disorders. Secondly, they are responsible for liaison with the cytogenetic and molecular genetic laboratories to arrange the appropriate investigations for the child and the family, and thirdly, and in parallel with this, they must counsel the family, explaining the diagnosis and its implications both for the child and for other family members (see Box 11.8). Such counselling must include information about the options available to the family, to allow them to make appropriate healthcare and reproductive decisions, always remembering that for each family member the decision is ultimately theirs alone to make on the basis of appropriate knowledge. This approach is known as non-directive counselling, and it is fundamental to ethical clinical genetic practice.

Box 11.1 Clinical genetics

- A family-orientated approach
- Two per cent of all births have a congenital malformation (many are genetic)
- The human genome has 20 000–25 000 genes

Box 11.2 Role of clinical geneticist

- Clinical assessment and diagnosis
- Identification of appropriate laboratory investigation(s)
- Family counselling

Modes of inheritance

Single gene disorders

Genetic disorders may arise as a consequence of mutations in single genes (single gene disorders), from the interaction of single genes with other genes and environmental factors (multifactorial inheritance) or because of aberrations involving whole chromosomes or parts of chromosomes (chromosome aneuploidy). Single gene disorders are usually inherited according to the laws of Mendel. In autosomal-dominant inheritance, the gene is located on an autosome, and only one of the two copies present is faulty. There is a 1 in 2 chance that the child of an affected person will inherit the faulty gene. Affected individuals in a family are often affected to different degrees (variable expression), and sometimes an individual may inherit a faulty gene but display no features of the disease (incomplete penetrance). Transmission of a genetic disorder from father to son implies autosomal-dominant inheritance. Transmission from father to daughter or from mother to son or daughter may also occur, but is also compatible with X-linked inheritance. In autosomal-recessive inheritance, both copies of the gene must be faulty for the disorder to arise. The affected child thus inherits one faulty copy from each parent, both of whom are therefore carriers of the condition. Autosomal-recessive disorders are more common where there is parental consanguinity, and tend to affect members of one sibship only, with no previous family history. In X-linked inheritance, the faulty gene is on the X-chromosome, and therefore tends to affect boys severely (as they have only one copy of the X-chromosome) and be transmitted by healthy females (who have a second, normal copy of the gene on their other X-chromosome).

Box 11.3 Modes of inheritance

- Autosomal dominant

- Autosomal recessive

- X-linked

- Mitochondrial

- Multifactorial

Occasionally, girls may be affected by an X-linked recessive disorder because of lyonisation. This is the process by which female embryos randomly inactivate one X-chromosome in each cell at around 12–16 days post conception. If the embryo happens to inactivate mostly the X-chromosome carrying the normal gene, then that female may manifest features of the disease. In addition to these forms of inheritance, some disorders arise because of mutations in genes encoded on the mitochondrial genome. These disorders are often very variable and affect many different systems of the body, and they are transmitted exclusively by the mother.

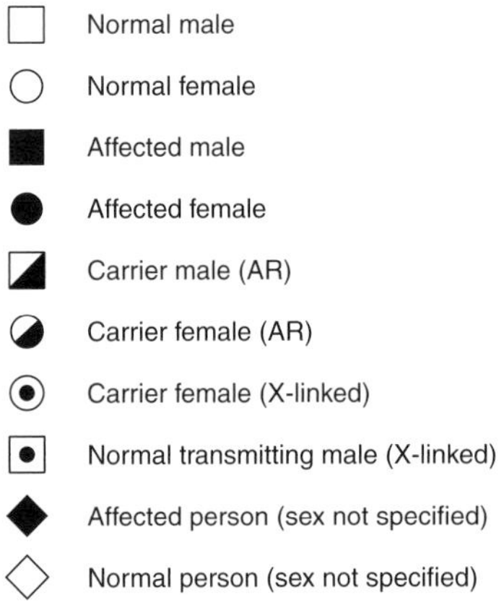

Figure 11.1 Symbols used in family tree (*see also* page 3). AR, autosomal recessive.

Multifactorial disorders

These arise from the interaction of many genes and environmental factors. Neural-tube defects (spina bifida, anencephaly) and facial clefting fall into this category. Recurrence risks for siblings are usually in the range 2–10%, depending on the disorder and its frequency in the population, and are much lower for more distant relatives.

Chromosomal disorders

These may involve the loss or gain of a whole chromosome (e.g. the lack of one X-chromosome in Turner's syndrome, or the presence of an extra chromosome 21 in Down syndrome), or the loss or gain of part of a chromosome. Additional material present on a chromosome may arise from duplication of a segment, or because of translocation of material from another chromosome. If part of a chromosome is missing, it is said to be deleted. Part of a chromosome may also be turned around or inverted. Inversions often have no effect on the carrier, unless a gene is disrupted at the inversion breakpoints, but may cause reproductive problems because of pairing difficulties between a normal and inverted chromosome at meiosis. Translocations may be familial or sporadic (*de novo*). When two chromosomes have exchanged material, but none of this has been duplicated or deleted, the translocation is said to be a balanced reciprocal translocation. A balanced translocation usually has no clinical effects on its carrier, but that individual may experience reproductive problems in terms of recurrent miscarriage or stillbirth, or the birth

of a disabled child if they transmit an unbalanced translocation (i.e. if they transmit one of the rearranged chromosomes but not the other) to their potential offspring (*see* Box 11.4).

Box 11.4   Chromosome disorders

- Chromosome loss or gain (e.g. Turner's syndrome)
- Duplication of segment
- Deletion of segment
- Inversion of segment
- Translocation (usually no effect if balanced)
- Non-disjunction (e.g. trisomy 21 in Down syndrome)

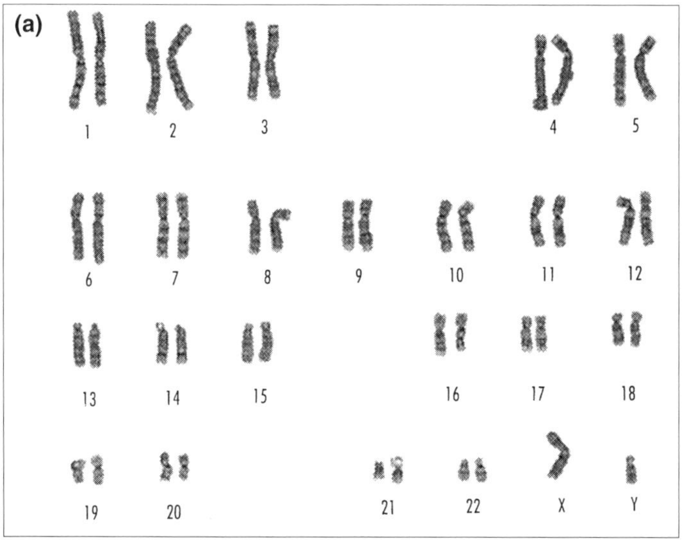

Figure 11.2   (a) Normal karyotype. (b) Balanced reciprocal translocation between 5 and 15.

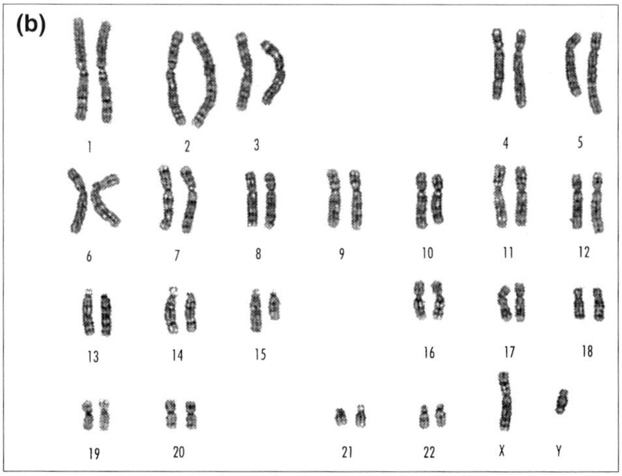

Marfan's syndrome (autosomal dominant)

Marfan's syndrome is a hereditary disorder of connective tissue with multisystem effects. The main features are tall stature, arachnodactyly (long fingers – literally 'spider fingers'), defect of the lens in the eye and a high risk of aortic dissection (*see* Box 11.5).

Box 11.5   Marfan's syndrome

- Autosomal dominant
- Up to 35% of cases have no family history
- Fibrillin gene on chromosome 15
- Skeleton (tall, scoliosis, arachnodactyly)
- Ocular (lens dislocation, myopia)
- Cardiovascular (aortic dilatation, aortic aneurysm)
- Prophylactic beta-blockers, aortic surgery
- Echocardiographic follow-up

Case study 1

Jenny (III.1), aged 12 years, presents with pectus excavatum, tall stature and a 6-month history of low back pain, particularly on sitting for long periods at school (*see* Figure 11.3). Examination reveals that her height is just above the 97th centile, and she has a very mild lumbar scoliosis. She has mild joint laxity, although she has never suffered a dislocation, her thumb and fifth finger overlap when wrapped around the opposite wrist (Walker–Murdoch wrist sign), and she can extend her thumb well beyond the ulnar border of the palm (Steinberg thumb sign) (*see* Figure 11.4). The latter two signs are indicative of arachnodactyly. Jenny also has a high arched palate. In the family history, her father (II.5) is tall and has myopia. His brother (II.2) died suddenly at work on his fishing boat at the age of 25 years. Another brother is tall but well, and two sisters are well. Their father died from a heart attack at the age 58 years, and is known to have had poor eyesight.

Jenny has many skeletal features suggestive of Marfan's syndrome. She has tall stature, arachnodactyly, scoliosis and a high arched palate. This does not of itself allow a diagnosis of Marfan's syndrome to be made. An echocardiogram is normal.

The family history of tall stature, myopia and sudden early death is highly suspicious. Investigation of the uncle's death certificate reveals that he died from a dissecting ascending aortic aneurysm. Clinical investigation of the father reveals that he too has skeletal features of Marfan's syndrome. This family history makes a diagnosis of Marfan's syndrome very likely.

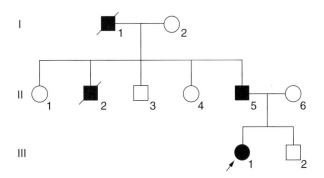

Figure 11.3 Jenny's family tree.

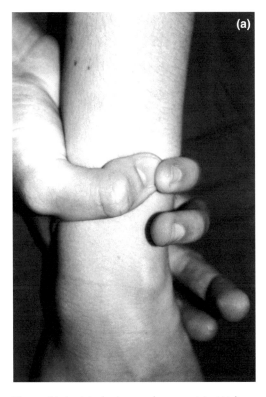

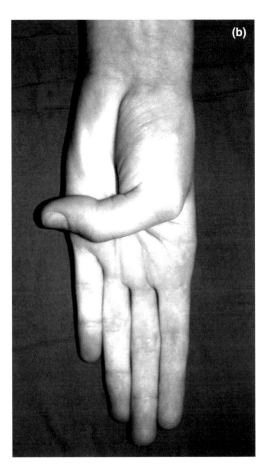

Figure 11.4 Marfan's syndrome. (a) Walter–Murdoch wrist sign (thumb and 5th finger overlap when wrapped around opposite wrist). (b) Steinberg thumb sign (thumb extends beyond ulnar border of palm).

Cystic fibrosis (autosomal recessive) (see *also* Chapter 5)

When a child is diagnosed as having cystic fibrosis (CF) there are many ramifications in the wider family. Cystic fibrosis is an autosomal-recessive disorder caused by mutations in a gene on chromosome 7 which encodes a membrane-bound chloride-ion channel. One in 25 people with no family history in the UK are carriers of a CF mutation. In an autosomal-recessive disorder, both parents are obligate carriers, there is a 1 in 4 chance that any child will be affected, and a 2 in 3 chance that any normal child will be a carrier. The family implications when cystic fibrosis is diagnosed start with the immediate family and then extend to the wider family. A major concern frequently expressed early on by the parents of the index case is whether their other child(ren) could be affected. It may be that there are no clinical features of cystic fibrosis, but if the sibling is younger, clinical features may not yet have developed (the average age at diagnosis was 3.5 years in one series, but is coming down as awareness of the condition increases and neonatal screening is introduced). Presentation may range from prenatal meconium ileus to recurrent chest infections in adult life. *See* Box 11.6 and Case study 2.

Box 11.6   Cystic fibrosis

- Autosomal recessive

- CF gene on chromosome 7 codes for a chloride-ion channel

- Four common mutations account for 85% of all mutations in Northern Europeans

- Over 400 mutations are known

- One in 25 Northern Europeans is a carrier

Case study 2

Anita (III.2), aged 13 years, has cystic fibrosis (CF) and was diagnosed before the CF gene was identified. Her mother is an only child, but her father has a younger sister, Jean (II.7), who has just married and would like a family. Jean is concerned about the risk of having a child with CF (*see* Figure 11.5).

Anita has been found to be homozygous for the DF508 deletion, the most common mutation in the Northern European population. As expected, both of her parents are heterozygous for this mutation (carriers). Anita's younger brother Andrew (III.3) frequently has a cough, and her parents ask for him to be tested. He has previously had a normal sweat test.

Anita's paternal aunt, Jean (II.7), has recently married and is now pregnant. When she learns that her niece has cystic fibrosis, she is keen to have carrier tests for herself and her husband.

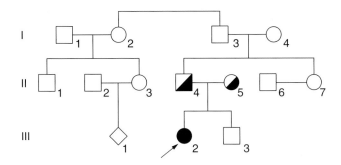

Figure 11.5 Anita's family tree.

X-linked disorders

Duchenne muscular dystrophy has a typical X-linked inheritance pattern, while fragile X syndrome illustrates the characteristics of an important class of genetic disorder, namely those due to unstable triplet repeat or 'dynamic' mutations. Different problems arise in genetic counselling as a result.

Duchenne muscular dystrophy (X-linked recessive) (see also Chapter 10)

Duchenne muscular dystrophy (DMD) is an X-linked muscle wasting disorder. Affected boys present with delay in learning to walk or with motor difficulties, including difficulty keeping up with children of the same age in walking or running and difficulty going up and down stairs. DMD is a progressive disorder associated with pseudohypertrophy of the calves (not always evident in the early stages). This means a swelling of the calf muscles which is not due to an increase in muscle strength. Respiratory muscle involvement leads to death by early adulthood. In about 60% of cases a deletion of the dystrophin gene at Xp21 is detectable by routine multiplex polymerase chain reaction (PCR) testing of lymphocyte DNA. The remaining cases have other types of mutation in dystrophin which are more difficult to detect. *See* Box 11.7 and Case study 3.

Box 11.7 Duchenne muscular dystrophy

- X-linked recessive

- Allelic with Becker muscular dystrophy

- Dystrophin gene at Xp21

- Around 60% of cases have a detectable deletion in dystrophin

- Two-thirds of mothers of an isolated case are carriers

- Female relatives' carrier status is determined by CK or DNA-based tests

---

Case study 3

Ben (III.2) was suspected of having DMD when his mother became concerned about his delay in walking. His clinical features (*see* Chapter 10), raised creatine kinase (CK) level and muscle biopsy findings confirmed the diagnosis. His mother already has one other child, but is pregnant again and wonders whether the pregnancy will also be affected, and whether it is possible to carry out prenatal diagnosis (*see* Figure 11.6).

There is no family history of DMD, but Ben's mother may still be a carrier of the disorder. Although Ben could be a new mutation, two-thirds of mothers of boys with DMD where there is no family history are carriers.

If Ben's mother is a carrier, there is a 1 in 4 chance that her pregnancy will be an affected boy, and a prenatal diagnosis could be made by DNA analysis of a chorionic villous biopsy or cultured amniocytes. If no deletion can be detected in Ben, carrier testing during pregnancy is not possible. Ben's mother could opt to terminate all male pregnancies, knowing that some or all of the male fetuses will actually be normal. We could also take a blood sample from Ben's healthy brother, and if the fetus is male, test using linked DNA markers to see whether it has inherited the same X-chromosome as Ben or as his brother. If it has the same chromosome as Ben, then it may be affected, but only if Ben's mother is a carrier.

As in all genetic disorders, the implications do not necessarily end with the nuclear family. Just as there is a 2 in 3 risk that Ben's mother is a carrier, there is a 1 in 3 chance that Ben's maternal grandmother (I.2) is a carrier, and also a possibility that Ben's maternal grandfather (I.1) has gonadal mosaicism for the dystrophin mutation/deletion. In either event, Ben's aunt Sally (II.3) may be a carrier, and there is a duty of care to offer to discuss these issues with the wider family and to arrange carrier testing should they so wish. Because of the relentless progression of DMD from an apparently healthy baby boy to a disabled child and then a dying teenager, families suffer immense emotional trauma which warrants sympathy and understanding from those involved in their management and counselling.

Fragile X syndrome (X-linked dominant)

Fragile X syndrome is the second commonest cause of learning difficulties after Down syndrome. It is an X-linked disorder which affects around 1 in 5000 liveborn males. Fragile X patients often have a characteristic behavioural and developmental phenotype (short attention span, speech and language delay, poor sensory integration, dysgraphia and dyscalculia). Physical features including macrocephaly (large head), prominent forehead and chin, prominent ears, post-pubertal macro-orchidism and sometimes joint laxity and mitral valve prolapse may be seen. X-linked disorders usually affect boys and are passed on through healthy unaffected women. In fragile X syndrome, affected females and normal transmitting males (male 'carriers') are often found because of the unusual characteristics of the unstable mutation which underlies the disorder. The syndrome takes its name from the appearance, first noted in 1979, of the X-chromosome in some cells of affected individuals when cultured under special conditions. The discovery in 1987 of the fragile X A gene and the presence of a triplet repeat expansion mutation within it revolutionised testing.

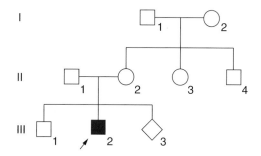

Figure 11.6 Ben's family tree.

Case study 4

James (IV.5), aged 2 years, attends the clinic for assessment of developmental delay and 'hyper-active behaviour'. He is found to have marked speech delay, mild motor delay and a short attention span. He has macrocephaly with a prominent forehead and mild joint laxity. His mother Carol reports that her brother, George (III.6), had similar speech and behavioural problems as a child, and that he still has poor communication skills as an adult. He lives at home with his parents and attends a day centre. His disability has been attributed to birth injury. Carol's older daughter, Kelly (IV.3), aged 8 years, was also late in learning to speak, but following speech therapy she attended a normal school. Because of learning difficulties, she has been kept back a year and receives learning support (*see* Figure 11.7).

The family history of an affected boy, an affected maternal uncle and a mildly affected girl suggests X-linked inheritance.

DNA testing of blood samples from James, Kelly, their mother Carol and their maternal uncle George was performed. It was found that James and George each have a large expansion (full mutation) of the triplet repeat region of the fragile X A gene, confirming that they both have fragile X syndrome.

Kelly has inherited a normal copy of the gene from her father, and a moderately large expansion of the gene (full mutation), which is displaying somatic instability, from her mother. Her mother has a normal copy and a mildly expanded copy (premutation). Kelly's mother is therefore an unaffected carrier of a small fragile X premutation, but Kelly has a full mutation and therefore her learning difficulties are probably due to fragile X syndrome, despite the fact that she is a girl. She has responded well to speech therapy, and is therefore clinically less severely affected than her uncle George. Girls are usually more mildly affected than boys even when the mutation size is similar, due to lyonisation. Making the diagnosis was very helpful to this family. They felt relieved of guilt that James's, Kelly's and George's problems were somehow due to bad parenting or to something the mothers had done wrong in pregnancy.

James's second cousin, Craig (IV.1), is an 8-year-old boy who, despite being kept back a year at school, is disruptive in class and has been very slow to develop reading and writing skills. The school feels that part of the problem is a lack of discipline at home, and the parents are very distressed by this.

DNA testing shows that Craig also has fragile X full mutation, confirming that he has fragile X syndrome. His disruptive behaviour is a consequence of his poor communication skills and short attention span. Appropriate schooling with specific attention to the characteristic learning difficulties of fragile X syndrome will improve both his progress and his behaviour. Making the diagnosis comes as a great relief to his parents and eases conflicts with the school. Looking at the family tree, you can see that Craig is connected to Kelly's branch of the family through his maternal grandfather (II.1). He is intellectually normal, and has a very small expansion of the gene, of premutation size. Premutations do not affect the individuals who carry them, and II.1 is therefore said to be a 'normal transmitting male'. The occurrence of such individuals can make the interpretation of family trees difficult at first glance, as they appear to contradict the rules of X-linked inheritance. DNA testing shows that this is not actually the case, but that the difficulty is caused by the variability and instability of the fragile X mutation when it is transmitted by a mother to her child.

When investigating this family you will have noticed that the family history was the key to finding the diagnosis – the behavioural and learning difficulties are non-specific and can only be seen to be compatible with fragile X syndrome in retrospect. When assessing a child with learning difficulties, always consider fragile X syndrome and take a family history, bearing in mind the difficulties illustrated by James's family.

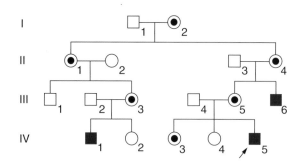

Figure 11.7 James' family tree.

Box 11.8 Genetic counselling

- Family implications — Genetic disorders affect families, not individuals

- Whose information is it? — Confidentiality of genetic information is crucial to avoid stigmatisation

- Conflict of interest — Family disagreements may cause problems if one part of a family will not permit disclosure of information that would be useful to another branch

- Social implications — Insurance and occupational problems can arise from prediction and diagnosis of genetic disease

- Responsibilities of health professionals — Non-directive counselling to allow informed choice; appropriate follow-up; aim for resolution of conflicts of interest

- Careful counselling, not indiscriminate testing

Further reading

- Bradley J, Johnson D and Rubinstein D (2001) *Lecture Notes on Molecular Medicine.* Blackwell Science, Oxford.

- Connor JM and Ferguson-Smith MA (1997) *Essential Medical Genetics.* Blackwell Science, Oxford.

- Turnpenny P and Ellard S (eds) (2004) *Emery's Elements of Medical Genetics* (12e). Churchill Livingstone, Edinburgh.

- Young ID (1999) *Introduction to Risk Calculation in Genetic Counselling.* Oxford University Press, Oxford.

Acknowledgement

Figures: Karyotypes courtesy of Dr D Couzin, Cytogenetics Laboratory, Department of Medical Genetics, Aberdeen Royal Hospitals NHS Trust.

Self-assessment questions

1   The following are single gene disorders:

(a) Duchenne muscular dystrophy   True/False

(b) cystic fibrosis   True/False

(c) sickle-cell disease   True/False

(d) cerebral palsy.   True/False

2   Antenatal detection is possible in the following conditions:

(a) cystic fibrosis   True/False

(b) Duchenne muscular dystrophy   True/False

(c) cerebral palsy   True/False

(d) spina bifida.   True/False

3   In an X-linked condition the following relatives of the affected person might
     also be affected:

(a) paternal grandfather   True/False

(b) maternal uncle   True/False

(c) mother   True/False

(d) cousin.   True/False

4   The following are true of Down syndrome:

(a) it is autosomal recessive   True/False

(b) it occurs only in males   True/False

(c) it only occurs if the mother is over 40 years of age   True/False

(d) it can be detected antenatally.   True/False

12 Emotional and behavioural problems

- Parenting and stress
- Simple behavioural management techniques for parents
- Common problems
- Sources of help

If they grow up not to love, honour and
    obey us
either we have brought them up properly
or we have not:
    if we have
there must be something the matter with
    them;
    if we have not
there is something the matter with us.

    (RD Laing (1970) *Knots.* Tavistock, London)

It is a depressing fact of life that, as parents, all of us pass on our emotional baggage to our children, no matter how hard we try not to. Good parents have learned to understand their own selves and are also able to empathise with their children – that is, be able to 'put themselves in their shoes'. This in turn requires a good theoretical understanding of the stages of emotional development of children (which parents will not automatically acquire) (*see* Box 12.1). Thus it is rarely the case that any emotional disorder in a child can be dealt with in isolation from the dynamics of his or her family or group of carers.

Box 12.1 Emotional development: key stages

Newborn: security comes from not having to wait too long to be comforted, fed or cuddled; being receptive to the baby's needs is crucial to their emotional and mental development.

Infancy: the parent and infant gradually learn to let go of each other; the baby gradually adjusts to being part of a wider community, and the parent must learn to let go and say no.

Early childhood: the child has to cope with a range of new experiences and confused feelings; this is a period of rapid development when the child struggles to acquire a range of new skills.

Starting school: it is normal for both parent and child to feel anxious when school life begins; the child is struggling with new relationships and emotions in a new environment and learning to accept new rules and boundaries.

Early adolescence: the child may feel very alone and insecure at this time; parents need to keep a cool head and be adaptable.

Late adolescence: both parent and child are developing more independent lives, and both need to let go and move on.

Source: Child Psychotherapy Trust.

Parenting and stress

Deprivation and health

The combination of poor housing, low incomes, uncertain health, insecure employment (coupled often, no doubt, with limited knowledge of parenting skills) offers a prescription for low-achieving, poorly behaved, disenchanted or alienated young people. It represents a 'prescription for anti-welfare' for children.

(P Wedge)

John Bowlby is credited with recognising that insecure attachment may result from such factors as maternal depression, lack of parenting and illness, or early institutionalisation, although one or two traumatic separations from a caring adult early in life do not usually result in long-term emotional damage. Some children are resilient to disadvantage, but frequent changes which prevent the formation of emotional bonds during the first 2 years (e.g. parent care followed by a series of foster carers) often cause serious emotional damage with an increased risk of later antisocial behaviour.

What seems to be important is that the child develops a sense of their own self-worth and a feeling of positive regard for a significant other person (usually a parent). Even in adverse circumstances these develop through positive involvement with the parents, other individuals outside the family, or interests and hobbies.

The most consistent parts of the environment of a baby or young child are the home and parents. Children need to feel loved, secure and valued, and to know the boundaries beyond which they should not go. This can be engendered in positive ways, through praise and encouragement in the main, with the occasional retribution for stepping 'beyond the mark'.

Where there is a lack of routine and consistent management, children can become difficult and out of control. This may occur in families where there is no social disadvantage and no pathological interaction. There may be lack of parental involvement because of excessive attention to work or television, or abuse of drugs or alcohol. Such families may care for their children physically, but do not give them 'quality time'. A child may not identify with such emotionally detached parents, will not want to please them, and may develop behaviour problems (conduct disorder). Conversely, some families apply extreme discipline but lack supportive warmth. These parents may be over-restrictive, hostile, ridiculing and sarcastic, causing the child to become anxious and withdrawn. The most serious sequelae occur when this translates into physical, sexual or emotional abuse.

Simple behavioural management techniques for parents (see Box 12.2)

Good parenting is very analogous to good teaching. The parent/teacher has a wealth of knowledge and experience to impart which might benefit the child, but there are some well-established ideals of good parenting.

Children should be as autonomous as their stage of development allows. They should not be punished for things that they could not have been expected to know. Conversely, they must be induced into learning that they are not alone in this world – that they have to 'share and share alike' and adopt the general social values that distinguish a civilised society from an uncivilised one. Educational theory teaches us that people (even adults) do not learn well by simply being told what is the right thing to do. People 'learn by their mistakes'. The best way to help a child to learn is to allow them to practise and make mistakes in a supervised environment, and to learn that the 'mistakes' result in a worse outcome for them.

There is no evidence that physical punishment of children is on balance in any way beneficial. It provides children with a model for bad behaviour that they are likely to copy. There are other ways of imposing order, but even these must be used fairly and consistently.

The most important thing is that the parent does not use withdrawal of love as an instrument of punishment. This is not justified because it is not true – with rare exceptions we do not cease to love our children because of what they do, and we should not play on their inbuilt insecurity by implying that. The first step is therefore to show affection and to reinforce the fact that 'mummy/daddy still loves you' while asserting that the present behaviour of the child is unacceptable for some given reason.

When using these methods it is important to achieve a balance such that *positive rewarding interactions are more frequent than negative ones*. Too much of the latter can only lead to rejection or rebellion. Also, if the only attention a child receives is through punishment, they will seek to 'be bad' more often. Thus, it may be important to concentrate on changing one or two aspects initially, and rewarding behaviours that are part

way towards the desired behaviour (putting away one toy in the box rather than all of them). This is referred to as 'shaping behaviour'.

Parenthood is about creating civilised, socialised, caring human beings who achieve whatever is their personal potential. It is essential that parents (and other adults) provide a good model. However, parents are only one (albeit the main) influence. At certain stages of child development the pressure on a child to conform to peer group culture may cause rejection of parental values.

Common problems

Sleep problems in babies

Under the age of 1 year it is a sound general rule that if a baby cries there is a good underlying reason for this – it is his or her main way of drawing attention to physical and emotional needs. Emotional needs are important even in the newborn. The normal baby rapidly becomes highly bonded to his or her mother. A baby has no concept of 'coming back' – separation is therefore their greatest anxiety. As far as they are aware, mother may have gone for ever when she goes to the bathroom. The needs of normal babies for intensive physical and emotional attention (particularly demanding for lone parents) underlie many of the complaints that mothers present to the primary healthcare team. Understanding of these complaints demands a good knowledge of the range of normal child development.

Box 12.2   Behavioural management techniques (principles of positive parenting)

- Reward desirable behaviour. An increase in positive behaviours leaves little room for negative ones.
- Ignore irritant but not serious bad behaviour.
- Time out helps the child to understand that their behaviour is not socially acceptable. It is not a withdrawal of love, but simply an opportunity to 'cool off'.
- Give positive behavioural reinforcement.
- Give an incentive. If the incentive is excessive, the child will perceive the desired behaviour to be of similarly excessive importance.
- Stop a treat. This technique needs to be carefully used to avoid breakdown of trust.
- Provide a diversion. This is particularly helpful and easier to achieve in young children.

As many as one in five mothers seek help for their baby's crying/sleeping problems, but these rarely indicate physical disease. Although there is an obvious relationship between crying and night-waking, video studies show that many babies are 'quiet wakeners' who do not disturb their parents. Night-waking is therefore more the rule than is perceived by parents. A few babies have patterns of particularly intense and prolonged crying, again almost always unrelated to physical disease (although this must be excluded). As babies develop other ways of communicating, crying becomes a more selective response to, for example, pain or loss of dignity.

In the first 2–3 months of life an average baby sleeps for about 15 hours a day, almost equally divided between day and night, sleeping for at most 4 hours and waking for perhaps 3 hours at a time. Rapid adaptation to a more mature pattern takes place by 3–4 months, when many babies sleep for a full 8 hours at night, although there has not yet been much reduction in the total amount of sleep. *See* Case study 1 and Box 12.3 for discussion of management.

Case study 1

A 22-year-old mother of Simon, a first baby of 10 weeks, complains to her GP that he is driving both parents mad because he won't sleep. He is difficult to settle, and he usually cries and wakes two or three times a night.

It seems that Simon has always been rather unsettled since his birth by Caesarean section. He does not always take his feeds well, but is otherwise developing normally. His mother is planning to go back to work in the next month, and is anxious that he gets into a good sleep routine by then, so she is more stressed than usual, and her husband is also anxious about the baby's crying. There is not a very good bedtime routine, and Simon often falls asleep while he is downstairs.

Examination shows no evidence of a physical problem. It is important to consider infection, teething (he is rather young for this) or hunger as causes of crying at night. It is worth taking a urine specimen to check for infection, and this proves to be negative.

The GP asks the health visitor to support the parents in managing a sleep programme in which they go into the baby's room and stay for a short period, but do not lift him when he cries. They try this over a holiday period, and when he is 14 weeks old they start him on solids. By the age of 16 weeks he is sleeping through the night with only the occasional wakeful episode.

Box 12.3   Management of a sleep problem

- Determine the pattern of the problem and possible stressors (e.g. chaotic household, argument between parents, recent illness).

- Ensure that there is a 'goodnight routine' with bathing, a quiet read and gradual settling on the baby's own bed.

- Do not reward unwanted behaviour (by staying with the baby for a long period after wakening).

- A sleep programme consists of visiting briefly to comfort the baby, but not staying long.

- It is not helpful to leave the baby crying for a long period, as distress will ensue.

- Encourage the natural development of a diurnal cycle by reducing daytime sleep and increasing daytime stimulation.

Food refusal in toddlers (see Box 12.4 and Figure 12.1)

In numerous aspects of his life the toddler, at a stage when he is acquiring many new capabilities and beginning to see himself as an independent person, can have this exciting new freedom curtailed by an adult. The toddler is dependent on adults for many things, but they cannot control his bodily functions, over which he retains complete autonomy. Many children assert their independence by refusing to eat, sleep or toilet train in the socially acceptable ways that their parents are trying to impose. This happens to a greater or lesser degree depending mainly on the personality traits of the child and the consistency with which parents 'set the limits'.

Box 12.4 Food refusal in toddlers

- Children at 2–3 years of age often seem to have a poor appetite.

- The rate of growth is much slower than in the first year.

- Parents become anxious when the child eats less, and they attempt to bribe or force them to eat.

- The child enjoys the attention and manipulates their parents at mealtimes.

- If growth is adequate, as it usually is, the parents should be reassured that intake is sufficient and that the child should be left to eat what they want, so long as a balanced diet is offered (toddlers never starve themselves).

Management

The first stage of management is to evaluate the child's nutritional state. The aim should then be to assist parents in making the meal an enjoyable event. This is done by giving praise for participation, even if little is eaten, and ignoring poor intake. The child should be offered a choice (but

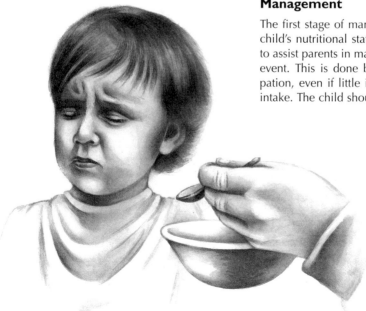

Figure 12.1 Food refusal.

not innumerable choices) and left to cope with the consequences if food is rejected. Offering 'healthy' snacks (e.g. fruit, yoghurt or cheese rather than crisps and sweets) is also sensible, as a small child's stomach may be quickly filled at a single meal.

The child should be fed at the same time and alongside other members of the family (preferably at the table), and should be offered small amounts of the foods that the adults are eating (including finger foods and lumps or pieces of food). Children sometimes develop a strong dislike of certain foods or textures (e.g. pieces of meat or carrot). If this is the case, the child should be given more of the foods that he is known to like (provided this gives a fairly balanced diet), and he may be offered the disliked food from time to time. However, the diet should always include some lumps and variation in textures (*see* Case study 2 and Box 12.5).

The 'terrible twos': challenging behaviour

This is a trying stage for many parents. The normal child has attained high mobility and all kinds of new skills which he wants to explore and try out. At the same time, at this stage he is entirely self-centred and incapable of seeing another person's point of view. He therefore cannot understand why he should not simply do anything he wants to do, and this can lead to apparently antisocial behaviour. Most parents have read about the so-called hyperactivity or hyperkinetic syndrome (see below) in one or other of the many childcare books written for parents. At the toddler stage, in the absence of developmental delay or other abnormality, it is usually impossible to distinguish true hyperactivity from normal extremes of variation and poor 'limit setting' by the parents. Many toddlers are very active, needing

---

Case study 2

Darren is 2½ years old. His mother, who is a few months pregnant with her second baby, says that he is driving both parents 'round the bend'. 'He won't do anything he's told, he won't eat his meals properly and he throws his food around and at people. We have a huge struggle getting him to eat anything sensible, and meals can take hours. We discourage snacks, to help him to eat his main meal.'

Ask the parents to write down everything Darren eats for 2–3 days. This may show that he is actually eating reasonably, or it may reveal excess milk consumption or that large amounts of sweets, crisps and biscuits are being eaten.

It turns out that Darren's growth pattern is normal and his intake is reasonable although it is not well balanced. His parents are supported to help him to eat independently, and if he throws food it is taken away. Snacks of banana and yoghurt are offered, and Darren enjoys these. Poor eating at mealtimes is ignored and the parents are encouraged to accept his limited eating habits. His grandmother points out that his mother was the same at his age. With the focus taken off having to eat, Darren begins to enjoy meals and his behaviour improves.

Box 12.5 Management of food refusal

- The child will win if there is a conflict, as it is not possible to force him or her to eat.
- Food refusal very rarely leads to malnutrition.
- Avoid drawing attention to poor eating.
- Eat as a family, and offer a small portion but take it away if it is not eaten.
- Offer sensible snacks between meals (e.g. fruit, cheese, yoghurt, sandwich, plain biscuit).

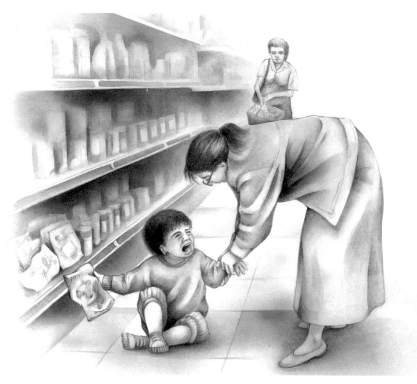

Figure 12.2   Child having a tantrum in a supermarket.

almost constant supervision to prevent accidents, and their attention span is very limited. Head banging is a less common variant of a number of comforting behaviours, such as rocking, masturbation and thumb sucking, that the normal child indulges in when tired, bored or unsettled. These behaviours can become abnormally fixed in retarded or autistic children, but disappear in the majority of children by the pre-school years.

Temper tantrums (*see* Figure 12.2) are normal and may be associated with breath holding. After refusing to eat, sleep or toilet train, refusing to breathe is the ultimate weapon in the child's armoury of assertive behaviours. Fortunately, few children carry independence this far, and the few who do usually stop this extremely disquieting behaviour after a few attempts, especially if the parents can steel themselves to respond calmly without the panic which the child intends to provoke. The doctor must distinguish these breath-holding attacks from loss of consciousness due to other causes, especially when they mimic convulsions (*see* Case study 3, Box 12.6 and Chapter 8).

Management

The parents need a more thorough understanding of child development, the great range of normal variation, and 'how the child's mind works' (i.e. empathy). Parents should provide a constant background of affection and be equally consistent in recognising and rewarding the child with 'quality time' for good behaviours. This is a crucial stage for development of socially acceptable behaviour. Excitable, highly active children do not like to be restricted. The parents should concentrate on modifying the most unacceptable behaviours, such as violence towards other children and excessive shows of temper, while trying to allow the child as much freedom as they safely can. Consistency is essential. If the child perceives a difference in management between the parents, he will exploit this. Temper tantrums and breath-holding attacks should be ignored, and the parents should be reassured that no harm will come from a brief episode of not breathing.

When managing difficult behaviour, the principles of positive parenting should be used and physical punishment should be avoided (*see* Boxes 12.2 and 12.7).

Case study 3

Darren's mother complains that he is also always 'on the go', 'into everything', often breaking things as he goes. He never seems to settle for even a few minutes, just going from one thing to another all the time. He won't go to bed, and he hardly seems to sleep at all, waking up at about 6 o'clock every morning. He used to bang his head on his cot for ages every night, but he seems to have stopped that now. 'Is he hyperactive, doctor?'

'He also gets terrible temper tantrums. If he doesn't get his own way he just throws himself on the floor and bangs his head with temper. Once, about a year ago, he got so annoyed he held his breath until he went blue and passed out. We had to call the doctor then, but she said it was all right and not to worry.'

Supporting parents in controlling their child's behaviour is a key task for the health visitor, who may do this through individual or group work. There is good evidence for the benefits of parenting groups which provide support as well as information.

A change in behaviour is always seen if parents are able to adopt a positive parenting model without the use of physical chastisement.

Box 12.6 Breath-holding attacks

- Normal developmental stage in under-fours.
- Child holds breath and may go blue, but always starts breathing again.
- It is important to distinguish breath holding from convulsions.
- Parents may be reassured that the child is not at risk.
- If breath-holding episodes are ignored, they gradually disappear.

Box 12.7 The case against physical punishment of children (smacking)

- It models behaviour not acceptable between adults.
- It may physically damage the child if repeated or excessive force is used.
- It encourages a violent nature if repeated.
- It is no more effective than other techniques.
- It relies on physical strength as a way of solving disputes.

School-age children: attention deficit hyperactivity disorder (ADHD)

A certain degree of overactivity is often normal in toddlers, and therefore the diagnosis of abnormal hyperactivity is not usually considered unless it persists into the school years.

A small percentage of children, mostly boys, may be unusually hyperactive, excitable and destructive, with a short attention span, constant restlessness and poor concentration. Many adults (again mostly men, and often successful people in business or professions) are similarly hyperactive and self-centred, with 'butterfly minds', and these traits may be passed on to their children, whether through heredity or via upbringing. Delineation of ADHD is therefore contentious and best defined by expert psychological assessment. ADHD is much more commonly diagnosed in the USA than elsewhere in the world, but the rate of diagnosis in the UK is rising rapidly.

The characteristic features of ADHD (*see* Box 12.8) are the triad of hyperactivity, impulsiveness and attention deficit. Diagnosis relies on the history and on information obtained from a variety of sources which should include the school. The symptoms should have started in early life and be pervasive (i.e. present in all situations).

In some children food additives can increase hyperactivity, and their removal may assist management.

Box 12.8 Characteristics of attention deficit hyperactivity disorder (ADHD)

Hyperactivity is thought to affect 3–5% of the school-aged population in the USA (ratio of 3 boys:1 girl)

- Poor sustained attention, easily bored, constantly shifting activity
- Impaired impulse control or delay of gratification
- Excessive task-irrelevant activity (fidgeting, unable to sit still)
- Difficulty in following through instructions
- Early onset (mean age 3–4 years)
- Problem less obvious in a one-to-one situation
- Normal IQ

Management

This includes the following:

- behavioural management and/or cognitive therapy
- dietary changes (see previous remarks)
- drug treatment (methylphenidate, dexamphetamine or atomoxitine).

Methylphenidate (Ritalin) is a stimulant that, paradoxically, does not increase activity in these children but may improve attention span, concentration, sleep and coordination. It should only be prescribed as an adjunct to psychological treatment. *See* Case study 4 and Box 12.9.

Case study 4

Ryan is 8 years old and has always had problems at school. He does not concentrate on his work, is always out of his seat, interrupts the teacher and talks all the time. His teacher says that Ryan cannot concentrate properly on his work and is falling behind. He cannot keep himself to himself and he annoys other children. At home he is constantly 'on the go' and does not seem to need much sleep. He is impulsive and seems to have no fears, so his parents have to watch him constantly.

Ryan is always flitting from one thing to another, seeming to have a very short attention span. Even when he is apparently settled (e.g. when drawing or watching television) he is always fidgeting. He seems impulsive and disinhibited, as shown by angry outbursts or tearfulness for no apparent reason. He also shows lack of awareness of 'personal space', always intruding on other people, and will often take apparently high risks when climbing and exploring.

Ryan's mother has read about food colourings being a cause of hyperactivity, and she has stopped giving him cola drinks, tomato ketchup and coloured sweets, but is not sure if this has made a difference.

Behavioural management has been used and has been of some benefit, but Ryan's mother finds that he is still very difficult to control and is anxious about his disruptiveness in school and his falling behind with his schoolwork.

He is referred for paediatric assessment and ADHD is diagnosed on the basis of long duration, severity of symptoms and occurrence both at home and at school. Behavioural management is emphasised, and Ryan is also started on methylphenidate. A dietitian referral is arranged to supervise the dietary exclusion of food colourants. A year later Ryan is progressing well at school and his mother says that although he is still very lively, he is manageable and learning to handle his excitable nature.

Box 12.9   Management of attention deficit hyperactivity disorder (ADHD)

- Diagnosis depends on the presence of symptoms since early life, severity and pervasiveness (i.e. it is present in every situation).

- Removal of food additives may be of benefit but should be supervised.

- Behavioural therapy is of benefit.

- Giving information to the school is essential.

- The disorder requires specialist supervision.

- Drug treatment may be of benefit to improve concentration, but there are potential side-effects.

Urinary and faecal incontinence (also known as wetting and soiling)

Incontinence of the bladder or bowel at an age when most other children have acquired an adult pattern of control is the most common problem at this age. It is usually yet another example of normal variation, although parents may find this difficult to accept. Even this normal delay in maturation may be a cause of emotional problems in the child. Conversely, gross or persistent antisocial behaviour (e.g. deliberate smearing of faeces on furniture or other people) may be a symptom of severe underlying psychiatric disorder. See Box 12.10.

Box 12.10   Definition of enuresis and soiling

Enuresis: involuntary passing of urine beyond the age of normal continence.

Primary enuresis: the child has never had a period of dryness.

Secondary enuresis: the child was dry for a significant period and then started wetting.

Encopresis (soiling): repeated involuntary or voluntary passage of stool into clothing or other places not intended, for a duration of at least 1 month, in a child aged 4 years or older (may be primary or secondary, as described above for enuresis).

Enuresis

Bedwetting is common and affects boys much more commonly than girls. See Box 12.11. It occurs in 10% of 5-year-olds and 5% of 10-year-olds, and there is often a positive family history. It is described as primary if it has always been present, and as secondary if there was an initial period of dryness. Secondary enuresis suggests an organic or emotional cause. Conditions which may underlie secondary enuresis are listed in Box 12.12.

Assessment is through careful history taking, physical examination and urinalysis. A physical cause is rare, but is more likely in the child who has daytime as well as night-time wetting.

Enuresis is distressing to the child, and this aspect of the condition should be recognised by the physician.

Box 12.11 Enuresis

- Most children are dry by the age of 3 years, but 10% of 5-year-olds have nocturnal enuresis.

- One in 20 children are still not completely dry by the age of 10 years.

- Male predominance.

- Wetting by day is associated with emotional difficulties.

- Enuresis is almost always functional.

- Organic causes are found in only 1 in 100 cases, and can generally be excluded by urine testing and culture.

- Management is by positive reinforcement, 'star chart's' for young children, and desmopressin/buzzer alarm in over-sevens.

- Tricyclic antidepressants should not be used because of side-effects and high relapse rate.

Box 12.12 Conditions which may underlie secondary enuresis

- Diabetes mellitus

- Urinary tract infection

- Diabetes insipidus

- Bullying

- Attachment disorder

At school age, the indignity and constant sense of failure engendered by enuresis may cause serious emotional problems and hinder other aspects of mature development. A punitive, blaming approach by the parents is very unhelpful, but fortunately is becoming increasingly rare with greater public awareness of the real nature of the problem. *See* Case study 5.

Management

It is most important to help the child to maintain their self-esteem. The approach must be highly positive, with no 'putting down' of the child. In pre-school-age children the parents may try lifting the child to go on his or her potty before they themselves go to bed, but little more should be done unless or until the problem persists into the school years. By the age of 5 or 6 years it is worth trying 'star charts' on which the child records his or her dry nights and is praised for them. Battery-driven pads or sensor alarms which buzz when electrical contact is made by small amounts of urine are the most successful method, but are not usually effective before 7 years of age. Desmopressin (antidiuretic hormone) nasal spray or tablets may be used at night for up to 2 months, usually in conjunction with an alarm. Desmopressin is also useful for short periods in situations where dryness is desirable (e.g. on holiday camps) and for helping to initiate the use of buzzer alarms.

In many areas, school nurses take the lead in management of enuresis and work closely with paediatricians.

Case study 5

Sam, a healthy 7-year-old, attends the clinic with his father. Although he can sometimes stay dry for several days, he wets his bed most nights and sometimes wets himself during the day. He finds this distressing and his mother tends to be annoyed because the sheets have to be washed almost every day. His father is a little more sympathetic because he himself was a 'bed-wetter' until the age of about 9 years and is still embarrassed about it. Sam has never been fully dry, but he does have the occasional dry night.

Physical examination is negative and the urine is clear to microscopy and urinalysis. It is agreed that a buzzer will be tried, and although at first it does not wake him, he perseveres and is dry at night within 3 months.

Faecal soiling (encopresis) (*see also* Chapter 4, page 63)

Bowel control is still precarious in most young-sters, and going to school often precipitates a lapse in control. However, by the age of 7 years almost all children are fully continent. As with enuresis, delay is generally thought to be matura-tional, and organic causes (e.g. Hirschsprung's disease; see Chapter 4, page 64) are exception-ally rare. Constipation, irregular bowel habit and faulty training are all predisposing factors. As faeces are even less acceptable than urine to most people, the potential for emotional distur-bance in the child is correspondingly much greater than with enuresis.

If the soiling has gone on for some time, it is likely that the lower part of the rectum has become stretched and insensitive. Parental anger or punitiveness may aggravate toilet refusal, lead-ing in extreme cases to rebellious behaviour and smearing or other provocative behaviour.

Leakage past a solid mass of faeces (constipa-tion with overflow) is the most common cause of soiling, and no real progress can be made until this mass is cleared (*see* Figure 12.3).

There should be a persistent effort to increase dietary fibre intake, but by this stage medication – usually lactulose (a stool softener) and senna (a laxative) are commonly needed, and occas-ionally even enemas or inpatient treatment.

Box 12.13 Differential diagnosis of soiling

Chronic constipation
- History of constipation in infancy
- Often painful defecation before potty training
- Large amounts of faeces in rectum
- No period of normal defecation

Primary behaviour disorder
- Constipation not a prominent feature
- Other behavioural disturbance
- Faeces often hidden, e.g. behind the sofa
- Often soiling is secondary, following a period of normal defecation

---

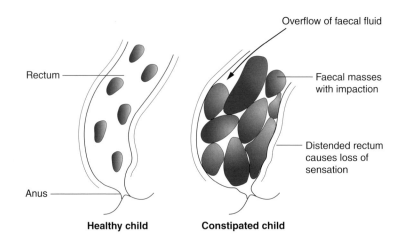

Figure 12.3 Mechanism of soiling in childhood. Leakage past a solid mass of faeces is the most common cause of soiling.

Prolonged and integrated physical and psychological management with a 'no-blame' ethos and small rewards for daily achievement needs to be maintained, often for as long as 2 years. *See* Box 12.13 and Case study 6.

Case study 6

Mark is a 7-year-old boy who soils his pants two or three times a day. According to his mother he was toilet trained at about 3 years of age, but often had accidents. The problem became much worse when he started school, and he has never really been clean since. He does not seem to know when to defecate, and his pants are found to be dirty three or four times each day. When he was younger he frequently screamed during defecation, and streaks of blood had been seen in his motion.

Mark does not seem to know when he is soiled, and he does not seem to care. He will not even go and try to defecate on the toilet now.

Mark's mother does not think he is constipated or 'bunged up'. She says 'If anything, he is really loose, it just seems to dribble out of him all the time'.

Mark's mother tries to persuade him to eat fruit and vegetables, but really he prefers to eat chips and burgers.

Abdominal examination reveals palpable faeces and a loaded colon, and many hard faeces can be felt in the rectum. Mark is treated initially with quite high doses of senna and lactulose which help to empty his loaded bowel, and his parents are given instructions on how to encourage him to go to the toilet regularly. A 'star chart' and incentives are used to encourage regular toileting, and when successful he is praised strongly for his achievement. Over the next few weeks Mark starts to go to the toilet and his soiling improves greatly.

Behaviour problems (conduct disorder)

Conduct disorder is the term given to difficult behaviour in older children that is not associated with an organic cause. It is more common in socio-economically disadvantaged families and in broken families where parenting skills are inadequate. Behaviour problems can lead to poor educational achievement, antisocial behaviour, lack of employment as an adult, and in some cases conflict with the police and the law. Non-compliance and temper tantrums are common in toddlers, who are developing their sense of self and testing for limit setting by their parents, and preventive work can be done at this stage. If difficulties persist beyond the toddler stage, the child may become outwith parental control. Children with abnormal disorders of conduct are generally 'externalisers' who direct their behaviours towards the environment. Boys outnumber girls by a ratio of 10:1.

A common causal factor is linked to the parent providing for the child's physical needs (and maybe having over-indulged the child with regard to material possessions) while providing poor limit setting and inconsistent management. The mother tries to win the child's affection by giving them what she thinks they want, but the child rejects the mother because they want attention, even negative attention, rather than material goods.

Almost always the parent has tried several punishments, but inconsistently, so that frequently they give in to the child's demands for the sake of peace, or the child receives a punishment that is out of all proportion to the misdemeanour. Periods of play between the parent and the child can be used to increase the amount of positive (rather than negative) attention for the child.

Many parents with problem children are having to cope with adverse social circumstances, and often they are single parents struggling to make ends meet. However, there are also parents who, because of this struggle or perhaps because of their own experience of parenting, attend mainly to physical well-being and are unaware of the concept of 'quality time' to be spent with their children. The father (if present) needs to be drawn into the treatment plan. Frequently parents feel that nothing can be done, and it can be quite difficult to persuade them to look to the more positive aspects of the child's behaviour and build on them. As the child with conduct disorder moves into the teenage years, antisocial conduct and risk-taking behaviour become more common and can result in the young person coming into contact with social services and the police. A preventive approach starting early in life will be much more effective than attempting to control a wayward teenager. *See* Boxes 12.14 and 12.15.

Box 12.14   Factors that assist in the development of prosocial and moral behaviour

- Reasonable parental control and limit setting
- Positive reinforcement of 'good' behaviour
- Attention and affection without over-indulgence
- Provision of a good model
- Non-punitive and non-aggressive approach
- Consistent management and ability to carry through threats/promises
- Ability to discuss and accept the child's developing autonomy
- Giving the child responsibility

Management

As with the younger child with behavioural problems, the management of conduct disorder involves positive reinforcement of good behaviour and the development of a positive parent–child relationship. Non-reinforcement (ignoring) and occasional 'time out' may be used for negative behaviours. It is important to offer the teenager choices and the gradual development of autonomy. There are agreed local and national guidelines for dealing with children who are considered to be at risk of emotional and/or physical abuse (*see* Chapter 14). *See* Case study 7.

Box 12.15   Behavioural problems/conduct disorder

- Child presents with oppositional behaviour and often with difficulties at school.
- They may be in trouble with the police.
- Behavioural problems are related to negative parenting and poor social circumstances.
- There is often lack of a father role.
- There is no organic psychiatric disturbance.
- Managed by social and educational support (multidisciplinary) and reinforcement of good behaviour.
- Parenting classes may be of great value if they are acceptable to the parents.

Case study 7

Mrs Reed, a mother aged 30 years, arrives with Rachel, reporting that she is 'at the end of her tether' with this 13-year-old girl who is increasingly defiant and rude, and does scarcely anything her mother asks.

Mrs Reed cannot understand how this has happened. 'I have always done everything for her, given her all the things she wanted and which I didn't have when I was her age, and she just takes liberties with me. The other night she didn't come home after school, and then when she did come in she didn't want the tea I'd made for her, even though it was her favourite.'

When asked what she has done about Rachel's behaviour in the past, Mrs Reed says 'I have tried everything – sending her to her room, turning off her television and smacking her – but it is all to no avail, she says she doesn't care anyway. At the moment she's gated for the next week'.

Mrs Reed states that she has little time for play. She has two other children younger than Rachel, and they are also a handful.

Her husband works long hours and is usually too exhausted at the weekends to spend time with the children. 'We're not badly off, though – we've seen that we have a nice house and, as I say, the children have everything.'

Rachel and her mother are referred to Denise, the school health adviser (school nurse), who has a special interest and training in assisting the parents of teenagers who have behaviour difficulties. She meets Rachel on her own and finds that she is being bullied at school in addition to feeling rather left out at home. 'My mother doesn't have any time for me and doesn't want to hear about my problems at school,' Rachel says. Denise helps her to draw up a contract which she can use in discussion with her mother about spending time together and Rachel being able to exercise choices. Denise then talks to Mrs Reed and suggests that she should think about the basic rules she would like to apply in relation to the time Rachel comes home and her helping in the house.

After this Rachel and her mother find it easier to talk together, and Rachel's behaviour begins to improve.

Pre-teenage and teenage children: eating disorders

Definition and prevalence

Anorexia nervosa is an eating disorder in which the child or young person (usually a girl) restricts their intake of carbohydrate and fat-containing foods by severe dieting in order to lose weight, leading to a body mass index of 17.5 kg/m^2 or less.

The prevalence of eating disorders in young people seems to be increasing, a recent figure being 0.7% for anorexia nervosa in teenage girls. There is some debate as to whether the increase is due to the media image of 'thinness' being desirable, since anorexia is rare in poor societies.

There are three diagnosable types of eating disorder.

1 *Anorexia nervosa.* This is characterised by low body weight with a body mass index of 17.5 kg/m^2 or less, which is sustained by undereating and/or frequent exercise. Amenorrhoea in girls is usual. There is preoccupation with body weight. As weight decreases, other features such as mood lability, depression, impaired concentration, obsessional features and loss of interest in other aspects of life increase.

Anorexia presents with a child who progressively reduces her food intake in order to lose weight. Often the child perceives herself as overweight although others do not share this view. The weight loss becomes addictive and the young person becomes averse to eating, although she may enjoy cooking as well as vigorous exercise.

2 *Bulimia nervosa.* The young person is of normal weight, but this is usually maintained by a binge/self-induced vomiting cycle. Some people use laxatives or a period of starvation to keep their weight at normal levels. The affected individual will usually be distressed by the loss of control after bingeing and, as with anorexics, there will be preoccupation with body image. Patients with this problem are usually slightly older than anorexic patients.

3 *Atypical.* Some individuals do not fit into either of the above categories, either because their bodyweight does not quite fulfil the criterion for anorexia or because there are other dominant features, such as excessive exercising. However, there is the same level of preoccupation with weight and body image.

There are a number of physical effects of anorexia in addition to amenorrhoea. These include feeling cold (cold hands), dry skin and sometimes downy body hair, stunted growth, cardiac arrhythmia, dizziness, glandular swelling (in bulimia) and muscle weakness. Endocrine, metabolic and other abnormalities (e.g. gastrointestinal and cardiovascular effects) may be found following investigation.

When treating the anorexic patient, appropriate help must be sought from the child psychiatry services. Some inpatient care may be needed, as the disease can be life-threatening. Gradual weight gain is necessary, but this cannot be achieved unless the patient is being helped to see that this is desirable. At the same time the young person's beliefs about weight and body image need to be addressed, usually by adopting a specific cognitive-behavioural approach. However, with younger patients there is some evidence to suggest that family therapy is most beneficial. There is also some evidence that antidepressant medication can be helpful in bulimic patients, as there is a reduction in the binge/vomiting cycle with improved mood. *See* Case study 8.

Case study 8

Jane's mother is very concerned about her daughter, who is becoming very thin and hardly ever eats. Normally a quiet girl, 12-year-old Jane screams and shouts at her mother whenever she raises the subject of eating. At the moment she seems to exist on a diet of pizzas, salad and coke.

Jane sees herself as quite fat, although she does not like to use the word. When her mother mentions her periods starting she just walks away, and she seems to abhor anything related to her body changing as she grows up.

Jane's mother is extremely worried and tries to give her daughter the things she wants (e.g. new clothes), and Jane promises that she will eat more. However, Mrs Brown says 'Whenever I mention food she screams and starts running up and down the stairs. I just don't know what to do'.

Jane shows many of the features of pre-pubertal anorexia (e.g. fear of puberty), as well as some features that are more common in older anorexics (e.g. distortion of body image, fear of fatness, excessive exercising).

She has great control over her mother, and the two of them are emotionally enmeshed to a high degree. This is typical of anorexic families, which are often dysfunctional, and family therapy (the most effective form of treatment for younger anorexics) is required.

Obesity

Box 12.16 Definition of obesity

Overweight $\quad\quad\quad$ BMI > 25 kg/m^2

Obese $\quad\quad\quad\quad\quad$ BMI > 30 kg/m^2

Body mass index (BMI) = weight/height^2

BMI centile charts should be used in children

Around 5–10% of schoolchildren are 20% or more above their ideal weight (*see* Boxes 12.16 and 12.17). Fat children usually become fat adults through a combination of inheritance and upbringing. The prevalence of obesity in western society is increasing rapidly due to children taking less exercise and engaging in more snacking. Both of these behaviours are hard to avoid in modern society.

Many overweight children have a familial pattern of comfort eating. Major trauma (often separation from a parent, or sexual abuse) may be a contributory factor, and low self-esteem is a common feature, as in bullying (*see* Figure 12.4).

Obesity is difficult to treat and requires an approach which takes the whole child into consideration, as mental health factors are of great importance. Treatment failure is common, which is depressing for the child. A population-based approach is desirable, based on school approaches to increasing exercise and reducing high-calorie snacking.

Management

This needs to focus on both the child and the family. With high motivation, regular small targets and an initial focus on no weight gain (especially with younger obese children, who will increase in height to compensate) some progress can be made, although relapse is common. Many fat children do not like to exercise (partly due to embarrassment), but physical activity should be encouraged. Swimming, walking and cycling are usually acceptable. Reducing the amount of television watching has been shown to be beneficial, particularly if it is replaced by a more active pursuit.

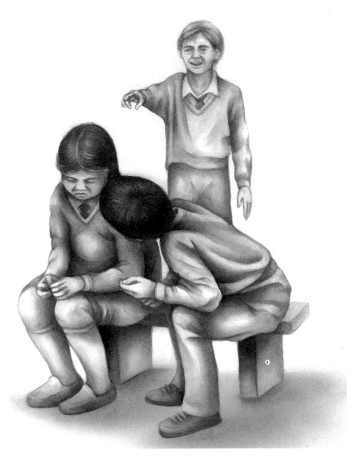

Figure 12.4   Overweight child being teased in the school playground.

Box 12.17   Obesity
- Becoming more common, probably because children are taking less exercise.
- Family factors (overweight, conflict between parents) and low self-esteem are common.
- Treatment is difficult, and requires a family- and psychologically oriented approach.
- All members of the family should follow the same dietary pattern.
- Increase the amount of exercise that the child takes if possible, and reduce television watching.
- Improving self-esteem is all-important.
- Aim to maintain the same weight, so as to regain a lower centile with growth.

Anxiety and phobias

There are many types of anxiety-based problems, ranging from generalised anxiety (including panic attacks) to specific phobias (e.g. dog phobia, spider phobia and needle phobia), which can all be treated effectively.

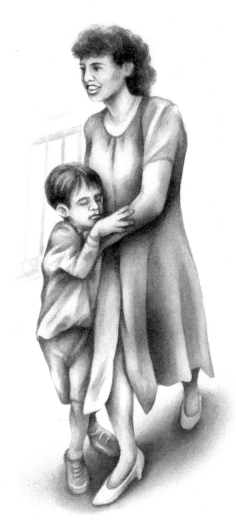

Figure 12.5 An anxious child clinging to his mother.

School refusal

School refusal (also known as school phobia) should properly be called *separation anxiety*, and is distinct from truancy. Truants usually show a bored, 'don't care' attitude rather than overanxiety. Often they are really lonely and miserable, tending to come from disorganised and uncaring families.

An anxious, introverted temperament predisposes the child to developing neurotic-type disorders (internalising problem) such as panic attacks, specific phobias, habit disorder or psychosomatic complaints. In cases of school refusal, the parent often has a problem with separation and is enmeshed with the child.

The problem needs to be tackled on two fronts – separation from the mother and gradual re-integration into school. Other factors include bullying (a common problem for which most schools now have a policy), domineering teachers or a large, unfriendly building.

Management

Collaboration between the school, educational psychologist, clinical psychologist or psychiatrist is usually necessary for cases of school refusal. For other types of anxiety, a combination of relaxation training and systematic desensitisation would normally be undertaken by a trained therapist. For psychosomatic and other physical complaints, relaxation training, lifestyle management, and withdrawal of inappropriate rewards for avoidance behaviour would be recommended. Specialist referral is recommended in most cases of school refusal and other anxiety neuroses, particularly if there are obsessive-compulsive elements. *See* Case study 9.

Case study 9

Susan has not been to school for about 6 months. The problem began soon after she started secondary school, when she was off with 'flu'. She was back in school again for a couple of days, but complained of nausea and stomach ache thereafter. There is nothing physically wrong with her, although she feels sick on most school days and has to stay at home.

She has always been well behaved at school, and is achieving well, but her parents moved house just before she joined the school and she was very clingy at first. Her mother does not work, is always around for her, and is involved with the Girl Guides, which Susan also enjoys.

Susan's mother has often tried to take her to school, but she only gets as far as the school gate and then runs home. The other children call her 'scaredy-cat' and try to trip her up. Susan does her schoolwork diligently at home and watches television with her mother in the afternoon.

A package of measures is devised to help her back into school, through the collaboration of the educational welfare officer, guidance teacher, school nurse and paediatrician. Initially Susan manages half-days only, but gradually this increases as her confidence improves.

Depression

Children and young people can be depressed, but this condition gets overlooked. The seemingly quiet and well-behaved child in a class may actually be depressed, as may a more boisterous and belligerent one. For some there is a psychosomatic component (fatigue, headache, etc.).

A depressed young person may not have the characteristics of a depressed adult, and can appear more as if they have behavioural problems or adolescent 'storm and stress'. Many children who are depressed are also school refusers, and some may harm themselves by taking an overdose, cutting or scratching themselves with a sharp object, or burning or bruising themselves (although self-harming behaviour is not necessarily a reflection of depression). If a young person has attempted suicide, is expressing suicidal thoughts or is self-harming, this should always be taken seriously and an urgent psychiatric opinion should be sought.

One study has shown that in children and young people aged 9–15 years the main components of depression are as follows:

1 depression, anhedonia (loss of ability to feel pleasure and enjoy life), fatigue and psychomotor retardation
2 negative thinking, which may be associated with thoughts of suicide
3 anxiety
4 anger-agitation.

See Box 12.18 and Case study 10.

Box 12.18   Features of depressive illness in children

• Feelings of hopelessness about the future and low self-esteem. Children younger than about 8 years cannot become depressed in this sense because they have not yet developed concepts of 'future' or of 'self'.

• Older children and adolescents can develop adult-like depressive illness, and this may be becoming more common.

• The prognosis for emotional disorders in childhood is not as good as was previously supposed. Vulnerability to relapses of affective disorder often persists well into adulthood.

• Academic failure is common.

• There may also be a real risk of suicide.

• Parents often fail to recognise the signs of depression.

• Depressed children usually have multiple problems.

• There is a strong family tendency to depressive illness.

• Most cases require specialist assessment.

Fortunately there is a very good CD–ROM available (see Further reading section on page 186) which can help both young people and teachers to recognise depression, and early intervention is often effective. Medication can help in many cases, but cognitive-behavioural therapy (CBT) by a competent therapist is also effective. If the depression is thought to have a hereditary component, a CBT approach alone is unlikely to result in sustained improvement.

Case study 10

Sally is an attractive but quiet 15-year-old who lives with her mother, stepfather and young half-sister, Becky, who is aged 2 years. Her mother has become increasingly concerned about Sally, who has become angry and irritable, snapping back at her mother's requests and not being helpful with her sister, whom she used to love. She will not go to bed in the evening, often not retiring until 10.30 or 11.00pm, saying that she cannot sleep anyway.

Sally works hard at school and has been achieving well, but although there have not been any negative school reports, her schoolwork has recently dropped off. She has also had a lot of absences in the last year with severe stomach aches such that she has had to stay in bed. Although she has one or two friends, she has not been seeing so much of them recently.

She is taken by her mother to see the family's GP, who is concerned that Sally seems troubled and not her usual bouncy self. The GP makes a referral to the local child and adolescent mental health team. Although quiet, Sally is able to talk about her feelings of unhappiness and just feeling 'dead inside'. She has thoughts of suicide, but says she would not do it because it would upset her mother. She feels that she is not part of the family any more, and she believes that her mother (whom she was close to and wants to please) is now too involved with Becky and her husband to notice. She has difficulty in sleeping, feels low and worries about her problems.

Sally is asked to complete the Children's Depression Inventory, on which she obtains a score indicative of depression, with high scores for anhedonia and depressed mood but not low self-esteem. She also has some anxiety symptoms.

In this case, Sally does not wish her mother to know how she is feeling about the family, and her wish for confidentiality is respected. Sally receives individual therapy (mainly CBT) both for her anxiety and for her depressive thoughts, and it is possible for her to address relationships within the family to some extent. With her permission it is possible to involve her mother at a later stage.

Autistic spectrum disorders

A range of developmental disorders is covered by this category, including childhood autism and Asperger's syndrome. The prevalence rate is thought to be somewhere in the region of 60 per 10 000. Children with an autistic spectrum disorder show impairment in the following areas.

- *Social development:* the child often seems aloof or odd, and interpersonal relationships are significantly impaired.

- *Language and communication:* there is both impaired and deviant language development, particularly with regard to semantics and pragmatics; sometimes there is gaze avoidance or unusual gaze.

- *Thought and behaviour:* there is rigidity of thought, 'demand for sameness', sometimes

including severe upset over change in routine, and delay or absence of 'pretend play'.

The difficulties are often severe and pervasive, and last throughout life. Children with an autistic disorder may have cognitive impairment (around 75% of cases). Many children with autism have no or very little speech (20–50%), and the usual age of onset is below 3 years.

Asperger's syndrome (AS) is the name given to a condition at the milder end of the autistic spectrum. It is thought to affect around 36 in 10 000 children. Common characteristics include difficulty in understanding non-verbal communication (picking up social cues), misinterpreting or taking literally what someone has said, having restricted and repetitive interests and routines, over-reacting to minor changes in routine, and difficulty in adjusting to new situations. This results in great difficulty in forming close relationships, and the young person may appear rude, unfriendly or odd. Children with Asperger's syndrome may be of average or above average IQ, but frequently show other psychological and behavioural problems.

Once the child is thought to have a pervasive developmental disorder, assessment by a specialist team is usually recommended. Children with these difficulties require a significant amount of professional input over a number of years to assist them and their parents in coping with the difficulties, and to provide support in the school setting.

Drug abuse

With the normal testing of the boundaries implicit in adolescence (*see* Chapter 23), risk taking and experimentation can lead to dangerous behaviours such as drug abuse (*see* Box 12.19). In addition to stimulants, opiates and cannabis, glue and solvent abuse (*see* Box 12.20) feature in adolescent risk taking because of the relative ease of accessibility.

Box 12.19   Drug abuse

- Abuse of drugs and other substances is a major health problem in adolescents.

- The average age of initial abuse is declining, and younger age of starting is correlated with higher likelihood of continued use.

- In some settings, abuse is almost 'normal'.

- Although abuse may be experimental and short-lived, it cannot be ignored because:
  - death can result even from initial use
  - psychologically vulnerable children may fail to develop healthy solutions to problems such as parental control, anxiety and low self-esteem if subtance abuse is used as a ready solution
  - drug use is systematically linked with other problem behaviours which are generally antisocial and damaging to the health or welfare of the child (e.g. theft and prostitution).

- The example set by adults (e.g. tobacco and alcohol use) may encourage experimentation with such substances.

Box 12.20   'Glue-sniffing'

- Inhalation of volatile hydrocarbons (e.g. sniffing glue or lighter fluid) is a common form of substance abuse that affects large numbers of young adolescents in all areas of the UK, both rural and urban.

- The immediate effects, which last for up to half an hour, are similar to those of alcohol intoxication.

- Polythene bags are commonly used to concentrate the fumes.

- Severe cerebral damage and death have resulted from asphyxia and/or the direct effects of the fumes (e.g. cardiac arrhythmia).

- Some solvents, particularly those used for the 'dry-cleaning' of clothes, may have severe acute toxic effects on the liver and kidneys.

- Chronic abuse may lead to severe and permanent renal, hepatic and neurological damage.

Box 12.21   Who does what?

Child psychologist:
• No medical training
• Specialist in assessment and formulation of emotional and behavioural problems based on psychological theory
• Specialist in psychometric assessment
• Treats children with behavioural problems using mainly cognitive-behavioural therapy, but may also use other approaches (e.g. play therapy, narrative therapy and family therapy)

Child psychiatrist:
• Medical training
• Specialist in mental illness
• Uses drug treatment as well as therapy
• May lead a mental health team
• Treats children with more complex and severe mental health problems (e.g. psychoses, depression, anorexia nervosa)

Sources of help

A child and adolescent mental health (CAMH) team includes a child psychiatrist, clinical psychologist, specialist nurse, occupational therapist and psychotherapist. Community paediatricians also work closely with CAMH teams (*see* Box 12.21).

Further reading

• Attwood T (1997) *Asperger Syndrome.* Jessica Kingsley, London.
• Baron-Cohen S and Bolton P (1993) *Autism: the facts.* Oxford University Press, Oxford.
• Bowlby J and Fry M (1990) *Child Care and the Growth of Love.* Penguin, Harmondsworth.
• Bryant-Waugh R and Lask B (2002) Childhood-onset eating disorders. In: CG Fairburn and KD Brownell (eds) *Eating Disorders and Obesity: a comprehensive handbook* (2e). Guilford Press, New York.
• Buchanan A and Clayden G (1992) *Children Who Soil.* John Wiley & Sons, Chichester.
• Carr A (1999) *Handbook of Child and Adolescent Clinical Psychology.* Routledge, London.

• Douglas J and Richman N (1988) *My Child Won't Sleep.* Penguin, Harmondsworth.
• Fairburn CG and Harrison PJ (2003) Eating disorders. *The Lancet.* **361**: 407–16.
• Green C (2000) *Toddler Taming: a parents' guide to the first four years.* Vermilion, London.
• Green C and Chee K (1995) *Understanding Attention Deficit Disorder.* Vermilion, London.
• Haddon M (2003) *The Curious Incident of the Dog in the Night-time.* Vintage, London. (A remarkable best-selling novel about a young person with Asperger syndrome, which portrays his view of life very well.)
• Myers B (1995) *Parenting Teenagers.* Jessica Kingsley, London.
• Richards C, Cannon N and Scott E (2002) *Depression in Teenagers.* CD-ROM produced by Lothian Primary Care NHS Trust. Available from Cathy Richards, Young People's Unit, Royal Edinburgh Hospital, Morningside Park, Edinburgh EH10 5HF; www.depression inteenagers.com

Self-assessment questions

1   The following are characteristics of a teenager in emotional development:
(a) strong desire for independence   True/False
(b) tendency to mood swings   True/False
(c) tendency to engage in risk-taking behaviour   True/False
(d) insecure attachment.   True/False

2   Positive parenting includes the following:
(a) close control over the child's behaviour   True/False
(b) use of corporal punishment   True/False
(c) unconditional positive regard   True/False
(d) rewarding wanted behaviours.   True/False

3   Management of food refusal will include:
(a) using a food diary to account for overall intake   True/False
(b) letting the child eat at a separate table   True/False
(c) not making an issue of eating particular foods   True/False
(d) monitoring the child's weight gain.   True/False

4   A child with attention deficit hyperactivity disorder has the following features:
(a) usually a girl   True/False
(b) high level of impulsivity   True/False
(c) often displays poor performance in school   True/False
(d) requires treatment with a tranquilliser.   True/False

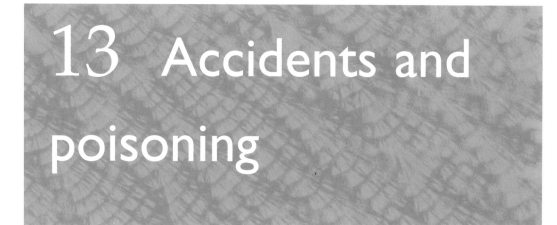

13 Accidents and poisoning

- Epidemiology of paediatric trauma
- Anatomy, physiology and psychology relevant to trauma
- Initial assessment and treatment
- Road traffic accident (head injury)
- Scalds
- Near drowning
- Poisoning

Epidemiology of paediatric trauma

Accidents will happen

It is impossible to completely avoid accidents in children, nor is it desirable. Children's desire to explore their environment will inevitably expose them to hazards. The best experience is learned experience – by finding out at first hand the unpleasant results of these hazards, the child learns to avoid them. The majority of accidents have no long-lasting effects (e.g. scraped knees, bumped head, etc.). Unfortunately, children may be exposed to accidents which result in severe morbidity or even death. Three to four children die each day from trauma, and approximately 10 000 children are disabled permanently every year in the UK.

Trauma is the commonest cause of death from the age of 1 year throughout childhood. It is a common perception that traumatic death is unavoidable. A true accident is an occurrence which appears to have no obvious cause. The majority of accidents that occur are not Acts of God, but have a definable cause. Many factors predispose children to accidents, and these may be anticipated. The injury resulting from the accident may be mitigated. For this reason, the term 'accidental injury' is preferred to 'accident'. Injury prevention strategies are an essential part of paediatric Accident and Emergency medicine (*see* Chapter 22).

Anatomy, physiology and psychology relevant to trauma

Children are not simply small adults. There are differences which lead to a different effect of injuries.

The small child represents a 'small target' when struck by an object such as a car. The energy transferred to the child dissipates over the smaller mass of the child, resulting in a higher concentration of force per metre squared compared with the same collision in an adult (see Table 13.1). The child's body has less elastic tissue and body fat to absorb this more intense energy which, combined with the closer proximity of organs, results in a high frequency of multiple-organ injuries.

As a general rule, with increasing age the bones become more brittle. For example, an elderly woman who falls on an outstretched hand is likely to break her wrist, as the force applied rapidly overcomes the inherent strength of the bone. The wrist breaks, absorbing the force. In a young adult the bone is more resilient and so transfers the force. Therefore the same mechanism of injury more commonly results in shoulder dislocation or clavicular fracture. In children the skeleton is incompletely calcified and so transfers the force more effectively, making fracture less likely.

In adults the bony skeleton usually fractures, resulting in dissipation of the energy applied, and this protects the underlying tissues and organs. Therefore it is unusual in adults to have underlying brain or lung damage in the absence of skull or rib fractures. However, this is not the case in children. The growing bone may easily transfer force to the underlying tissues and not fracture (e.g. rib fractures are rare in children, but pulmonary contusion is relatively common). Therefore the unwary may underestimate the severity of a child's injury in the absence of traditional markers of severity in adults (e.g. skull fracture, etc.).

The child's body proportions vary with age. For example, the relative contributions to the total body surface area change with age. At birth, the head accounts for approximately 20%, decreasing to 10% by the age of 15 years. The ratio of body surface area to weight increases with age, so young children lose heat much more rapidly, which may compound the effect of the initial injury.

The infant has a higher metabolic rate and oxygen consumption, which results in the respiratory rate being highest at birth. Therefore airway obstruction results in severe hypoxia more rapidly in children, leading to metabolic acidosis.

Physiological parameters must be interpreted according to the age of the child. A systolic blood pressure of 90 mmHg, respiratory rate of 30 breaths/minute and pulse rate of 120 beats/per minute may indicate severe physiological compromise in an adult, but may be perfectly normal for a 4-year-old child.

The ability to compensate for fluid loss is more efficient in children. A child may lose up to 25%

Table 13.1 Effects of injury: differences between child and adult

Injury	Adult	Child
Heavy impact	Energy dissipates Low frequency of organ injuries	Less mass for energy to dissipate High frequency of multiple organ injuries
Fall	Bone less resilient Force not transferred, hence peripheral fracture	Bone more resilient Force is transferred through bone Fracture less likely (e.g. shoulder dislocation)
Major trauma	Bony skeleton fractures Energy dissipates Underlying tissues protected	Growing bone transfers force to underlying tissues Injury common in absence of fracture

of their circulating volume before measurable change occurs in physiological parameters, compared with 10% in an adult.

Capillary refill time is a useful way of measuring peripheral vasoconstriction. The skin of the hand or foot (held at the same level as the heart) is squeezed firmly for 5 seconds. The resultant blanching normally clears in less than 2 seconds. If blanching is prolonged, this may indicate decreased peripheral perfusion. Anatomical injury should be used to assess initial fluid resuscitation. For example, a child with bilateral femoral fractures will have significant fluid loss even if their blood pressure and pulse are normal. Fluid resuscitation must not be delayed. Once the child becomes hypotensive, death may be imminent (see Table 13.2).

The smaller size of the child means that drug dosages, fluid replacement, etc. must be scaled down appropriately, as should resuscitation equipment (e.g. intravenous lines, endotracheal tubes, etc.). There are various charts which may help in this assessment using the child's age or height, which is useful when actual weighing of the child is impractical due to their injuries (see Figure 13.1).

Children react differently from adults in response to injury. Many children are frightened simply by the hospital environment. The parents

Table 13.2   Clinical signs of blood loss in children

Blood loss	< 25%	25–40%	> 40%
Heart rate	Mild tachycardia	Marked tachycardia	Tachycardia or bradycardia
Blood pressure (systolic)	Normal	Normal or falling	Marked drop
Pulse volume	Normal/reduced	Mildly reduced	Markedly reduced
Capillary refill time	Normal/increased	Mildly increased	Markedly increased
Skin	Cool, pale	Cold, mottled	Cold, deathly pale
Respiratory rate	Mild tachypnoea	Marked tachypnoea	Sighing respiration
Mental state	Normal/agitated	Lethargic	Reacts to pain or unresponsive

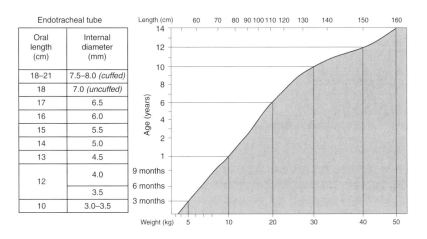

Figure 13.1   Paediatric resuscitation chart.

must be present when the child is assessed, as children look to their parents for reassurance. The doctor must appear confident and in control, which will reassure both the parents and the child. Remember that fear may alter a child's physiological parameters, causing increased respiratory rate, blood pressure and heart rate. However, one should never assume that such alterations are due to fear until organic causes have been excluded.

Parents should accompany children at all times.

Initial assessment and treatment

The traditional method of assessment of patients, beginning with history taking and then examination, followed by investigation, is not employed in the severely injured or unwell child. The general approach to the child *in extremis* has four phases (*see* Box 13.1).

> **Box 13.1** Assessment of severely injured child
>
> 1 Primary survey
>
> 2 Resuscitation
>
> 3 Secondary survey
>
> 4 Definitive treatment

Primary survey

The primary survey is a rapid assessment of the patient's overall state. Its purpose is to identify rapidly any life-threatening conditions and treat them immediately. *See* Box 13.2.

Airway with cervical spine control

The cervical spine is immobilised while the airway is assessed by talking to the patient. The 'trauma handshake' is used. While the head is immobilised the attendant asks 'How are you?' in order to determine the reaction to verbal stimulus and thus the conscious level.

Breathing with ventilation if required

A rapid assessment of the respiratory system is made in order to identify life-threatening conditions such as tension pneumothorax, open chest wound, etc. If the patient is not breathing, assisted ventilation may be required.

> **Box 13.2** Primary survey
>
> **A**irway with cervical spine control
>
> **B**reathing with ventilation if required
>
> **C**irculation with haemorrhage control
>
> **D**isability
>
> **E**xposure

Circulation with haemorrhage control

The aim during the primary survey is to assess the circulation rapidly and to preserve the remaining circulating volume until resuscitation is under way.

Disability

This involves a rapid mini-neurological assessment consisting of assessment of the pupillary response and conscious level. The pupils are rapidly inspected for size, equality and responsiveness to light.

The Glasgow Coma Scale is commonly used to assess conscious level, but takes too much time in the initial phase. Therefore the AVPU system (*see* Box 13.3) is used for rapid assessment.

> **Box 13.3** AVPU system
>
> **A**lert
>
> **V**ocal – responds to vocal stimulus
>
> **P**ain – responds to painful stimulus
>
> **U**nconscious

Exposure

To complete the primary survey, the child is undressed completely to ensure that no injuries, rashes, etc. are missed. Do not leave the child exposed for prolonged periods of time, to avoid hypothermia and also embarrassment.

Resuscitation

The resuscitation phase may follow the primary survey, but is often performed simultaneously. A high concentration of oxygen is administered, intravenous access is achieved to obtain blood for cross-matching, and other appropriate tests and fluid resuscitation are commenced.

Blood pressure, pulse, temperature and respiratory rate may be formally measured and recorded with various monitors being applied. Initial X-rays may be taken in the resuscitation area.

Splinting of fractures, administration of antibiotics and tetanus prophylaxis should take place now if required. As soon as respiratory and circulatory functions are secure, pain relief must be considered and administered safely. Intramuscular, oral and rectal routes may be ineffective if fluid loss is present, as absorption will be minimal in the presence of compensatory vasoconstriction. Analgesia should only be administered intravenously or intra-osseously in small doses, which are titrated against the patient's response (i.e. give small amounts and assess the effect before proceeding to give more).

Secondary survey

A secondary survey is the taking of a full history and the performance of a top-to-toe examination. This is undertaken once resuscitation is established and ongoing. If the child has a life-threatening condition that requires immediate intervention (e.g. surgery), the secondary survey may have to be postponed, but must not be forgotten.

A more complete history is obtained either from the patient or from the accompanying parents or adults. A useful *aide-mémoire* is *AMPLE* (*see* Box 13.4). A thorough examination is then carried out, including examination of the back. If a spinal injury is suspected, the patient must be turned in a rigid position which avoids any twisting of their spine. This is called the *log roll*

Box 13.4   Secondary survey: AMPLE

Allergies

Medications

Previous illness/injury

Last ate or drank

Environment in which the injury occurred or illness developed

---

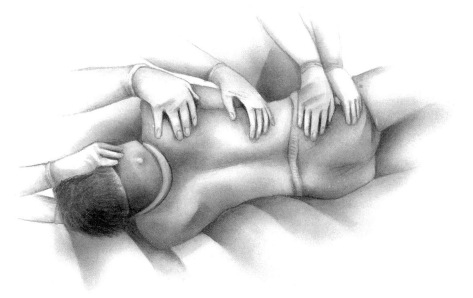

Figure 13.2   The log-rolling procedure.

(*see* Figure 13.2). All orifices must be inspected (e.g. ears, rectum). Once the examination is complete, all findings must be documented. Further investigations indicated by the examination should be carried out at this time. Once these are complete, a definitive treatment plan can be devised for the patient.

Definitive treatment

Definitive care takes place when the patient undergoes treatment for their illness or injury (e.g. surgery for fractured limbs, renal dialysis for kidney failure, etc.).

The shorter the time from insult to definitive care, the better the outcome.

The above system should be employed for all patients who present with emergency conditions and accidents. The majority will not require immediate intervention, but this system ensures that those who do are not overlooked. *See* Case study 1 for an example.

Road traffic accident (head injury)

The mechanism of injury is important, as it allows the prediction of patterns of injuries. There is no need to memorise various different injury patterns,

---

Case study 1

It is the summer holidays, at about 8pm in the evening, and Paul (aged 6 years) and his older brother are returning home on their bicycles. Neither of them is wearing a helmet. While crossing the road to reach their house, Paul is struck by a motor vehicle travelling at 45 miles an hour in a built-up area. Paul's father witnesses the accident and immediately bundles Paul up, enlisting the aid of a neighbour to drive him to the Accident and Emergency department, which is only half a mile away. The father runs into reception carrying Paul.

Paul is rushed into the resuscitation area accompanied by his father, and a rapid primary survey is undertaken. The 'trauma handshake' is performed. Paul is moaning incoherently and does not respond to verbal stimulation. An obvious head wound is noted, with blood around the right ear.

The astute doctor seeks out anticipated injuries. This is particularly vital in children, who are less likely to volunteer information about the sites of pain. For example, Waddell's triad describes the injuries sustained by a child pedestrian when struck by a car. A child is small, so the car bumper strikes the femur. The child's thorax on the same side strikes the bonnet. The kinetic energy delivered to the child's small target catapults them down the road, landing on the contralateral side of the skull. Obviously if the mechanism is known, these injuries may be sought out directly.

The airway is inspected and found to be clear. There is no evidence of airway obstruction. The respiratory rate seems to be very rapid. The trachea is central and there is obvious bruising to the left side of the chest and abdomen. Surgical emphysema is felt on the left side, and breath sounds are decreased on the left. Paul's pulse is rapid and of low volume. He appears pale and has a capillary refill time of 6 seconds. He responds to painful stimulation of his sternum by grasping the doctor's hand with his right hand. The pupils are equal but sluggish. The nursing staff begin to remove his clothing.

Resuscitation is commenced by immobilising the neck with a cervical collar, tape and sandbags, and administering oxygen. Intravenous access is obtained with difficulty and blood is taken for cross-matching. Paul's weight is estimated by measuring his length with a tape measure, which allows rapid conversion to weight using standard tables. Monitors are used to measure his heart rate, blood pressure and oxygen saturation. His pulse is 140 beats/minute, his blood pressure is unrecordable, and an oxygen saturation monitor is unable to detect a signal peripherally. Initial X-rays are taken in the resuscitation room of cross-table cervical spine, chest and pelvis. The chest X-ray shows no rib fractures but a pneumothorax on the left. Therefore a chest drain is inserted. While fluid is given intravenously, the secondary survey begins. Details of the injury are obtained from the father. Paul was struck on his left-hand side by the car, and was thrown approximately 7 metres (20 feet) before landing on the road. Examination reveals a scalp laceration to the right side of the head, with blood coming from the ear. There is bruising along the whole of the left side of his torso and a deformed left thigh. On 'log-rolling' the patient, no injury is found. The first bolus of fluid is completed and the primary survey is repeated. The airway is still clear, the respiratory rate is decreasing to 35 breaths/minute with equal air entry, the saturation monitor is now reading 96%, and the systolic blood pressure is detected at 60 mmHg, with a capillary refill time of 5 seconds. The fluid bolus is repeated. While this is being performed, local anaesthesia is instilled around the left femoral nerve and the left leg is splinted.

Further X-rays are taken, and these confirm that the lung has re-expanded and that there is a femoral shaft fracture. Paul's blood pressure, oxygenation, respiratory and pulse rates and capillary refill times are now returning to normal and he is coherent. A blood transfusion is commenced. He undergoes an ultrasound scan of his abdomen in the resuscitation room which shows fluid in his abdomen, possibly from a tear of his spleen. A computerised tomography (CT) scan of his abdomen is arranged. A pelvic X-ray should always be taken, as pelvic fracture may result in torrential bleeding. (Clinical signs of pelvic fracture are notoriously unreliable.)

A CT scan confirms a splenic tear, but Paul's condition remains stable. Therefore surgery is not required. He has good perfusion and urinary output, and is admitted to the general surgical ward. His femoral fracture is treated by splintage. He makes a slow but steady recovery. He is finally discharged from follow-up 3 months after the accident with full mobility.

as a good description of the mechanism of injury combined with the application of common sense is all that is required.

The long-term outcome is dependent on rapid, effective and complete resuscitation with early institution of definitive management. However, in children it is not simply a case of achieving physical recovery, but also of ensuring that growth and psychological development continue normally. Following traumatic episodes, children frequently revert to an earlier developmental stage (e.g. a 5-year-old may act like a 3-year-old). A head injury may have a prolonged effect on a child's learning abilities. Follow-up by a paediatrician with involvement of the school health service will be required, and extra help provided in school if necessary. The lasting emotional trauma to the parents should also be recognised and managed with skilled counselling.

Scalds

Burns and scalds are the second commonest cause of accidental death in children in the UK after road accidents. The majority of deaths occur at home, and are usually the result of house fires.

Scalds do not lead to death but are common and very damaging to children (*see* Figure 13.3).

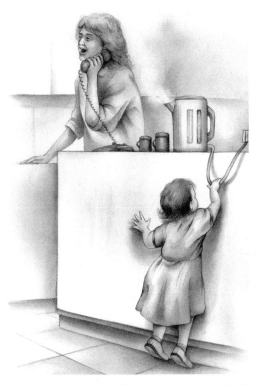

Figure 13.3   Child pulling flex with risk of boiling water pouring on to head.

The cause of death in fires is normally asphyxiation combined with carbon monoxide or other toxic gas poisoning.

Approximately 60 000 to 70 000 attendances per year at Accident and Emergency departments in the UK are due to burns and scalds in children, with approximately 10–15% of cases requiring admission. Around 70% of cases occur in pre-school children, the most common age being between 1 and 2 years.

Assessment of the burn involves several factors. First, the surface area is estimated. Children's relative proportions vary with age. Wallace's rule of nines used in adults does not apply in children. Specialised charts for children of different ages are available (*see* Figure 13.4) and should be used

(a)

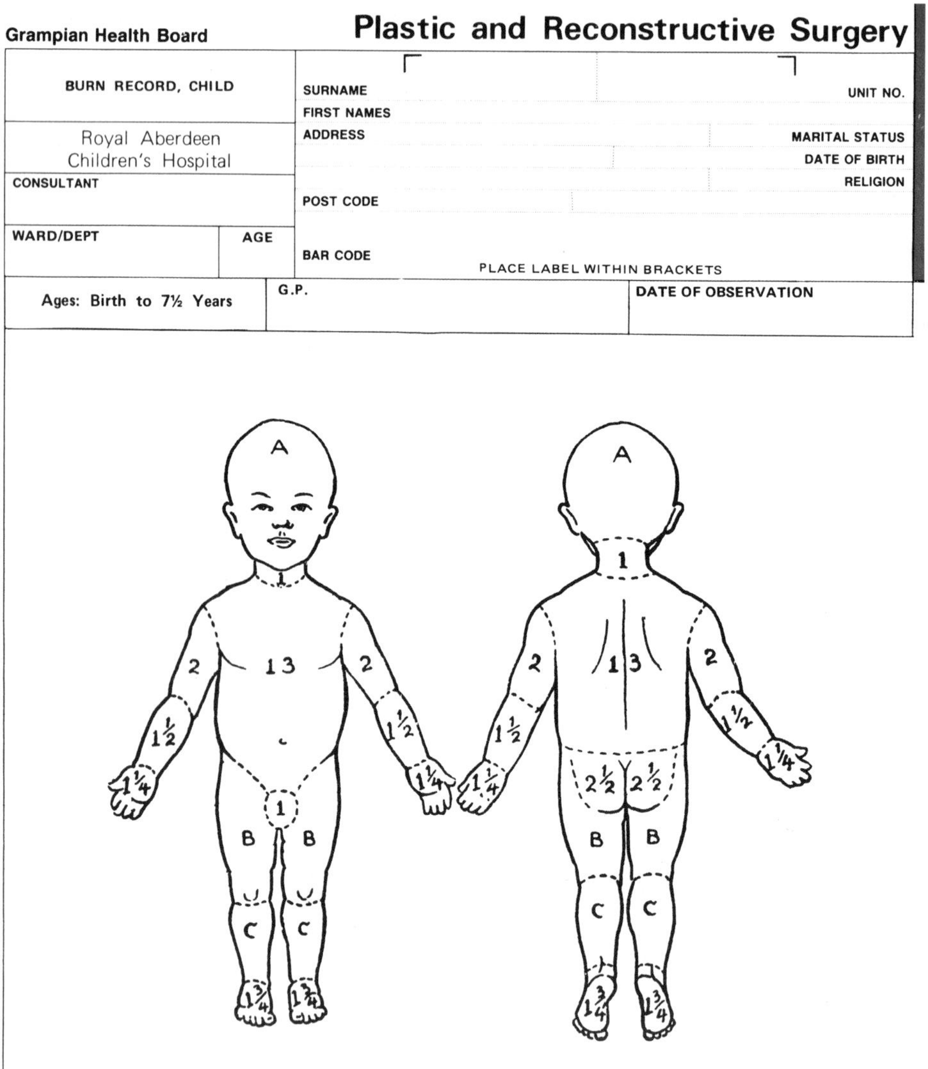

Area	Age 0	1	5
A = ½ of Head	9½	8½	6½
B = ½ of One Thigh	2¾	3¼	4
C = ½ of One Leg	2½	2½	2¾

RELATIVE PERCENTAGES OF AREAS AFFECTED BY GROWTH

Figure 13.4   (a) and (b) Burn/plastic surgery charts.

to estimate the burned area. If none are available, an estimate may be derived by using the patient's palm and adducted fingers to represent 1% of the body area (*see* Figure 13.5). Secondly, the depth of the wound must be assessed. Burns are either superficial, partial or full thickness (*see* Figure 13.6).

A superficial burn affects the epidermis only, resulting in erythema and no blister formation. This simple erythema should not be included in the surface area assessment.

(b)

Grampian Health Board

Plastic and Reconstructive Surgery

BURN RECORD, ADULT	SURNAME / UNIT NO. / FIRST NAMES
HOSPITAL	ADDRESS / MARITAL STATUS / DATE OF BIRTH
CONSULTANT	RELIGION / POST CODE / OCCUPATION
WARD/DEPT. / AGE	BAR CODE / PLACE LABEL WITHIN BRACKETS
Ages: 7½ Years to Adult	G.P. / Date of Observation

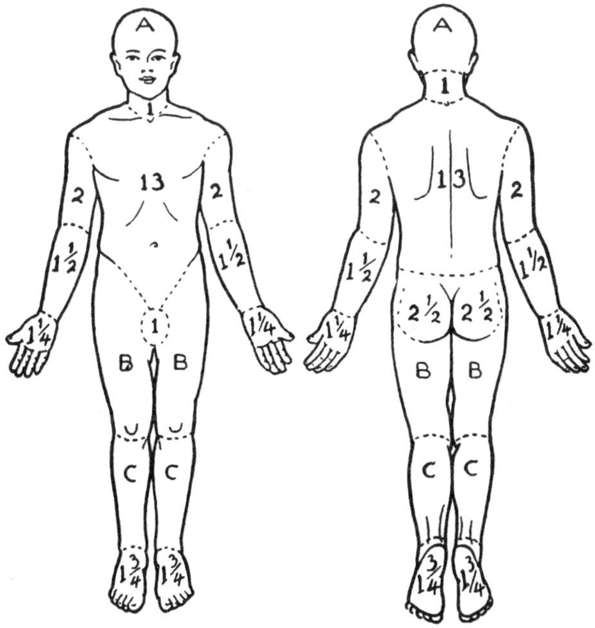

RELATIVE PERCENTAGES OF AREAS AFFECTED BY GROWTH

Area	Age 10	15	Adult
A = ½ of Head	5½	4½	3½
B = ½ of One Thigh	4¼	4½	4¾
C = ½ of One Leg	3	3¼	3½

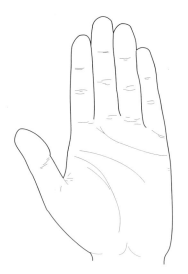

A partial-thickness burn results in some damage to the dermis. Blistering occurs, but sensation is usually retained.

A full-thickness burn damages the epidermis, dermis and perhaps even deeper structures. The skin appears white and charred, and is painless.

As a general rule, full-thickness burns in excess of 5% or combined burns in excess of 10% should be referred to a burns unit. Smaller burns in significant areas (e.g. the face, sole of the foot, or over the joints) should also be referred.

Case study 2 describes a child with a severe scald.

Figure 13.5 Palm represents 1% of body surface area.

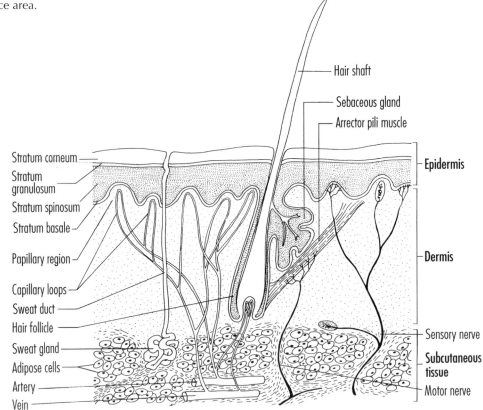

Figure 13.6 Skin layers.

Case study 2

Ailsa, aged 18 months, is an inquisitive toddler and an only child. Her mother is boiling water in an electric kettle but does not realise that the flex is hanging over the edge of the work surface (*see* Figure 13.3). She leaves the cooking area briefly to answer the telephone. She hears Ailsa scream and returns to find that she has pulled the kettle full of boiling water over herself. There is a large laceration on her forehead. Her mother rapidly removes all of Ailsa's clothes and puts her under the cold shower. She then wraps her in a blanket and drives directly to the Accident and Emergency department. The important factors in determining the severity of the burn are the temperature of the stimulus and the duration of contact. It is important to have an estimate of the temperature (e.g. if a hot drink had milk in it, this would reduce the temperature). If a child's clothes are soaked in hot water, the clothes hold the heat against the child, increasing the duration of contact. Those children who are unable to remove their own clothing will sustain a more severe burn.

First aid involves removing all clothing and cooling the affected area rapidly under cold water for 5 minutes. The burned area should have nothing applied to it. There are many 'old wives' tales' about applying butter and other substances, but these have no benefit and may even be detrimental. The child should be wrapped in clean linen, such as a pillow case or tea towel.

Ailsa is immediately taken to the resuscitation area and a primary survey is performed. She is screaming hysterically. A cervical collar is applied and oxygen is given. The airway is clear, the respiratory rate is 45 breaths/minute, pressure is applied to the wound and the pulse is estimated to be 160 beats/minute with a capillary refill time of less than 2 seconds.

Ailsa has intravenous access established rapidly and blood sent for various investigations. Intravenous morphine is given at an initial dose of 0.1 mg/kg. Initial fluid resuscitation is commenced with crystalloid solution.

Ailsa is comfortable and sleeping with her mother holding her hand. Her blood pressure, pulse, respiratory rate and oxygen saturation are stable. The area of the burn is mainly over her face, neck, chest and arms. The percentage burn is estimated to be approximately 15% combined partial and full-thickness burns. The fluid replacement required is calculated and the flow rate adjusted accordingly. The burns are now covered in clingfilm and a clean warm blanket is placed over Ailsa. She is then transferred to the nearest burns unit after consultation with the duty plastic surgeon.

Ailsa does well in hospital, but requires skin grafting for full-thickness burns on her face and upper chest. This involves multiple operations over a period of several years.

Near drowning

Drowning is death from asphyxia associated with submersion in a fluid.

Near drowning occurs if any recovery (however transient) occurs following a submerging incident.

Drowning is the third commonest cause of accidental death in children in the UK after road accidents and burns. The highest incidence occurs in under-fives in private swimming pools, baths, ponds and land waterways. Coexisting disease such as epilepsy, diabetes and ingestion of alcohol increases the risk of drowning.

First aid involves removing the child from the water rapidly. The airway is assessed and cleared of all material, taking care not to manipulate the neck excessively. Breathing is then checked for 5–10 seconds. If it is absent, 5 rescue breaths are immediately given. A major pulse is then sought and, if absent, external cardiac massage is commenced, with 20 cycles of 1 ventilation to 5 compressions being given per minute. In this situation, basic life support should not be interrupted and must never be abandoned before reaching hospital, as even in apparently desperate cases the prognosis may be good (*see* Case study 3, Figure 13.7 and Box 13.5).

Never abandon pre-hospital resuscitation of a drowned child.

Prevention of drowning requires that all children should be taught to swim at an early age, all private swimming pools should be securely fenced and covered when not in use, and public facilities should be supervised by qualified instructors.

Case study 3

Rajinder (aged 3½ years) is the second son of four in the family of a wealthy businessman. The family has a large house just outside town with its own outdoor swimming pool. It is October and someone has inadvertently left the gate to the swimming area open. When Rajinder's mother calls the children in for lunch, Rajinder does not appear. His mother finds Rajinder face down floating in the swimming pool. She is unable to swim, so she dials 999 and calls her neighbour for help. Her neighbour pulls Rajinder from the pool but finds fluid in the airway, which he drains by turning Rajinder on to his side. He is apnoeic, so the rescuer gives five rescue breaths. There is no evidence of a major pulse, so five compressions are given with the heel of one hand, one finger breadth above the xiphisternum. The neighbour continues to give basic life support at a ratio of one ventilation to five compressions until help arrives in the form of a paramedic closely followed by an ambulance crew. The ambulance crew continues basic life support, and the paramedic intubates the child, ensuring that the neck is not manipulated. Intravenous access is impossible. A cardiac monitor is applied, which shows possible ventricular fibrillation. Basic life support is continued and Rajinder is transferred to the nearest Accident and Emergency department. On arrival in Accident and Emergency, a primary survey is performed again. Rajinder is being ventilated with a secure cervical spine. There is still no pulse, so external cardiac massage is continued. The monitor trace continues to appear like ventricular fibrillation. The child's weight is estimated using an Oakley chart. Defibrillation is attempted immediately. After delivery of the first three shocks the child is further assessed. He feels cold and is peripherally vasoconstricted. Therefore intravenous access is impossible and an intra-osseous needle is inserted. Blood is drawn and sent for a full blood count, urea and electrolytes, and a blood glucose stick is performed. Adrenaline is given at a dose of 10 mg/kg initially. The child continues to be in ventricular fibrillation, and therefore a further three shocks are given and the adrenaline dose is repeated.

Cardiopulmonary resuscitation continues at all times except to allow defibrillation. Following defibrillation, a rectal temperature is obtained with a low-reading thermometer, and is found to be 29°C. Attempts are made to rewarm Rajinder. All of his wet clothing is removed, and warm blankets are applied as well as an overhead heater. Using a blood warmer, intravenous fluids are given at 37°C and the ventilator gas is heated to 42°C.

After 20 minutes of resuscitation and warming, Rajinder spontaneously regains cardiac output but continues to require ventilation. His temperature is now 32°C. Intravenous access is now possible. Blood gases and arterial blood gases are drawn. In addition, X-rays of the cervical spine, chest and pelvis are taken. A 12-lead electrocardiogram (ECG) is also performed. Rajinder is transferred to the intensive-care unit for further monitoring and care. His mother wishes to know the prognosis.

Up to 70% of children survive near drowning if basic life support is provided at the scene. Of those who survive having required cardiopulmonary resuscitation, approximately 70% make a full recovery and 25% have only a mild neurological deficit. The remaining 5% will be severely disabled or in a permanent vegetative state.

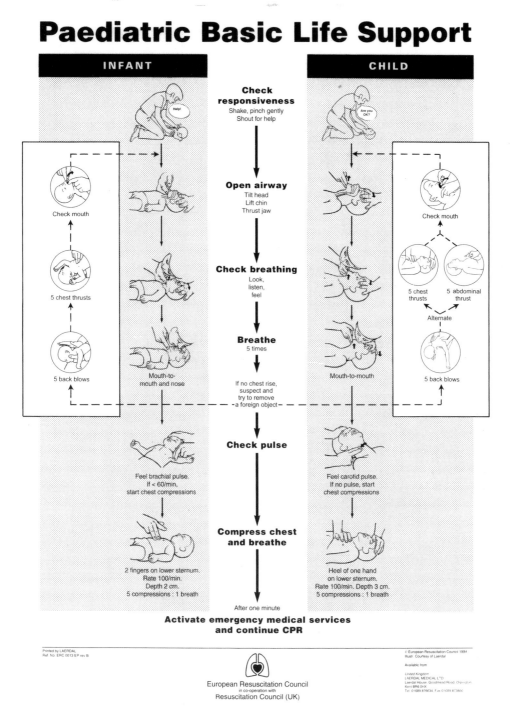

Figure 13.7   Basic Life Support chart. Reproduced by kind permission of the European Resuscitation Council. (Available from Laerdal Medical Ltd, Orpington, UK.)

> **Box 13.5** Poor prognostic factors in near drowning
>
> - Time to first gasp > 40 minutes
> - Immersion time > 8 minutes
> - Absence of hypothermia
> - Persistent coma (no sedation)
> - pH < 7.0, PO_2 < 8.0 kPa (despite treatment)

Poisoning

Suspected poisoning is an extremely common presentation in children, accounting for over 50 000 presentations to Accident and Emergency departments each year, with 50% of cases being admitted. Deaths are uncommon and usually due to tricyclic antidepressants or household products. The commonest cause of poisoning resulting in death is carbon monoxide in house fires. The introduction of child-resistant containers has significantly reduced mortality from accidental poisoning, but 20% of children under 5 years of age are capable of opening them. The vast majority of poisonings in children are accidental in nature, most commonly occurring in the 2–3 years age group, in whom curiosity usually leads to ingestion. In addition, many modern drugs resemble sweets. Accidental ingestion occurs more frequently when there is disruption to the household (e.g. moving house, a new baby, etc.). Deliberate overdose does occur, but usually in teenagers. These patients will require psychiatric referral as well as medical attention for the overdose. Recreational drug abuse is an increasing problem among teenagers, the biggest culprit being alcohol. Very rarely, the poisoning may be iatrogenic or may be deliberate on the part of the parent, either as part of a non-accidental injury pattern or to gain access to hospital in the case of fabricated or induced illness (see Chapter 14, page 207).

Identification of the poison is of paramount importance if the child is not unwell. Wherever possible, remains of the poison should be obtained. Obtaining the drug bottle will allow identification of the substance.

An estimate of potential quantity may be made by counting the remaining tablets. The largest potential overdose should always be assumed to have been taken. The time from ingestion should be assessed if possible.

Treatment of poisoning (see Box 13.6 and Case study 4)

If the drug is considered to be toxic enough to require removal, and the time since ingestion is relatively short, removal may be indicated. However, gastric lavage is rarely indicated, and should only be initiated by a senior paediatrician.

Neutralisation of the toxin may be achieved by giving an agent to bind the toxin in the gut or by intravenous administration of a specific antidote. Activated charcoal acts by binding with the toxin in the gut, and is effective on a wide range of drugs, including tricyclic antidepressants and digoxin. If gastric lavage has been employed, it may be instilled down the tube at the end of lavage.

> **Box 13.6** Treatment of acute poisoning
>
> - General supportive measures
> - Reduction of exposure to the drug
> - Neutralisation of the drug
> - Increased elimination of the drug

Products or drugs which are likely to be harmful to children are listed in Box 13.7.

> **Box 13.7** Substances harmful to children in overdose
>
> *Drugs*
> - Digoxin
> - Diphenoxylate (Lomotil)
> - Iron
> - Paracetamol
> - Salicylates
> - Tricylic antidepressants
>
> *Chemicals, etc.*
> - Alcohol
> - Bleach
> - Paraffin

Box 13.8 Poisons information centres

The following single number for the UK National Poisons Information Service directs the caller to the local poisons information centre where information is available on all aspects of poisoning, day and night:

0870 600 6266

There are several national poisons information centres in the UK which may be consulted with regard to the management of various individual substances (*see* Box 13.8). It is impossible to remember the management of all poisons, and the centres maintain large databases on a range of substances, including household products and plants.

Case study 4

Daniel, aged 2 years, is staying with his grandparents while his mother is in hospital after the birth of his younger brother. His grandparents find him in the bathroom before his bedtime with an open bottle of his grandmother's tablets which she uses for her depression. The tablets look like Smarties and are scattered across the floor. Daniel's grandmother has no idea how many tablets were in the bottle. The grandparents immediately take Daniel to the local Accident and Emergency department.

On arrival at hospital, the tablet involved is identified as a tricyclic antidepressant, and Daniel had last been seen 20 minutes before being found in the bathroom. It is assumed that if any ingestion occurred, it did so within 1 hour.

There is no objective evidence of ingestion, but in view of the potential toxicity of tricyclic antidepressants, Daniel is given activated charcoal which he drinks reluctantly. He is admitted for cardiac monitoring and observation.

The following day he is well and is discharged home. Written advice is given to the family with regard to the safe storage of drugs.

Further reading

- British Medical Association (2003) *Advanced Paediatric Life Support. The practical approach* (3e). British Medical Association, London.
- Capehorn A, Goldsworthy L and Swain A (1998) *A Handbook of Paediatric Accidents and Emergencies: a symptom-based guide.* Elsevier Science Health Division, Oxford.
- Mills K, Morton R and Page JG (1995) *A Colour Atlas and Text of Emergencies* (2e). Mosby-Wolfe, London.
- Muir IFK, Barclay TL and Settle JAD (1987) *Burns and Their Treatment* (3e). Butterworth, Sevenoaks.
- Resuscitation Council UK; www.resus.org.uk

Self-assessment questions

1 A primary survey includes:
(a) taking blood for urea and electrolytes   True/False
(b) taking a family history   True/False
(c) asking 'How are you?'   True/False
(d) checking capillary refill time.   True/False

2 The commonest causes of trauma in a child in the UK are:
(a) road traffic accident   True/False
(b) falling out of a tree   True/False
(c) falling in the home   True/False
(d) falling into a private swimming pool.   True/False

3 Scalds in a child:
(a) do not require analgesia   True/False
(b) should be run under cold water for longer than 15 minutes   True/False
(c) should be covered with clingfilm   True/False
(d) have their area assessed by Wallace's rule of nines.   True/False

4 Poisoning in children:
(a) is treated by gastric lavage in most cases   True/False
(b) is not usually life-threatening   True/False
(c) is commonest in pre-school children   True/False
(d) may be associated with non-accidental injury.   True/False

14 Child abuse and neglect

- Children at risk
- Clinical presentations of injury
- Growth patterns
- Emotional deprivation
- Sexual abuse
- Behavioural markers
- Evaluation of the abused child
- The case conference
- Prevention strategies

There are few situations in the life of a medical student or doctor which are more difficult or painful than those which arise when deliberate injury or preventable misery of a child is presented within a health context. The physician should be aware that his or her contact with a child or family may prove to be the watershed event that helps to change the future for both.

An open-minded and non-judgemental approach is essential. Anger, horror or disbelief are natural and unavoidable emotions that may be overwhelming, but they may also impede the development of the rapport and compassion which should accompany our dealings with families. It is important that the physician does not feel isolated or burdened by an undue sense of responsibility. Extensive statutory structures have been created precisely because such situations are rarely simple and none of them may be wholly resolved by medical intervention alone.

Children at risk

Child abuse and neglect occur in all sectors of society. Studies show that they are more prevalent where there is disadvantage or stress within communities. These situations include families in which mothers are young and unsupported, or have had unrewarding or damaging childhoods themselves. Parents who have endured abusive childhoods may lack the role models that lead to good child care. They may have poor insight into the needs of their child, or into their own needs.

They may choose unsuitable or violent partners, and they may not have the resilience to cope with the violence, poverty and neglect which their partners bring into their households. Poverty, debt, poor housing and loneliness may be part of a spectrum of stress that leads to falling standards of care.

An understanding of these complexities is essential if a child's well-being is to be established within the family and solutions found. There are very few parents who seek to harm their children deliberately, and it is always important to view the presentation of abuse in a child as a marker of serious family distress. Evaluation of the child alone will not bring the answers to that child's needs. Criminal and civil legal processes should only be invoked with care and forethought.

The outcome of all of these processes is shared in a *child protection case conference,* which will be attended by the parents. The case conference has powers to place the child on the Child Protection Register (*see* Box 14.1 and page 218).

Means of protecting children are through the courts by child protection orders (*see* Box 14.2) and through decisions of the case conference (*see* Box 14.3).

Box 14.1 The Child Protection Register

This register is maintained by social services and is a record of children who are at risk of child abuse. A child may be entered on the register as a result of a decision by a case conference (*see* page 218). The register may be consulted at any time by a health professional who is worried about the possibility of abuse of a child.

Box 14.2 Protection orders

Emergency Protection Order
Under the Children Act (1989), section 44, a court may make an order if it is satisfied that there is reasonable cause to believe that a child is likely to suffer harm. It gives parental responsibility to the local authority in addition to the routine carer. Such an order may only last for 8 days. The court may extend it for a further 7 days.

Police Protection Order
Section 46 allows the police to prevent the child's removal from hospital for a period of up to 72 hours.

Box 14.3 Case conference decisions

1 To place the children on the Child Protection Register

2 To remove the children from their parents under a Care Order

3 To place the children in foster care with the parents' agreement with no Order

4 To return the children to their parents under a Supervision Order

5 To return the children to their parents with no Order

Clinical presentations of injury

- *Non-accidental injury.* Physical abuse of children is the most overt form of child abuse, detected by the assessment of visible injury and the finding of hidden trauma (e.g. fractures). There are several features which should lead the doctor to suspect non-accidental injury (*see* Boxes 14.4 and 14.5).

- *Accidental injuries* are common once a child is mobile. The rough-and-tumble of play is likely to account for a small number of minor bumps and bruises. Such injuries are usually seen over bony prominences in the young child (e.g. the parietal bone, chin or nose, and the knees and shins of more mobile youngsters). Bite marks may be inflicted by another child, and scratches and abrasions may be acquired during play with pets or sharply contoured toys.

- *Inflicted injuries* should be suspected if multiple soft tissue sites are involved, particularly the buttocks or the back of the thighs. Injuries to the abdomen, genitals, chest wall, inside of the mouth or the ear lobes should cause concern.

- *Instrumental trauma* (which includes adult human bites) can be recognised by its characteristic shape and pattern. Tears to the upper lip and frenulum occur either by direct blows or by forced feeding, or by having a pacifier roughly jammed into the mouth. Pinch marks and squeeze marks often appear as multiple oval bruises resembling fingertips. Bruises to the neck may be due to choke injuries, and linear petechial haemorrhages may be caused by twisting of a child's collar, or by pulling a child up off the ground by their clothing. There may also be linear bruising from implements (*see* Figure 14.1).

- *Induced-illness syndrome,* formerly known as Munchausen's syndrome by proxy (MSP), is a rare and unusual form of abuse that should be suspected if a child presents repeatedly with features of illness which have no apparent cause. In this very serious type of abuse a parent induces symptoms which may require hospitalisation (*see* Box 14.6).

Box 14.4   Physical abuse or non-accidental injury

Physical abuse or *non-accidental injury* is defined as actual bodily trauma to a child which has been deliberately inflicted. Such an injury may include bruising, fractures, bites, burns and scalds, or the administration of toxic substances.

Box 14.5   Features that suggest non-accidental injury

- The appearance of the injury does not reflect the history given:
  - because of its appearance and age
  - because of the developmental stage of the child
  - because the injury represents a known pattern of deliberate injury (e.g. a hand or belt mark).

- There are multiple injuries of several ages.

- The history is inconsistently offered.

- The injury is not explained: 'I just found him like this'.

- There is a delay in seeking medical care.

- There are other worrying factors or clinical signs.

Box 14.6   Induced illness syndrome

This is a complex form of child maltreatment in which a child's carer (usually the mother) deliberately and repetitively fabricates or induces symptoms in the child in order to bring him or her to medical attention. Examples include deliberate administration of salt, or the introduction of blood or sugar into urine or stool samples. Children may suffer prolonged hospitalisations before diagnosis. They may also undergo painful tests and procedures and be required to accept unnecessary and potentially harmful drug treatments.

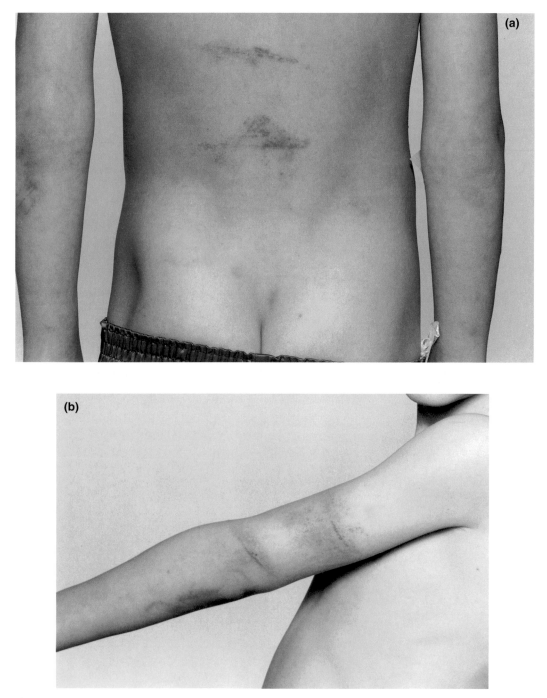

Figure 14.1   (a) and (b) A 9-year-old who has been beaten with a billiard cue. The pattern of injury is linear, supporting the history.

Not all children need to be admitted to hospital for investigation of suspected abuse. Indeed admission should be avoided if at all possible, as it only adds to the child's emotional distress. The investigations may proceed with the child in a safe place either within the extended family or in foster care.

Case study 1

John is a 2-year-old boy who is brought to your attention because of a bruised ear. It is 10pm and John's 19-year-old mother, Lisa, has attended with two children. She also describes persistent crying in the younger sibling, Maria, who is 10 months old. Maria's father, Gary, who is not John's father, does not come into the department, but waits outside in the car park. You examine Maria and find that she is physically healthy but looks thin. Her clothing is somewhat scanty and she has severe nappy rash. John appears tired and pale. You note linear yellowish bruising over his buttocks and upper thighs. John's mother tells you that he bumped into a door a week ago: 'He is always bumping into things and bruises easily'. She is anxious to leave, and tells you that her partner will not countenance her stay. You attempt to engage with Maria's father and bring him into the department. Gary is hostile, verbally abusive, and tells you that unless the children need emergency treatment he will not let them stay. The findings in John also indicate a recent injury over the ear that is incompatible with the history given. The linear bruising is compatible with contusion from a belt repeatedly applied, and a mark on his arm looks like a human bite mark (*see* Figures 14.2 and 14.3). Maria is poorly cared for and appears to be failing to thrive. Both John and Maria appear to be children at risk, and there is a strong suspicion of non-accidental injury to John.

Immediate referral is made to the social services and the police. Following the children's admission to hospital, a child protection investigation takes place. At the case conference it is agreed that John's injury was caused deliberately. Lisa admits to the violence in the home and has separated from her partner. The children are now in her sole care. She has always found Maria difficult to feed, but is managing better with the help of the health visitor. It is agreed that her children will be placed on the Child Protection Register under the category 'Physical abuse', and that the situation will be reviewed in 3 months' time.

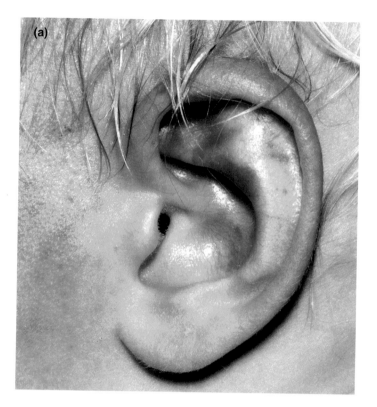

Figure 14.2 (a) and (b) Ear bruising in a 2-year-old.

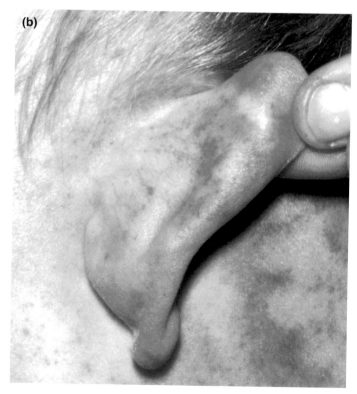

(a)

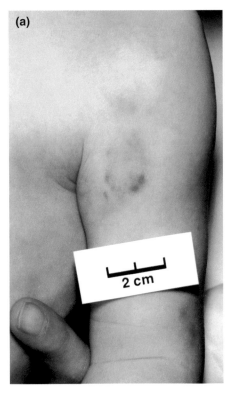

(b)

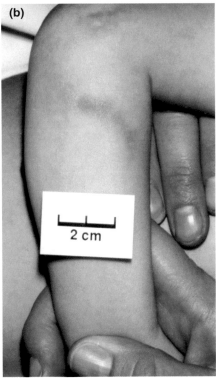

(c)

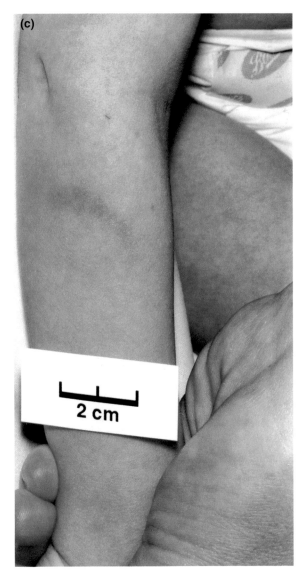

Figure 14.3 (a), (b) and (c) Bites on the upper arms and forearm (the same child as in Figure 14.2).

The shaken baby syndrome

Infants and children under the age of 2 years may present with multiple injuries associated with violent shaking events. Many of these injuries may not be evident on initial examination. They are commonly a result of the shearing forces of rapid uncoordinated accelerating and decelerating forces. The child is picked up around the chest, shoulders or neck, and the rib-cage is firmly held or squeezed. Violent shaking in a young baby with poor muscle tone results in repeated hyperextension of the neck and spine and uncoordinated flailing of the limbs. These forces result in rupture of vessels in the conjunctiva and retinae and bridging veins in the brain. Tears of the falx cerebri may occur. Lateral rib fractures due to compression, or posterior rib fractures due to shearing forces, are also noted. The growing ends of the long bones are particularly susceptible to these forces, and chip or separation fractures occur at the metaphyses. Such fractures are virtually pathognomonic of deliberate injury, and are rarely if ever seen in accidental injuries (*see* Box 14.7 and Case study 2).

Box 14.7 Shaking injury

- Conjunctival and retinal haemorrhages
- Rib fractures
- Metaphyseal fractures
- Subdural haematomas
- Bruising to chest wall
- History of persistent crying
- Unconscious infant with convulsions or anaemia

Case study 2

Jenny is 8 weeks old. You are called urgently to the home at 2am. Jenny's father tells you that he woke to offer Jenny her feed, and found her pale, unconscious and limp.

Jenny's parents, John and Alison, are in professional jobs, and Jenny is cared for during the day by her grandmother. You have had no previous worries about her care.

When you arrive at the home, you find Jenny very ill. Focal fits started 10 minutes before you arrived. On examination, Jenny is not febrile. She is twitching on the left side, and looks very pale. There are no other findings, apart from a small conjunctival haemorrhage in the right eye.

Her parents tell you that she has been fractious all evening, but perfectly well, and there were no other symptoms. In hospital, Jenny is found to have a right subdural haematoma, and on skeletal survey a metaphyseal fracture of the right distal tibia is found. The paediatrician has involved social services, and the police are investigating the origin of these injuries. Jenny is placed in intensive care and makes progress, but is likely to have residual neurological handicap. There are signs of a developing left hemiparesis.

The social services department arranges a case conference which you attend. Information about the family is shared, and you are told that after initial denial by both parents, Jenny's mother has acknowledged shaking Jenny roughly on the night of her admission because she had refused a feed and was crying incessantly. She has told the investigating workers of her own exhaustion and feelings of depression, and is asking for help.

Jenny has suffered severe physical abuse. Shaking a baby is not an uncommon response to prolonged crying, when a parent can become extremely stressed. However, it can be extremely damaging to the infant. Fortunately, Jenny's mother has recognised this and is therefore likely to accept help. As a result of extensive publicity, most parents are aware of the adverse effects of shaking a baby, but this will not entirely prevent such abuse occurring. Fortunately, Jenny made a complete recovery and escaped neurological sequelae. She was sent to stay with her grandparents while her mother was assessed, and she went home after a month with the agreement that Alison would receive more support and would also involve both her mother and John in Jenny's care in future.

Non-accidental burns

Burns and scalds also occur as a result of deliberate immersion in hot water. This type of non-accidental injury has a characteristic appearance (*see* Figure 14.4 and Box 14.8).

(a)

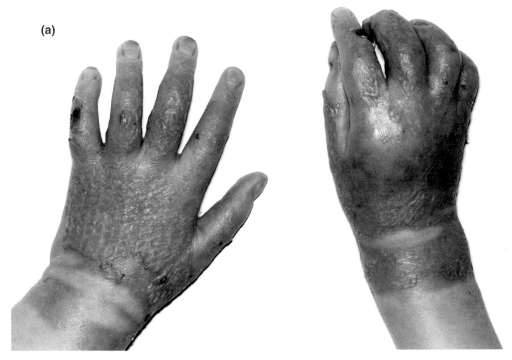

Figure 14.4   (a) and (b) Classic pattern of deliberate immersion scalds in a 22-month-old. Note the clean demarcation lines and the bands of dorsal sparing where the wrists were held hyperextended – the expected reaction to such a painful process. (Figure continued overleaf)

(b)

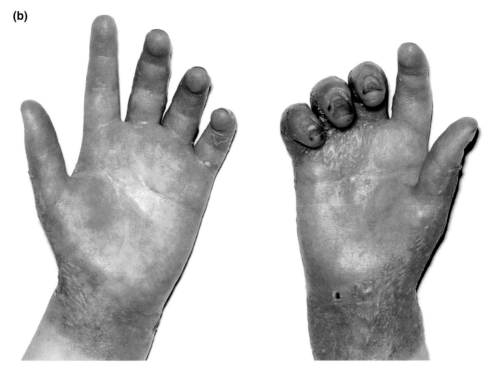

Figure 14.4   *Continued.*

Box 14.8   Burns and scalds (*see also* Chapter 13, page 195)

- Accidental burning in childhood is not uncommon, and up to 80% of cases occur within the home.

- Such injuries are more frequent in the winter months, and at times of the day when stress in the family is at its highest.

- Accidental injuries relating to spills of hot liquids from kettles, pans or cups may be extensive and severe, but most often are small, involving the upper limb, chest wall and shoulder.

- Flow is rapid and the fluid cools as it flows. The findings are therefore of scalds of variable depth with splash marks and a 'trickling' effect.

- Immersion scalds are characteristic (*see* Figure 14.4), with a clear demarcation line and usually with the involvement of the distal part of the limb.

Growth patterns

Physical growth is one of the most objective markers of the health of a child. Careful and serial analysis of weight and height progress in children provides important clues to poor or deteriorating health.

'Failure to thrive' was a descriptive term developed to describe apathetic, wasted children living in long-term state institutions. The term 'growth faltering' is now often used to describe children who fail to grow for no apparent reason, and where it is suspected that psychosocial factors are critical (*see also* Chapter 4, page 61).

Box 14.9 Neglect

This is failure to provide essential care of a child (e.g. food, warmth, or protection from danger), or indifference to or denial of a child's physical, medical and educational needs.

However, it is most important to recognise that growth in children is influenced by calorie intake, calorie absorption, rest, exercise, hormonal influences and metabolic requirements in disease and health. Trauma and neglect in children will impact on their growth through a combination of these influences. The withholding of food from an infant will result in a clearly observed failure to gain

weight, which is rapidly correctable by adequate replacement. On the other hand, an abused child may fail to grow because of abnormal food intake mediated by apathy and anorexia, which is difficult to resolve without therapeutic intervention other than food. The unhappy child may be stunted in height without necessarily demonstrating a serious fall in weight achievement. Neglect may coexist with organic disease states, and severely neglected children are predisposed to more low-grade infection and ill health (*see* Box 14.9).

The chart shown in Figure 14.5 is taken from *A Child in Trust*, a public enquiry report into the death of Jasmine Beckford on 5 July 1984. She was then 4½ years old, and was in the care of the local authority from the age of 20 months.

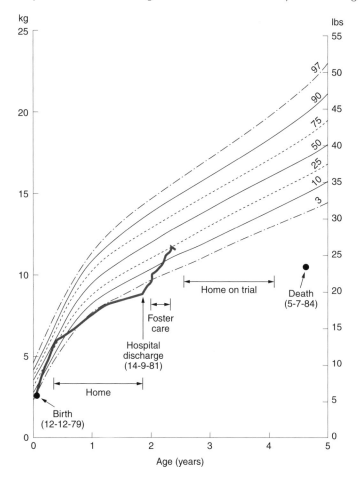

Figure 14.5 The weight chart of Jasmine Beckford, who died of neglect in 1984. It shows good weight gain in hospital and foster care, and weight fall-off at home. (*From A Child in Trust*, public enquiry report into the circumstances surrounding the death of Jasmine Beckford, London Borough of Brent, 1985.)

She was admitted at that age with a femoral fracture. After a period of 7 months in foster care she was returned to the care of her parents. At the time of her death, over 2 years later, she weighed less than she did in foster care, and had suffered numerous soft tissue and bony injuries in the weeks and months leading up to her death.

Emotional deprivation

A disturbing manifestation of child abuse is the child who presents with emotional deprivation.

This results from inadequate parenting and lack of individual loving care which is severe enough to impact on the child's well-being. The child may present either with 'acting-out' behaviour (when the child has found that being very difficult is the only way to gain attention) or with silent withdrawal. In either case, skilled intervention is needed to listen to the perspective of the child and to rectify the situation, as there are likely to be long-term emotional consequences. This type of child abuse can be hard to identify and very difficult to correct.

Case study 3

Sarah, a 6-year-old, has been noted at school to be withdrawn and isolated. Previously bright and bubbly, she has recently tended to be clingy towards her teacher. She has wet herself on two occasions, and has once fallen asleep during a lesson. Her single-parent mother has recently become pregnant to a new boyfriend, Stuart. Sarah shows anxiety at the end of the day and is sometimes fearful and refuses to go home when her mother's boyfriend comes to collect her. Her teacher asks you to see Sarah, and an appointment is made. However, Sarah's mother does not bring her to school on the day of the appointment. The family's GP tells you that Sarah's mother is not attending antenatal appointments. She is now 21 years of age, and was 15 years old when Sarah was born. She has lost the support of her own mother because of a family row. The health visitor reports that Sarah's mother and Stuart drink heavily and that the home is visited by several of Stuart's acquaintances, who stay there at night and sometimes take care of Sarah.

When you visit Sarah's mother and Stuart, they speak to you on the doorstep and tell you that they have no concerns. They are angry that the school staff have involved you, and tell you of their intention to keep Sarah away from school and find another placement for her.

Your information suggests that Sarah is at risk. Social services should be involved, and if possible this should be with the agreement of the family. Their confidence should be gained so that they are prepared to share their difficulties, but if this does not happen then child protection procedures may be needed.

At this stage, however, there is little specific evidence of abuse, and it may be that Sarah's interests are best met by a non-confrontational, friendly approach and by sharing information with the new school health and educational staff so that there is heightened vigilance. She may be given special attention. Staff must be alert to any distress and should listen to her with care.

Several months after Sarah's problems were brought to your attention, the police investigate an allegation made by another young child, who is Stuart's daughter from a previous liaison. She is 11 years old and has felt able to talk about sexual molestation by Stuart, which went on for several years before he left her home.

The strategy is now much clearer. Given the previous concerns about Sarah's behaviour, a case conference should be called. This will provide a forum at which Sarah's mother's views may be sought again. Stuart will be advised to leave the home, at least for a period, while investigations are under way, and this period should be used to involve Sarah and her mother in therapeutic work that is directed at uncovering any fears Sarah may have.

Sexual abuse

The fact that sexual exploitation of young children occurs has been recognised for many centuries.

For child sexual abuse to occur, two pre-conditions need to exist. First, there must be an individual who is predisposed to sexually abusing children. Such a person needs to have access to a child and needs to overcome their inhibitions. This is more likely to occur if alcohol or drugs are involved. However, as the second precondition is usually fulfilled, such influences are unnecessary. The second precondition is the vulnerability of the child victim. Factors that influence a child's vulnerability include developmental immaturity, susceptibility to coercion, absence of a protective parent, and poor experiences of nurturing. Most child protection workers recognise that although isolated, unpredictable, sexually traumatising events occur in the lives of children, in the majority of children sexual abuse occurs as part of a spectrum of adverse experience. It is also true that the perpetrator of abuse is most commonly an individual known to the child, often someone in a position of trust. *See* Case study 3 and Box 14.10.

Behavioural markers

Children who are subjected to non-accidental trauma and/or sexual abuse, and those who live in emotionally depriving environments, are highly likely to suffer significant developmental damage, even when there are no permanent physical sequelae. Observations of such children may reveal certain behaviours that appear characteristic. A withdrawn, apathetic state, or alternatively a hyper-alert, still child who smiles little, a baby whose feeding is anxious and gulping in nature, loss of appetite, and pallor are all features which should arouse the gravest concern. Emotionally neglected children may display self-stimulatory behaviours such as rocking or head banging. The sexually exploited child may display inappropriate boundaries of behaviour (e.g. seeking to touch or stroke adult carers, or engaging in compulsive masturbation or simulated sexual activity with toys or peers).

Box 14.10   Recognition of sexual abuse

- A child may make a direct statement to a peer or adult about abuse. Such statements should always be taken seriously.

- Children rarely, if ever, lie about such matters. Indeed, when such statements are thought to be unfounded, the gravest concern should exist about the reasons for and background to the child's statement.

- Children may present with changes in behaviour, or with disturbances in conduct, school progress or peer interaction. These may be non-specific (e.g. depression, anger, anxiety) or more specific (e.g. self-harming or sexualised behaviour).

- Physical symptoms include urinary and stool incontinence as a direct outcome of trauma, and vulvo-vaginal infections, including sexually transmissible disease.

- On rare occasions, the situation may present with acute symptoms of genital bleeding, bruising and swelling.

Evaluation of the abused child

An understanding of aetiology and family systems that predispose to abuse should underpin the clinical approach to suspected child abuse.

Communication with the family should be in depth and with the intention of obtaining a wide perspective. Pre-judgement, anger or hostility will impede such an approach. The best way to ensure a proper evaluation is to adopt a systematic approach to the investigation of child abuse (*see* Box 14.11).

> **Box 14.11** Investigation of child abuse
>
> - Full family history, including social supports, physical and developmental examination, and diagrams including measurement and dating of all injuries
>
> - Coagulation profile
>
> - Growth charting
>
> - Skeletal survey – healed and fresh fractures
>
> - Developmental assessment
>
> - Swabs for semen detection (sexual abuse)
>
> - Swabs for trace material and items of clothing (sexual abuse)
>
> - Screening for sexually transmitted disease (sexual abuse)
>
> - Reconstruction of events (e.g. a home visit may be helpful in cases of non-accidental burns)

Management of child abuse

In 1991, the Department of Health produced a document entitled *Working Together Under the Children Act 1989* to guide professionals towards proper arrangements for child protection. This document was revised in 1999. All health districts and individual hospitals and health units should have procedural guidelines accessible to all professionals. Each local authority has an area or district child protection committee. This is a body made up of representatives from health, social services, police, education and voluntary bodies, whose role is to design a strategy for child protection practice for the area that it serves. In 2003, the report of an inquiry into the murder of a child, Victoria Climbie, indicated that a radical review of training and inter-agency working is needed. The report by Lord Laming recommends new structures to widen the onus of responsibility for child protection. The Government has since issued a Green Paper entitled *Every Child Matters*, which outlines its responses to these concerns.

The case conference

The case conference provides a forum for the development of an understanding of an individual child's needs and the way forward to secure that child's safety and future good care. The views and knowledge of various professionals and carers are sought in a discussion which should be open and frank, and which should include the child's parents and other adults who may have contributed or wish to contribute to his or her upbringing.

The responsibility for calling such a conference rests with the social services department, and is influenced by guidelines laid down by the Department of Health. When a doctor, health worker or any other agent suspects abuse or is concerned about a child's care, notification of that concern is the start of the process leading to a case conference.

The objectives of the case conference are crystallised into outcomes described as 'decisions' (*see* Box 14.3). One of these is the 'decision to register'. The Child Protection Register (CPR) is a central list held by the social services department in each district. The list records the names of children who are deemed to be 'at risk'. There are firm criteria for deciding whether a child is at risk of harm (*see* Box 14.12).

The CPR will provide information to concerned professionals when requested to do so (e.g. by a doctor dealing with an injured child in an Accident and Emergency department). A child whose name is placed on the CPR with or without legal sanctions remains on it up to such time as sufficient change in his or her circumstances occurs. Once a child is on the CPR, regular reviews take place to reassess the continuing need for registration, and a care team meets regularly to provide for needs. Table 14.1 shows the number of

> **Box 14.12** Categories used in the Child Protection Register
>
> - Actual physical abuse or future potential physical abuse
>
> - Actual emotional harm or potential for future emotional harm
>
> - Actual or future risk of sexual abuse
>
> - Actual neglect or risk of neglect

children on the CPR nationally (in England and Wales) in 2001 and 2002.

Table 14.1 Number of children on the Child Protection Register in different categories (2001 and 2002)

Type of abuse	2001	2002
Neglect	12 900	10 100
Physical abuse	7300	4200
Sexual abuse	4500	2800
Emotional abuse	4800	4500

Source: Department of Health Statistics (2002) *Registration Data for Years Ending March 2001 and March 2002 (England)*.

Prevention strategies

Child maltreatment is a societal issue that is rooted in complex interpersonal relationships and the often unpredictable coming together of a series of environmental factors. At a simple level, one may consider three strands to a prevention process.

Primary prevention

Strategies to prevent abuse involve a clear understanding of potential danger. For an individual child, this could mean the early provision of support to a young mother, sensitivity to the stresses of poverty and unemployment in a family, or material and befriending provision for children and parents in distress. At a community level, examples of primary prevention include programmes such as the 'Don't Shake the Baby' campaign, prevention of under-age pregnancies, and early parentcraft education in secondary schools. There is now much emphasis on programmes to promote positive (violence-free) parenting, and health visitors are key health professionals in this exercise, since they have access to every parent. The new Government 'Sure Start' initiative is an example of a widely acclaimed approach to helping parents. There is an organisation in the UK (EPOCH, End Physical Punishment of Children) which is seeking legislation to ban corporal punishment in the home, a move

that has so far been successfully carried through in five European countries.

Secondary prevention

This refers to early detection of abuse, particularly emotional abuse, scapegoating and neglect. All primary healthcare services have a role in such detection, and most child protection agencies are heavily involved in such work. The National Society for the Prevention of Cruelty to Children (NSPCC), which was established in the late nineteenth century, has done much to bring to public attention the fact of abuse taking place in our midst, and their facility to assist members of the public in reporting abuse anonymously is an example of secondary prevention. 'Childline' is a free telephone helpline specifically to help children to report abuse experienced by themselves or by friends.

Tertiary prevention

This refers to the rehabilitation of children who have been maltreated. Compensatory nurturing, high-quality tailored mental health services, and early acknowledgement of damage and of need may allow some children to grow into adults who can fulfil the needs of their own children. The availability of proper resources both within the criminal justice system and within psychotherapeutic health services and social service systems could make it possible to treat some people who maltreat children, and to reduce their potential to cause harm in the future.

Further reading

- Addcock M, White R and Hollows A (1991) *Significant Harm*. Significant Publications, London.

- Department of Health (1989) *Working Together Under the Children Act*. HMSO, London.

- Department of Health (1999) *Working Together to Safeguard Children*. The Stationery Office, London.

- Hobbs CJ, Hanks HGI and Wynne JM (2002) *Child Abuse and Neglect: a clinician's handbook*. Churchill Livingstone, Edinburgh.

- Newell P (1989) *Children Are People Too. The case against physical punishment.* Bedford Square Press, London.

- End Physical Punishment of Children (EPOCH); www.epoch.org and www. childrenareunbeatable.co.uk

- Every Child Matters (Green Paper); www. dfes.gov.uk/everychildmatters

- *The Victoria Climbie Inquiry: Report of an Inquiry by Lord Laming, January 2003.* The Stationery Office, London.

Self-assessment questions

1   With regard to physical abuse:

(a) bruising on the legs would suggest non-accidental injury   True/False

(b) bruising of different ages on different parts of the body would suggest
non-accidental injury   True/False

(c) a retinal haemorrhage in a baby is suggestive of a shaking injury   True/False

(d) a cigarette burn on a child is highly suggestive of abuse.   True/False

2   Neglect:

(a) implies a deficiency of physical care   True/False

(b) is commoner in low-income than in high-income families   True/False

(c) is a category for registration of child abuse   True/False

(d) poor weight gain is an objective feature.   True/False

3   Sexual abuse:

(a) occurs in boys as well as in girls   True/False

(b) the perpetrator is most often a member of the family   True/False

(c) is often accompanied by emotional abuse   True/False

(d) may present with sexualised behaviour.   True/False

4   The case conference:

(a) is presided over by a magistrate   True/False

(b) may be attended by parents   True/False

(c) is set up by health services   True/False

(d) is legally empowered to register a child with regard to abuse.   True/False

15 Growth and the endocrine system

- Normal growth and puberty
- Measuring growth and pubertal development
- Problems of linear growth
- Neonatal sexual ambiguity
- Diabetes mellitus

Normal growth and puberty

Growth and development go hand in hand. The most rapid phase of longitudinal growth is in the mid-trimester fetus (see Figure 15.1). Thereafter, rapid growth in infancy slows down through early childhood before a doubling of growth rate at puberty, followed by virtual cessation of growth when the epiphyses of the long bones fuse in the mid-teen years. Growth is so rapid in the first few months of life that weight increase is often used as a marker of linear growth. After 6 months of age, increase in length is measured in its own right, and height is measured after 2 years.

The main influences on growth in fetal and early postnatal life are nutritional rather than endocrine, with hormonal factors becoming progressively more important from infancy onwards. Severe psychological deprivation can adversely affect growth both in infancy and during childhood (see Chapter 14, Figure 14.5).

Sexual differentiation and development of the endocrine system occur in fetal life towards the end of the first trimester. Androgens from the fetal testis stimulated by placental chorionic gonadotrophin and luteinising hormone (LH) and follicle-stimulating hormone (FSH) from the developing pituitary are important in the developing fetus in imprinting a male pattern on the indifferent female-type precursor (see Figure 15.2).

After birth the gonadal hormone axis enters a quiescent phase until the onset of puberty. The first sign of puberty in girls is breast bud development, occurring on average just before 11 years of age, and in boys it is 3 ml testicular size, found shortly after 12 years.

The peak height velocity of the pubertal growth spurt is just before 12 years in girls and 14 years in boys, making the average 12-year-old girl briefly taller than her male peer. Menarche at an average age of 13 years is a late event in female puberty, after which the average girl grows only

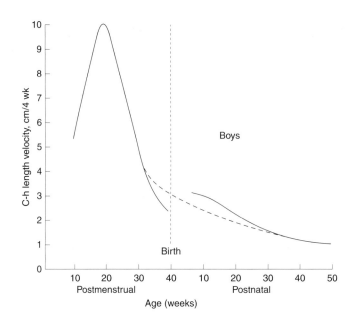

Figure 15.1   Velocity curves for growth in body length in the prenatal and early postnatal period in boys: (———), actual length and length velocity; (– – – –), theoretical curve if no uterine constriction occurred. (Based on several sources of data and reproduced from Tanner JM (1989) *Fetus into Man* (2e). Castlemead Publications, Welwyn Garden City.)

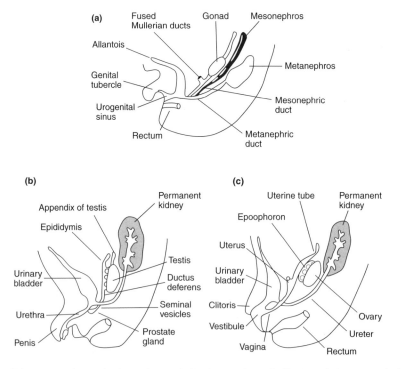

Figure 15.2   Diagrammatic sagittal sections of the internal genitalia (a) of the 8-week fetus, and at 13 weeks fetal age in (b) the male and (c) the female fetus.

6 cm. The hormonal contribution to the pubertal growth spurt is partly due to androgens from the adrenal cortex in both sexes and from the testis in boys, but more important is increased growth hormone production under the influence of sex steroids.

Variations in the timing of puberty are wide. Early pubertal development (precocious puberty) is defined as before the age of 8 years in girls and 9 years in boys. Early development in girls from the age of 6 years and sometimes younger is relatively common, and is usually due to constitutional factors, whereas early development in boys is much more likely to be due to organic disease of the adrenal gland, testis or hypothalamus. Delayed puberty is common in boys (a tendency often inherited from the father), but occurs less often in girls (where again the mother may have passed the menarche late). A boy who shows no signs of puberty at 14 years of age, or a girl at 13 years, warrants specialist assessment. A 14-year-old boy with few or no signs of puberty may suffer psychological stress on this account, and may also be at lifelong risk of low bone density and other effects of late onset of androgen surge.

Measuring growth and pubertal development

Accurate and careful measurement of height or length (*see* Figures 15.3 and 15.4) is important, and requires an accurate measuring device. Shoes, bulky socks and hair slides need to be removed. In the vertical position (height), the heels, buttocks and shoulder blades should touch the measure with the feet together and upward pressure exerted on the mastoid processes to achieve a stretched height. Infants and very young children can be measured in the supine posture (length).

Growth measurements on an individual child need to be compared with standard norms for the child's peer group by plotting the results on a growth chart that shows normal centiles for that group (*see* Figure 15.5). Similar charts are available for other countries. Worldwide racial and genetic variation in growth shows that, for example, the Hausa of Nigeria and the Dutch are among the tallest populations in the world. Populations from the Far East are shorter, but there has been a considerable secular trend towards taller stature in Japan in recent decades, possibly due to dietetic factors.

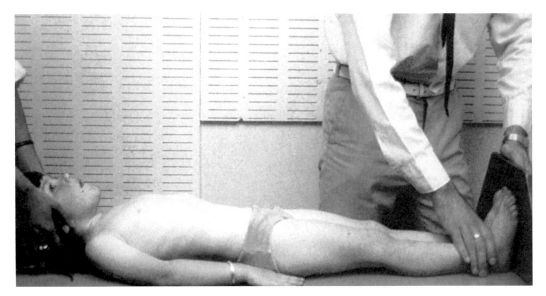

Figure 15.3   Length measurement.

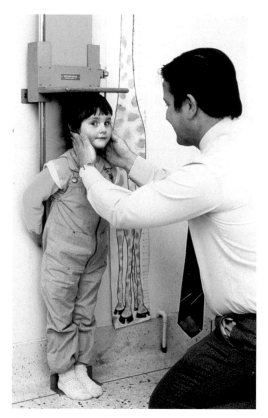

Figure 15.4   Height measurement.

Pubertal development is described according to Tanner stages (*see* Table 15.1). Testicular size is measured by comparison with a standard set of beads of graded volumes, known as an orchidometer.

Problems of linear growth

Tall stature

It is important to remember that the expectations of a child are very dependent on his height. Thus although a short child may suffer on this account within his peer group, less is expected of him than of a child who is tall for his age and also expected to have the intelligence and maturity of a child several years older. This particularly affects the early developing girl, who may appear physically like an 11-year-old at the age of 7 years.

Tall stature is usually due to tall parents or early puberty. Organic conditions are rare (*see* Box 15.1).

Short stature

The common causes of short stature are shown in Box 15.2. Basic information that is needed to make a growth diagnosis includes parental heights, birth weight, the timing of parental puberty, and social background. It is extremely important that height is measured accurately, and on more than one occasion, in order to distinguish short stature from progressive growth failure.

Growth assessment must be accompanied by careful explanation, reassurance and counselling of parents about their child's likely progress in height. Particularly in the case of constitutional delay in puberty in boys, a child who at the time is much shorter than his peers may turn out to be of normal adult height.

Table 15.1   Stages of puberty

Girls

Sexual maturity rating (SMR) stage	Pubic hair	Breast
1	Preadolescent	Preadolescent
2	Sparse, lightly pigmented, straight, medial border of labia	Breast papilla elevated as small mound, areolar diameter increased
3	Darker, beginning to curl, increased amount	Breast and areolar enlarged, no contour separation
4	Course, curly, abundant but amount less than in adult	Areolar and papilla form secondary mound
5	Adult feminine triangle, spread to medial surface of thighs	Mature, nipple projects, areolar part of general breast contour

Boys

Sexual maturity rating (SMR) stage	Pubic hair	Penis	Testes
1	None	Preadolescent	Preadolescent
2	Scanty, long, slightly pigmented	Slight enlargement	Enlarged scrotum, pink texture altered
3	Darker, starts to curl, small amount	Longer	Larger
4	Resembles adult type but less in quantity, course, curly	Larger, glans and scrotum increase in size	Larger, scrotum dark
5	Adult distribution, spread to medial surface of thighs	Adult size	Adult size

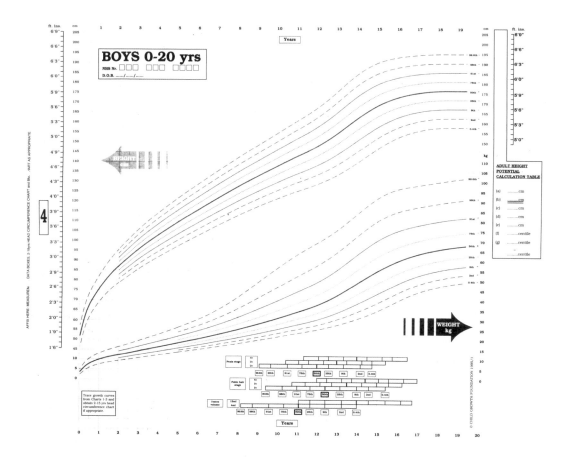

Figure 15.5   UK 9-CENTILE growth chart. (Available from Harlow Printing Ltd, South Shields, UK.)

Box 15.1   Causes of tall stature

- Constitutional (tall parents)
- Early puberty
- Thyrotoxicosis
- Marfan's syndrome
- Sex chromosome abnormalities, such as XYY and XXY
- Homocystinuria
- Growth-hormone-secreting pituitary adenoma

Box 15.2   Causes of short stature

- Constitutional (short parents)
- Psychosocial deprivation
- Delayed puberty
- Intrauterine growth restriction
- Organic disease (see below)

Growth failure

Growth failure occurs when a child's height or length falls progressively further from the median. Different causes tend to predominate at different ages (*see* Box 15.3). The commonest problem in the growth clinic is apparent growth failure in a 12- to 14-year-old boy with delayed puberty, but he will regain his former height centile later in his teens. (For information on growth faltering in infancy, *see* Chapter 4, page 61.)

Box 15.3   Some causes of growth failure

Infancy
- Growth hormone deficiency
- Dyschondroplasia
- Down syndrome

Mid-childhood
- Hypothyroidism
- Turner's syndrome
- Chronic renal failure
- Crohn's disease

Early teenage delayed puberty
- Craniopharyngioma

Any age
- Psychosocial deprivation
- Severe asthma and severe eczema

Neonatal hypothyroidism is detected by universal screening (in the UK), involving the measurement of thyroid-stimulating hormone (TSH) in blood spots taken on a filter paper card (*see* Chapter 17, page 268). Thyroxine is not needed in the fetus, but from birth to 2 years of age it is required for brain growth, so diagnosis and treatment of hypothyroidism in a neonate with an absent thyroid gland or abnormal thyroxine metabolism prevents learning difficulty. On the other hand, children with hypothyroidism (usually due to auto-immune thyroid disease) diagnosed *after* the age of 2 years have normal intellect. Treatment consists of daily thyroxine by mouth for life (*see* Case study 2).

Hypothyroidism can also present with growth failure in mid-childhood. As treatment takes effect, body weight decreases and height increases together with the general level of activity. Paradoxically, hypothyroid children tend to over-achieve at school, in contrast to thyrotoxic children, who commonly do badly at school. Treatment of moderate or severe hypothyroidism can lead to school problems for a year or two due to difficulties in concentration.

Classical *growth hormone deficiency* may present in the newborn with hypoglycaemia, or in infancy or early childhood with growth failure. Children who have been treated with cranial irradiation for cancer may lack growth hormone due to pituitary damage. Other groups who may benefit from growth hormone treatment include children with Turner's syndrome and those with chronic renal failure. Growth hormone is given by daily injection and is expensive. It may be of short-term benefit in improving growth rate in children with constitutional short stature and with delayed puberty, but it does not significantly improve adult height in these conditions.

Case study 1

Rob, aged 7 years, is the youngest child of a family of five. He is the shortest in his class, at school entry measuring 103 cm at 5½ years (3rd centile). A further measurement of 111.8 cm is taken at 7.1 years (3rd centile). His parents are unhappy with the explanation that he is just going to be short, because his four older brothers (aged 16–24 years) range in height from 172 to 177 cm. They ask their school nurse and GP for a second opinion.

Rob was of normal birth weight, and there is no suggestion of social problems. Parental puberty occurred at the normal time, and Rob's father is 172 cm tall and his mother is 150 cm tall. Calculation of mid parental height (*see* Table 15.2) shows this to be 168 cm, with a target centile range of 158–178 cm (0.4–50th centile).

Rob eventually proves to have an adult height of 163 cm, and it is concluded that he is a child of constitutional short stature who takes after his mother, whereas his older brothers take after their father in height (*see* Figure 15.6).

Table 15.2 Calculation of mid parental height (MPH)

(a)	= father's height	172 cm
(b)	= mother's height	150 cm
(c)	= sum of (a) and (b)	322 cm
(d)	= c/2	161 cm
(e)	= d + 7 cm (MPH)	168 cm (*subtract* 7 cm for a girl)
(f)	= mid parental centile [nearest centile to (e)]	9th centile
(g)	= target centile range (MPH ± 10 cm)	158–178 cm 0.4–50th centile

This calculation is not applicable if either of the natural parents is not of normal stature.

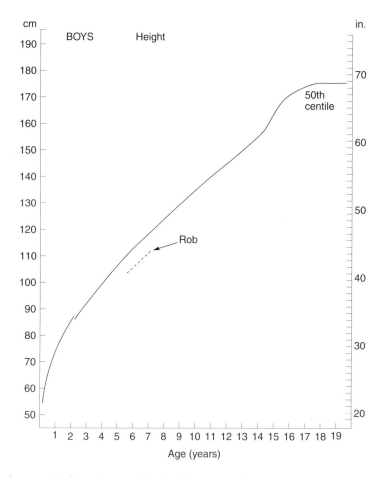

Figure 15.6 Rob's growth chart, showing his height at 5.5 and 7.1 years. Note that he is growing at a normal pace along the 3rd percentile.

Case study 2

Kirsty is 122.5 cm tall at the age of 9.2 years (3rd centile). Her mother has noticed that she has been gaining weight over the past year or two. Comparison with the measurement at 7.3 years (121.8 cm) shows that she has fallen away in height through two major centile lines (25th and 10th) on the growth chart. She is rather pale, and has dry scurfy hair and a small smooth goitre. Blood is taken for analysis of thyroid function and thyroid antibodies, confirming the suspicion of auto-immune hypothyroidism.

In Kirsty's case the thyroid underactivity may have been developing for 4 or 5 years. She has primary hypothyroidism, in which total thyroxine or free thyroxine levels in the blood will be low, with high pituitary thyroid-stimulating hormone (TSH) levels because of lack of negative feedback.

Neonatal sexual ambiguity

When a baby's sex cannot be immediately ascertained at birth by inspection of the external genitalia, it is vital not to make a guess. Gender assignment should await the results of investigations and discussion with a team that is expert in the management of sexual ambiguity. It is important to carry out investigations quickly, and these include an urgent karyotype, serum 17-hydroxyprogesterone levels and pelvic ultrasound scan. Sexual ambiguity at birth is an unusual and complex problem.

A virilised female due to 21-hydroxylase deficiency *congenital adrenal hyperplasia* is the commonest cause (*see* Box 15.4 and Case study 3). However, an undermasculinised male may need much more complicated endocrine, genetic, radiological and surgical investigation, but a diagnosis must be vigorously sought and the sex of rearing agreed within a few weeks. The multidisciplinary team involved may include a neonatologist, paediatric surgeon, paediatric endocrinologist, radiologist, clinical geneticist and child psychologist.

Box 15.4   Congenital adrenal hyperplasia

- Lack of the enzyme 21-hydroxylase

- Incidence: 1 in 10 000 live births

- Cortisol deficiency leads to adrenocortical hyperplasia and excess circulating androgens

- Inheritance is autosomal recessive

- Treated with hydrocortisone (glucocorticoid) and fludrocortisone (mineralocorticoid)

- Risk of adrenal salt-losing crisis as in Addison's disease due to intercurrent stress or infection

---

Case study 3

Flora was born by normal delivery at full term, but at first it was not clear which sex she should be assigned. She had a 2 cm long phallus, a small apparent vaginal opening, and rugose genital folds with no palpable gonads.

The karyotype was reported as 46,XX, and 17-hydroxyprogesterone levels were greatly elevated. Pelvic ultrasound and a genitogram showed a normal infantile uterus and vagina. A diagnosis was made of congenital adrenal hyperplasia and Flora was started on hydrocortisone and fludrocortisone, and arrangements were made for corrective plastic surgery later in infancy and for genetic advice.

Diabetes mellitus

Insulin-dependent diabetes mellitus (IDDM, also called type 1 diabetes) is due to failure of insulin production. Its incidence varies between populations, from less than 10 to over 30 cases per 100 000 children per year, but appears to be increasing worldwide. Type 2 diabetes, which is largely related to obesity and the 'metabolic syndrome', used to be confined to adults, but is now increasingly found in association with severe childhood obesity.

Polyuria and polydipsia in any child should be assumed to be diabetes mellitus until proved otherwise. Urinary tract infection (*see* Chapter 20) should always be excluded, and if the urine is negative for glucose then it may be appropriate to investigate for *diabetes insipidus*, in which there is a deficiency of production of antidiuretic hormone by the pituitary. However, *habit polydipsia* is much more common among young children than diabetes insipidus.

Childhood IDDM usually presents in a previously well child with a short history of polyuria and weight loss, but should be remembered in children with secondary enuresis or acute abdominal pain, and it can present for the first time with acute ketoacidosis. A blood glucose concentration of > 12 mmol/l confirms the diagnosis, and no other diagnostic tests are necessary. There should be no delay in starting insulin, as severe ketoacidosis may develop rapidly (e.g. due to viral infection).

Initial education involves the whole family (parents adapt to the diagnosis of a serious chronic disease less well than does their child) and the diabetic hospital and community team (*see* Table 15.3). Newly diagnosed diabetic children may be managed at home rather than in hospital if they are not dehydrated, drowsy or have ketoacidosis. It is important to remember the serious psychological impact of the diagnosis of diabetes on parents, who often need a great deal of support and counselling over the first days and weeks. The affected child quickly realises that diabetes does not prevent them from doing any of the activities of their peer group, and will usually adapt to the diagnosis much more rapidly than the parents.

The diabetic child is managed with at least two insulin injections a day. Unlike the non-diabetic, in whom blood sugar levels rise and insulin appears in the blood after a meal, the diabetic takes insulin beforehand so that the body thinks it has been fed. The main aspect of the diabetic lifestyle, apart from regular insulin injections and capillary blood glucose tests, is frequent food intake to catch up with the exogenous insulin (*see* Figure 15.7). A common insulin regimen is a daily injection of mixed short-acting insulin (lasting around 6 hours) and medium-acting insulin (lasting around 12 hours) at breakfast, short-acting insulin at teatime, and medium-acting insulin at bedtime – that is, three injections a day in total. Increasing numbers of children are being managed with multiple daily injections and subcutaneous insulin pumps.

The aim of diabetic management is to make the child and their family self-sufficient in coping with most problems of diabetic control. Children

Table 15.3   Education at diagnosis of diabetes

Inform	Teach	Demonstrate	Provide
Consultant in charge of children's diabetic clinic	Insulin injection	Induced hypoglycaemia by missing a meal and if necessary giving extra quick-acting insulin	For hypoglycaemia: Glucose tablets Glucose gel Glucagon for injection
Dietitian	Capillary blood glucose testing		For intercurrent ketosis: Urine ketostix Quick-acting insulin
Diabetes nurse specialist	Urinary ketone testing		

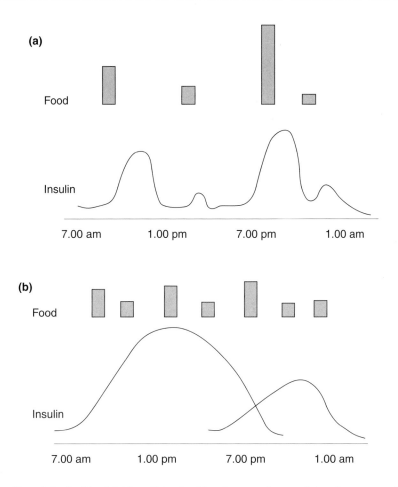

Figure 15.7   The diabetic life. (a) Non-diabetic. Blood sugar rises and insulin appears in the blood-stream after a meal. (b) Diabetic. Insulin is taken before meals so that the body thinks it has been fed.

become involved with their own diabetes from 5 years onwards, and should be doing their own capillary blood tests and giving their own injections under supervision by 8 years of age, though not becoming completely independent in their diabetic management until the age of 15 years. Children as young as 5 years can understand the effect of food, insulin and exercise on blood sugar level (*see* Figure 15.8), and how an event involving exercise, excitement and perhaps forgetting food intake (e.g. a holiday or a football match) can be managed with either planned taking of extra food, or less insulin beforehand. The routine of a diabetic child involves sugar and a Talisman or a diabetic identity card to be carried at all times. Any absence from base for more than a few minutes requires food to be

available, and for absences of more than a few hours insulin must be carried in case a snack or an injection time becomes due. Insulin resistance can be a problem during the pubertal growth spurt, due to additional production of growth hormone. Increased doses of insulin are required during these years, and control of diabetes becomes more difficult. Although diabetes can present at any age in childhood, the peak incidence is at 12–14 years, when diabetes is more likely to become an issue of adolescent rebellion (*see* Chapter 23).

Intercurrent illness requires careful management, and insulin should be continued despite loss of appetite. It is also important that a child with diabetes learns how to recognise hypoglycaemia, so that they will know what to do when it happens subsequently.

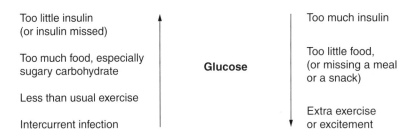

Too little insulin (or insulin missed)		Too much insulin
Too much food, especially sugary carbohydrate	**Glucose**	Too little food, (or missing a meal or a snack)
Less than usual exercise		
Intercurrent infection		Extra exercise or excitement

Figure 15.8 Basic factors in control of glucose levels in a diabetic child.

Box 15.5 Diabetes mellitus

- The commonest endocrine condition of childhood

- Child diabetes is nearly always type 1 (requires insulin)

- Peak incidence at 12–14 years of age

- Involves a progressive destruction of pancreatic islet cells, usually over several years

- Concordance of 35% in identical twins

- The incidence of type 1 diabetes in children in developed countries has increased strikingly over the past 40 years

- Population screening and prevention of diabetes may develop in the future

---

Box 15.6 Management of intercurrent illness in diabetic children

- Continue normal insulin at usual dose and times.

- Test more frequently.

- If capillary blood glucose concentration is > 20 mmol/l, test urine ketones. If urine ketone level is 16 mg/ml or above, give extra Actrapid insulin, one-sixth of the total daily dose. Check again after 3–4 hours and repeat this dose if indicated.

- Take carbohydrate-containing fluids if solids are not tolerated (e.g. fruit juice or ordinary diluted juice).

- Persistent vomiting is an indication for hospital admission.

In general, children with diabetes do well at school and in settling into work. Only a very few careers (e.g. airline pilot, uniformed services) are not open to people with diabetes.

A recent large study conducted in the USA, namely the Diabetes Control and Complications Trial, demonstrated conclusively that better diabetic control over the years in young adults (as represented by lower levels of haemoglobin A_{1c}, an index of the average blood sugar level over the previous few months) led to fewer complications. This was balanced by an increased number of hypoglycaemic episodes. Screening for complications of diabetes should start in the children's diabetic clinic, and includes regular measurement of blood pressure, retinal examination, and testing for urinary microalbumin (as a screen for nephropathy), coupled with meticulous care of the feet (where microvascular disease often presents) and advice about smoking.

Box 15.5 summarises childhood diabetes and Box 15.6 the management of intercurrent illness in diabetic children.

Case study 4

Andrew, aged 9 years, presented with a 3-week history of polyuria, polydipsia and weight loss. He was a previously healthy boy with no family history of diabetes.

His random capillary blood glucose concentration was 21.2 mmol/l, and his urine was strongly positive for ketones. This is diagnostic of diabetes mellitus. Andrew was started on twice daily mixed short- and medium-acting insulin and was quickly brought under control. On his second day in hospital his breakfast was not given after his insulin, so that a mild hypoglycaemic episode could be experienced.

Andrew will be expected to carry with him a high-calorie snack to eat should a 'hypo' develop. His parents were given glucagon to inject in the event of a severe episode.

Andrew was discharged after 3 days, he and his parents having been fully educated about diabetes and how to administer the insulin himself. He learned this quickly. The diabetic liaison nurse visited Andrew's home and school to make sure that everyone knew about the condition, and she passed on information to the school health service.

Further reading

- Court D and Lamb W (1997) *Childhood and Adolescent Diabetes*. John Wiley & Sons, Chichester.

- Raine JD, Donaldson MDC, Gregory JW and Savage MO (2001) *Practical Endocrinology and Diabetes in Children*. Blackwell Science, Oxford.

Self-assessment questions

1   In childhood diabetes:
(a) microangiopathic complications are never seen   True/False
(b) newly diagnosed children can be managed at home if they are well   True/False
(c) less insulin is needed during puberty   True/False
(d) cerebral oedema can complicate ketoacidosis   True/False
(e) the incidence is increasing.   True/False

2   Growth failure:
(a) is usual in Down syndrome   True/False
(b) may result from psychosocial deprivation   True/False
(c) is always reversible with growth hormone treatment   True/False
(d) may be a sign of hypothyroidism   True/False
(e) often accompanies delayed puberty.   True/False

3   Short stature:
(a) investigation is required for all children below the -4 SD line   True/False
(b) may be screened for at school entry   True/False
(c) if familial may be diagnosed by measuring the parents   True/False
(d) should be treated with growth hormone even if no cause is found   True/False
(e) can be detected in the first year of life.   True/False

4   Hypothyroidism:
(a) is screened for in the Guthrie test   True/False
(b) is related to iodine deficiency in the UK   True/False
(c) requires lifelong treatment   True/False
(d) is associated with Down syndrome   True/False
(e) is associated with diabetes.   True/False

16 Haematology and oncology

- Basic haematology
- Nutritional anaemia
- Sickle-cell disease (haemoglobinopathy)
- Bruising and petechiae (thrombocytopenia)
- Bruising (coagulation factor deficiency)
- Lymphadenopathy
- Abdominal mass

Basic haematology

The blood system connects with every organ and working mechanism of the human body and is responsible for the oxygenation of, transmission of chemical messengers to and excretion of waste products from all tissues. Thus blood is fundamental to health and disease. Accessing it for analysis is one of the easiest tests to carry out. The levels of public awareness of the importance of blood is high, although even concepts such as anaemia are not well understood and should be carefully explained both to the parents and to the child. Children themselves, while disliking blood tests, are fascinated by the subject of the blood, and accurate information will be well received.

Haematopoiesis

In the embryo, the initial site of haematopoiesis is the yolk sac. From there haematopoietic stem cells migrate to the liver and spleen, which are the main sites of blood formation in the fetus, and finally to the medullary cavity of the bones, which is the main site of haematopoietic tissue in extra-uterine life.

Bone-marrow stem cells have the characteristics of self-replication, division and differentiation (see Figure 16.1). The production of circulating blood cells is under the control of a variety of cytokines (growth factors). Erythropoietin is the main growth factor controlling red cell production, chronic hypoxia being the main stimulus to erythropoietin production by the kidney. The production of white cells and platelets is controlled by a variety of cytokines ('colony-stimulating factors'

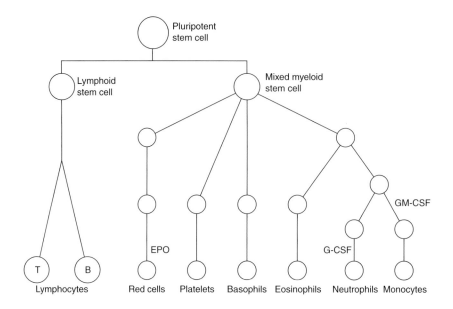

Figure 16.1   Diagram of the bone-marrow pluripotent stem cell and the cell lines arising from it. The growth factors with demonstrated clinical efficacy are shown. Epo, erythropoietin; G-CSF, granulocyte colony-stimulating factor; GM-CSF, granulocyte macrophage colony-stimulating factor.

and interleukins). The importance of cytokines lies not only in their physiological control of haematopoiesis, but also in their therapeutic potential. Many cytokines can be produced by recombinant DNA technology, and their therapeutic role is now becoming clearer. The role of erythropoietin in improving the anaemia of chronic renal failure is established. Granulocyte-colony-stimulating factor (G-CSF) is useful for promoting the recovery of neutrophil counts after chemotherapy and bone-marrow transplant, and in the management of patients with severe congenital neutropenia.

These controlling factors in haematopoiesis mean that the number of red cells, white cells and platelets in the circulating blood remain within defined 'normal' limits in health. Peripheral blood is one of the most easily sampled tissues of the body. As a result, the normal ranges for the blood count have been established for different age groups. In adults, the normal range for the blood count is stable over the years, whereas in children there is considerable variation with age. This is seen in particular with regard to haemoglobin and red cell volume (mean corpuscular volume or MCV) (see Figure

16.2), but there is variation in the proportion and number of white cells, with lymphocyte predominance being normal at a young age and neutrophil predominance at older ages. Platelet count remains much the same. It is important to remember that although a test result may be 'abnormal' (i.e. lie outwith the defined normal range) this does not necessarily indicate the presence of disease. Many other blood tests also show age-related variation.

The haemoglobin in red cells is composed of two alpha chains and two 'non-alpha' chains, forming a tetrameric molecular structure with a varying affinity for oxygen binding. During later fetal life the main form of haemoglobin is fetal Hb (HbF, alpha-2, gamma-2), which has a relatively high affinity for oxygen. Within a short period after birth, HbF production 'switches' to production of adult Hb (HbA, alpha-2, beta-2), which has a lower oxygen affinity that is more suited to extrauterine life (see Figure 16.3).

As in other branches of medicine, the clinical assessment of a patient starts with the history, as will be emphasised in the case studies. The family history can be of particular importance because of the significant numbers of hereditary forms of

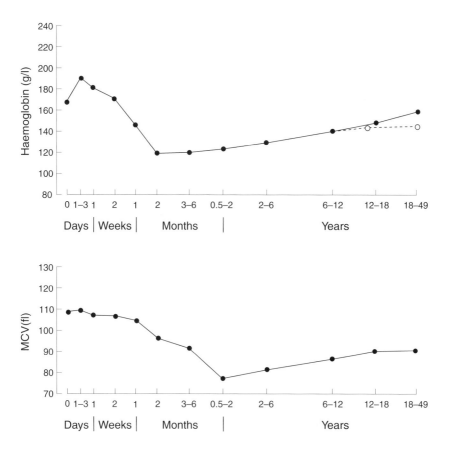

Figure 16.2   Normal ranges for haemoglobin concentration and mean cell volume (MCV) of red cells, from birth to adult life. The broken line on the right shows the values for adult females.

anaemia and haemorrhagic disorders (*see* Box 16.1).

Physical examination should assess features such as pallor and other signs of anaemia, the character and distribution of bruising, the site and nature of lymphadenopathy, the presence of hepatomegaly or splenomegaly, and abdominal masses. There should be assessment for pre-existing disease (e.g. the characteristic facial appearance of a child with Down syndrome, where there is an increased incidence of leukaemia).

The clinical effects of blood disorders are shown in Box 16.2.

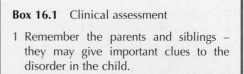

Box 16.1   Clinical assessment

1 Remember the parents and siblings – they may give important clues to the disorder in the child.

2 Do not consider the haematological disorder in isolation – there may be important effects on the growing child.

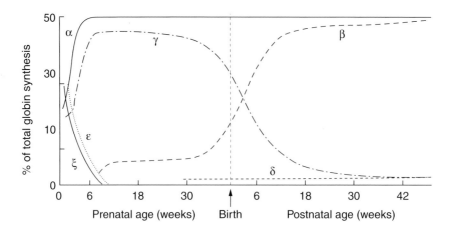

Figure 16.3 Pattern of haemoglobin chain production in the fetus and in the first year of life.
α = alpha; β = beta; δ = delta; ε = epsilon; γ = gamma; ζ = zeta.

Box 16.2 Clinical effects of blood disorders

- *Anaemia*: symptoms due to reduced oxygen delivery to tissues.
- *Polycythaemia*: sludging of the circulation.
- *White-cell abnormality*: risk of infection.
- *Platelet abnormality*: risk of bleeding; possibly thrombosis.
- *Haemostatic factor abnormality*: imbalance of haemostatic mechanism; risk of bleeding or thrombosis.

Nutritional anaemia

Iron-deficiency anaemia (IDA) is the commonest nutritional deficiency in the UK, as well as the commonest blood disorder. The prevalence in the UK is 12–20% between the ages of 12 and 24 months. Toddlers are the age group most commonly affected, due to low iron intake in the early months of life. IDA is also relatively common in teenagers following the growth spurt.

IDA is often asymptomatic. As in Case study 1, the presentation may consist of a clinical appearance of pallor (*see* Box 16.3). When symptoms appear they include tiredness, shortness of breath on exertion and (more subtly) developmental delay. Mood is also considered to be affected, and there is a lowered resistance to infections.

Box 16.3   Presentation of iron-deficiency anaemia

- Pallor (distinguish between skin pallor and mucous membrane pallor)

- Tiredness

- Shortness of breath

- Developmental delay

- Depression of mood

- Increased risk of infection

Diagnosis of iron-deficiency anaemia

The diagnosis of anaemia is relatively easy due to the accessibility of blood for testing. The level of haemoglobin defines the presence or absence of anaemia, and the red cell indices and microscopic appearance of red cells show a characteristic picture (*see* Box 16.4).

Box 16.4   Diagnosis of iron-deficiency anaemia

Reduced haemoglobin concentration (men, < 135 g/l; women < 115 g/l)

Reduced mean cell volume (< 76 fl)

Reduced mean cell haemoglobin (29.5 ± 2.5 pg)

Reduced mean cell haemoglobin concentration (325 ± 25 g/l)

Blood film (microcytic hypochromic red cells with pencil cells and target cells)

Reduced serum ferritin* (men, < 10 μg/l; postmenopausal women, < 10 μg/l; premenopausal women, < 5 μg/l)

Reduced serum iron* (men, < 14 μmol/l; women, < 11 μmol/l)

Increased serum iron and total binding capacity* (> 75 μmol/l)

* Local laboratories may have their own standards.

Children do not like to have blood samples taken, and the simplest method is a capillary sample from a finger prick. This is adequate for screening purposes, but a venous sample is required for diagnosis. This can be readily obtained if an anaesthetic cream is applied to the skin before venepuncture.

IDA can occur in several other conditions as well as in simple dietary deficiency. These are listed in Box 16.5.

Box 16.5   Non-dietary causes of iron-deficiency anaemia

- Coeliac disease (*see* Box 4.4, page 57)

- Intestinal bleeding (e.g. Meckel's diverticulum, or hookworm in endemic areas)

- Other bleeding disorder (e.g. peptic ulceration)

- Ingestion of cow's milk

- Thalassaemia may present with a blood picture of iron-deficiency anaemia

Management of iron-deficiency anaemia

Iron deficiency is a description, not a diagnosis. In the management of a patient with IDA it is essential to identify and correct the cause (e.g. dietary advice, gluten-free diet in cases of coeliac disease, or excision of the Meckel's diverticulum). The iron deficiency is specifically corrected by giving an adequate course of iron replacement.

Iron is usually given in the form of sodium iron edetate (Sytron), which is a liquid preparation that is more likely to be tolerated by children. It is necessary to ensure that the treatment has corrected the anaemia, and the expected improvement in haemoglobin level would be 1 g/dl per week. Once the haemoglobin concentration has returned to normal, it is important to continue the iron treatment for a further 2–3 months to build up the iron stores in the bone marrow.

Dietary correction is desirable although not always easy, due to toddlers' finicky food preferences. Iron-containing foods are listed in Box 16.6.

Boxes 16.7–16.10 review other characteristics of anaemia.

Box 16.6   Dietary sources of iron

Haem: red meat, liver, hamburgers, sausages, pork, chicken, turkey

Non-haem: egg yolks, wholemeal bread, fortified breakfast cereal, pulses, dark green vegetables, dried fruits

Note: vitamin C (e.g. as orange juice) taken with an iron-containing meal will promote the absorption of iron from non-haem sources.

Case study 1

Paul, aged 2 years, is a first child. His parents were not concerned about his health, but when his grandmother came to visit she was worried that he was very pale. She encouraged his parents to take him to his GP. Paul's mother indicated that he had been well, with no change in his energy level and no increased frequency of infections. On reflection, she felt that he was probably paler than 3 or 4 months ago. From the time he was a baby it had always been difficult to get him to settle at night, and he usually had a bottle containing cow's milk to get him to sleep. He was described as a 'picky' eater, and consumed at least 500 ml (1 pint) of cow's milk a day. He took little in the way of solid food, and had not been breastfed. There was no history of obvious blood loss or jaundice, and no family history of anaemia.

On examination, Paul was strikingly pale but lively. There was no bruising or purpura, no enlargement of the lymph nodes, liver or spleen, and no abnormality on abdominal examination. The GP measured his haemoglobin concentration on a capillary haemoglobinometer, and it was found to be 7.0 g/dl.

In view of the low haemoglobin level, the GP requested a full blood count. This showed a haemoglobin level of 7.2 g/dl, a mean corpuscular volume (MCV) of 55 fl, and mean corpuscular haemoglobin (MCH) of 20, with the blood film confirming a severe hypochromic microcytic anaemia with rod forms, the white cells and platelets appearing normal. The picture was diagnostic of iron-deficiency anaemia.

Paul was treated with iron, and his haemoglobin level rapidly returned to normal. It seemed that the main reason for his anaemia was his early introduction to cow's milk and his poor dietary intake of iron-containing foods. Dietary advice was offered, emphasising in particular the use of vitamin C or orange juice to promote the absorption of iron from the diet. A final check of his haemoglobin level in the surgery 6 months later showed that it remained within the normal range.

Table 16.1 Factors that affect iron content at birth

	Increased	Decreased
Tissue iron	High birth weight Haemolytic disease	Low birth weight
Blood volume	High birth weight Late cord clamping Materno-fetal transfusion Feto-fetal transfusion	Low birth weight Early cord clamping Haemorrhage from cord Feto-maternal transfusion Feto-fetal transfusion
Cord haemoglobin	Growth retardation Maternal anaemia Maternal hypoxia	Preterm infant Haemolytic disease

---

Box 16.7 Differential diagnosis of anaemia

- Iron deficiency
- Blood loss (e.g. epistaxis, rectal bleeding, especially Meckel's diverticulum)
- Blood dyscrasia (e.g. aplastic anaemia, haemolytic anaemia, leukaemia)
- Haemoglobinopathy (e.g. sickle-cell disease)
- Other congenital disorders (e.g. spherocytosis, thalassaemia)

Box 16.8 Approach to anaemia

1 *Is the child anaemic?*
   Knowledge of 'normal' ranges

2 *What type of anaemia?*
   Morphological diagnosis

3 *What is the mechanism?*
   Pathophysiological diagnosis

Box 16.9 Serum ferritin levels

Low
- Iron deficiency

Normal/increased
- Thalassaemia
- Haemoglobinopathy
- Sideroblastic
- Secondary

Box 16.10 Causes of iron deficiency

- Low birth weight
- Early introduction of 'doorstep' cow's milk
- Late introduction of iron-containing solids
- Malabsorption (e.g. coeliac disease)
- Bleeding from intestines (e.g. Meckel's diverticulum)
- Chronic infection

Sickle-cell disease (haemoglobinopathy)

Haemoglobinopathies and thalassaemias are inherited disorders of globin chain production. Although these disorders occur in all ethnic groups, they are most common in non-Caucasian populations. In thalassaemias there are a number of mechanisms that result in decreased production of a normal globin chain (e.g. alpha chains in alpha-thalassaemia and beta chains in beta-thalassaemia). A haemoglobinopathy results from the production of normal amounts of an abnormal globin chain (e.g. HbS in sickle-cell disorders). Generally in both thalassaemias and haemoglobinopathies, the presence of one abnormal gene (heterozygous state) tends to result in minor, often asymptomatic disease, whereas the presence of two abnormal genes (homozygous state) results in severe, potentially life-threatening disease. Thalassaemic disorders are associated with a hypochromic microcytic red-cell picture, but haemoglobinopathies may have either hypochromic microcytic or normochromic normocytic indices. The ethnic origin of the patient can give a clue to the likely underlying disorder (e.g. beta-thalassaemia in Mediterranean races, alpha-thalassaemia in Asians, and sickle-cell disorders in Afro-Caribbean races).

The pathogenesis of sickle-cell disorders results from the insolubility of HbS at low oxygen tensions, so that when HbS is deoxygenated it polymerises to form strands known as 'tactoids'. This results in the characteristic sickle cells that are seen in the blood film (see Figure 16.4), these cells losing the normal deformability of the biconcave red cells and causing microvascular obstruction. Depending on which part of the circulation is involved, there can be neurological symptoms, pain of tissue infarction (e.g. in the bones of the hands), abdominal or chest pain, and pain from splenic enlargement. The clinical course of a patient with sickle-cell disease is punctuated by different types of 'crises', the majority of which are precipitated by infection, resulting in hypoxia and often aggravated by dehydration.

The aim of management of a child with sickle-cell disease is to decrease the number and severity of crises, thus reducing long-term problems with growth and development. Bone-marrow function is supported by supplemental folic acid. As infection is an important precipitating factor in crises, it is important to try to prevent infections if possible. Pneumococcus is a common infecting agent, and patients should be on prophylactic penicillin and immunised with pneumococcal vaccine.

Education of the parents, and subsequently of the child, in avoiding situations which may lead to a crisis is a central aspect of management.

Box 16.11 summarises sickle-cell disease and Box 16.12, its management. Case study 2 describes a typical case.

Box 16.11   Sickle-cell disease

- Sickle-cell trait is symptomless.

- Sickle-cell anaemia does not present until HbF is replaced by HbS.

- Presenting features are anaemia, abdominal pains, limb pains and swelling of fingers.

- Pneumococcal infection is common.

- Skull X-ray is characteristic.

- Child is stunted in later years.

- Splenomegaly is marked in early years, but disappears later.

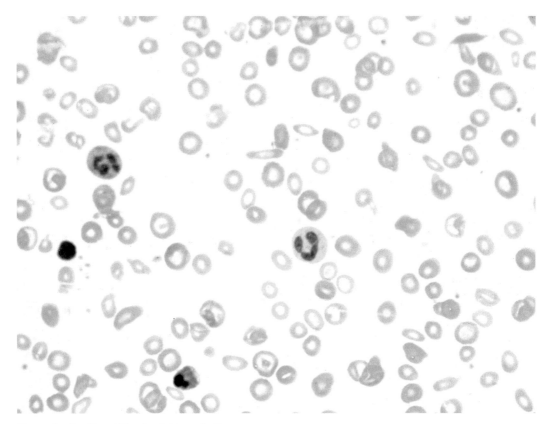

Figure 16.4   Blood film in sickle-cell disease.

Box 16.12   Management of sickle-cell disease

- Blood transfusion may be required for anaemia.
- Pain relief and correction of dehydration in crisis.
- Splenectomy if there is evidence of hypersplenism.
- Folic acid to support bone-marrow function.
- Pneumococcal vaccine and penicillin prophylaxis.
- Genetic counselling.

Case study 2

John presents with anaemia at 2 years of age. His parents are from Nigeria, and his mother was known to be a carrier of the sickle gene, but his father had been tested previously and was reported to be normal. At birth John appeared well, but he is now significantly anaemic with characteristic sickle cells on the blood film. Haemoglobin electrophoresis showed bands of HbF and HbS with no HbA. John also had a period of jaundice which responded to phototherapy.

He appears to have sickle-cell disease in which both genes controlling beta-chain production are abnormal and there is no production of normal adult haemoglobin. His father was tested again and was shown to be a carrier of the HbS gene. There was thus a 1 in 4 chance of any child being affected by sickle-cell disease, and a 1 in 2 chance of a child being a carrier. This was important with regard to advising the parents about planning future pregnancies and offering antenatal testing if this was acceptable (*see also* Chapter 11).

John was started on prophylactic penicillin and folic acid supplements. He was seen regularly at the clinic, and was immunised against pneumococcus as well as receiving his routine immunisations. His parents were told about the signs of infection and other possible crises to look for, and were given open access to the hospital.

Bruising and petechiae (thrombocytopenia)

Thrombocytopenia (a low level of platelets in the blood) leads to the appearance of petechiae, namely small red spots caused by bleeding at the end of capillaries, which do not blanch on pressure. There may also be rather easy bruising.

One of the major considerations in a child with bruising/petechiae is that these symptoms might be due to *non-accidental injury* (*see* Chapter 14, page 206). Therefore when taking the history it is necessary to assess whether the bruising or other evidence of bleeding is consistent with that history.

Box 16.13   Differential diagnosis of purpura

- *Capillary damage*: meningococcaemia, bacterial endocarditis, scurvy, Henoch–Schönlein purpura.

- *Congenital capillary defect* (e.g. Ehlers–Danlos syndrome).

- *Thrombocytopenia*: idiopathic thrombocytopenic purpura, leukaemia, aplastic anaemia.

- *Abnormality of platelet function.*

The assessment of a child with a bleeding disorder requires a basic understanding of haemostasis (*see* Boxes 16.13 and 16.15). The major components of normal haemostasis are intimately related in a dynamic process (*see* Box 16.14), and any single part may show abnormality, the commonest being abnormalities of platelets or coagulation factors. There are different clinical presentations of these.

Box 16.14   Components of normal haemostasis

1 Reaction of the vessel wall

2 Formation of the platelet plug

3 Activation of coagulation to form fibrin

4 Fibrinolysis

Idiopathic thrombocytopenic purpura (*see* Box 16.16, Figure 16.5 and Case study 3)

Idiopathic thrombocytopenic purpura (ITP) usually follows an infection, and tends to affect two age groups. In the younger age group (2–5 years) the incidence is the same in both sexes, and in the majority of children the disease remits with no long-term problems. In school-age children, the majority of children affected are girls, and the disease has a tendency to become chronic and to merge with adult auto-immune disease (see Table 16.2).

There are still controversies about the management of ITP in children, the main ones being the need for bone-marrow examination and the need for any form of treatment. In the presence of a normal haemoglobin concentration and white cell count, it is highly unlikely that the thrombocytopenia could be due to bone-marrow infiltration by diseases such as leukaemia. Many clinicians prefer to perform a bone-marrow examination to exclude this possibility, and it is advisable to do so if treatment with steroids is indicated. ITP in children tends to recover spontaneously with no major risk of serious haemorrhage. If it is decided that treatment is indicated, the initial choice is to give a short course of prednisolone, not lasting for more than 2–3 weeks, usually leading to a prompt recovery of the platelet count. In children it is rarely necessary to consider other forms of treatment, such as intravenous immunoglobulin, splenectomy or other more potent immunosuppressive agents, unless the thrombocytopenia becomes chronic.

Box 16.15   Comparison of bleeding in platelet and coagulation disorders

Platelet disorder
- Purpura
- Easy bruising
- Bleeding from mucosal surfaces (e.g. gums, nosebleeds)

Coagulation disorder
- Easy bruising
- Bleeding into joints and muscles
- Internal bleeding

Box 16.16   Idiopathic thrombocytopenic purpura (ITP)

- Acute onset following upper respiratory tract infection

- Presents with bleeding or purpura

- Rarely, there may be intracranial haemorrhage

- Normally remits spontaneously, but may become chronic

- Steroids are used in severe cases

Table 16.2   Idiopathic thrombocytopenic purpura (ITP)

	Acute	*Chronic*
Age	Younger (< 5 years)	Older (> 5 years)
Sex	Girls = boys	Girls > boys
History	Short (days)	Long (weeks)
Seasonal	?Winter/spring	No
Preceding infection	Frequent	Rare
Platelet auto-antibodies	Not implicated	Implicated
Proportion	85%	10%

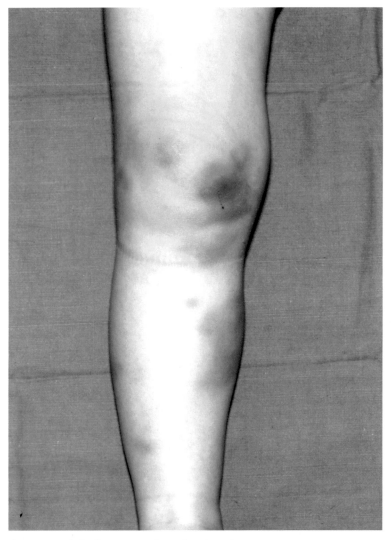

Figure 16.5 The bruises in idiopathic thrombocytopenic purpura (ITP) are typically of different ages and can be extensive.

Case study 3

Alison, aged 3 years, presented to the Accident and Emergency department with a 3-day history of easy bruising. Her mother had noted bruising on various areas of Alison's body, many apparently without obvious trauma. On the morning of attendance there had been bleeding from the gums after Alison brushed her teeth.

Alison's mother reported that Alison had an infection about 2 weeks earlier, with vomiting and diarrhoea. This had settled, but then the bruising started. There was nothing else of note in the history. In particular, no drugs had been taken and there was no history of a bleeding disorder in the family.

On examination, Alison appeared well and contented in her mother's presence. She was afebrile, and there was a purpuric rash on her face, neck and trunk. On various parts of her body there were bruises of different ages, these being most marked on her arms and legs (see Figure 16.5). In her mouth there were purpuric spots and some blood blisters on the buccal mucosa. There was no significant lymphadenopathy, hepatomegaly or splenomegaly, and examination of the cardiovascular and respiratory systems was normal. There were no haemorrhages on fundoscopy.

Alison's blood count showed a normal haemoglobin concentration and white cell count, but the platelet count was markedly reduced at $10 \times 10^9/l$. The coagulation screen and urea and electrolytes were normal. Examination of the blood film confirmed the severe thrombocytopenia, but no immature white cells were seen and there was no red cell fragmentation (which is found in haemolytic–uraemic syndrome; see Chapter 20, page 317).

A bone-marrow aspiration was performed, which showed normal red cell and white cell production with an increased number of megakaryocytes. No abnormal cell population was present. A diagnosis of ITP was made and Alison was started on oral prednisolone, and after 2 days there were no new bruises and her platelet count had risen to $27 \times 10^9/l$. She was allowed home to continue the prednisolone for 2 weeks, and to take part in normal activities. In an older child there would be restrictions on physical activities such as contact sports until the platelet count had recovered to near-normal levels. Alison was seen for review after 2 weeks of treatment, when all of the bruising and purpura had resolved and her platelet count was normal at $245 \times 10^9/l$. It was still normal at the 6-month follow-up.

Henoch–Schönlein purpura

Another important condition which can present with purpura is Henoch–Schönlein (or anaphylactoid) purpura (*see* Figure 16.6 and Box 16.17). This condition is thought to be a hypersensitivity reaction to infection, and it leads to a purpuric rash, mainly over the buttocks and the back of the legs. There is associated renal involvement, although this is not inevitable. Normally the course is towards spontaneous resolution.

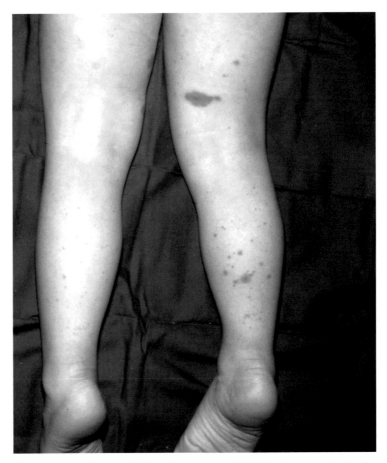

Figure 16.6 Henoch–Schönlein purpura (HSP) bruises are typically over the buttocks and the back of the legs, and are more discrete.

Box 16.17 Henoch–Schönlein purpura

- Often a preceding history of sore throat
- Rash is highly characteristic – purpura on buttocks and on extensor surfaces of legs and arms, but face is spared (except in infants, in whom the disease is rare)
- May be painful swollen joints
- Haematuria is common, with glomerulonephritis in 20% of cases (*see* Chapter 20, page 309)
- Normally recovers completely, but a small number of cases develop long-term renal problems

Bruising (coagulation factor deficiency)

Bruising in a child with no satisfactory history of how this might have occurred should raise the possibility of non-accidental injury. If the bruises are of abnormal appearance and follow a history of injury, this would be suggestive of an underlying *bleeding tendency*. This always requires investigation (*see* Box 16.18). The clinical manifestations of a bleeding disorder due to deficiency of a coagulation factor depend on the level of that factor (*see* Table 16.3). In severe cases there can be spontaneous bleeding into joints and muscles, and excessive bruising and bleeding resulting from relatively minor trauma.

Diagnosis of a bleeding disorder involves identification of abnormalities in the coagulation screening tests and performing appropriate assays for specific factors. If a diagnosis of haemophilia A is confirmed, it may be possible to identify the specific gene mutation in that patient and their family. This is useful for genetic counselling and identification of female carriers in the family.

If the mother is a carrier, further family studies should be undertaken (*see* Figure 16.7).

Table 16.3   Clinical manifestations of haemophilia A or B

Coagulation factor activity (% of normal)	Clinical manifestations
< 2	Severe disease
	Frequent spontaneous bleeding episodes from early life
	Joint deformity and crippling if not adequately treated
2–5	Moderate disease
	Post-traumatic bleeding
	Occasional spontaneous episodes of bleeding
5–20	Mild disease
	Post-traumatic bleeding

Box 16.18   Investigation of bleeding tendency (*see also* Figure 16.8)

- Full blood count with platelets
- Prothrombin time (PT) (measures extrinsic pathway)
- Thrombin clotting time (TCT) (measures extrinsic pathway)
- Activated partial thromboplastin time (APTT) (measures intrinsic pathway)
- Specific factor assays

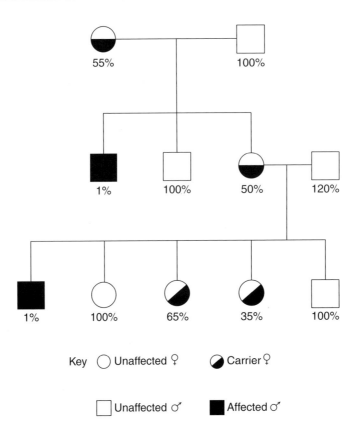

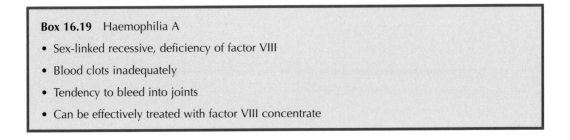

Figure 16.7 A typical family tree for haemophilia A, showing the X-linked mode of inheritance. The figures refer to the percentage of factor VIII which is carried: 100% is normal and 1% is an affected case.

Box 16.19 Haemophilia A

- Sex-linked recessive, deficiency of factor VIII
- Blood clots inadequately
- Tendency to bleed into joints
- Can be effectively treated with factor VIII concentrate

Haemophilia

The specific management of a child with haemophilia starts with educating the parents in how to recognise the signs of internal bleeding, particularly as it affects joints and muscles, and how to report for treatment.

The treatment of an episode of bleeding involves giving factor VIII replacement in order to achieve a high enough level in the blood to stop the bleeding. Until recently, the main source of factor VIII concentrate was obtained by processing plasma given by blood donors, and this carried the risks of transmission of viral infections. The gene for factor VIII has been cloned, so recombinant factor VIII concentrate is now available. This is not a plasma-derived product, and the risk of transmission of viral infection is virtually eliminated. Recombinant factor VIII concentrate is now the treatment of choice for severe haemophilia, but has significant cost implications. In patients with severe hemophilia A, prophylactic therapy involves the administration of factor VIII concentrate on alternate days in order to maintain a high enough level of factor VIII in the blood to substantially reduce the frequency of severe bleeding episodes and thus decrease the likelihood of long-term joint damage. Boys with moderate or mild haemophilia may be treated with desmopressin (DDAVP) to raise the factor VIII level, and do not need factor VIII concentrate. The management of haemophilia is summarised in Box 16.20 and Case study 4.

Box 16.20   Management of haemophilia

- Education of parents and child

- Early treatment of bleeding episodes

- Treat any bleeding episode with factor VIII replacement

- Prophylaxis with factor VIII concentrate may be given at home

---

Case study 4

The parents of Norman, aged 5 months, were concerned about the fact that bruises were appearing on his body without obvious injury. He could roll around in his cot, but it seemed doubtful that this would be sufficient to cause the bruising. Could his 3-year-old sister be hitting him because of jealousy?

Norman had been born at full term, and there had been no obvious bruising or bleeding either related to the delivery or at separation of the umbilical cord. His routine immunisations had not resulted in bruising, although there may have been some swelling after the injections. There was no family history of any bleeding disorders.

On examination, Norman was found to have a number of bruises on his trunk and one bruise on his right hand. The bruises were raised and had a firm central area. There were no purpura, and there was no enlargement of the lymph nodes, liver or spleen. All of his joints appeared normal.

Initial investigation showed a normal blood count, and in particular a normal platelet count. It was deemed appropriate to assess the coagulation mechanism (*see* Figure 16.8). The coagulation screen showed a normal prothrombin time (PT) and thrombin clotting time (TCT), suggesting that the extrinsic clotting pathway and the ability to convert fibrinogen to fibrin were normal. The activated partial thromboplastin time (APTT) was prolonged at 115 seconds (normal range 35–45 seconds), consistent with an abnormality in the intrinsic clotting pathway. Specific assays of factors VIII and IX showed that the factor VIII coagulant level (VIII:C) was 1%, with a normal factor IX level. A diagnosis of severe haemophilia A was made.

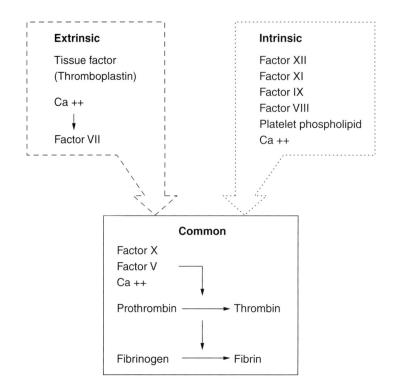

Figure 16.8 The coagulation cascade and its laboratory assessment.

Lymphadenopathy

When assessing a child with lymphadenopathy, one of the most difficult decisions to make is whether the lymphadenopathy is reactive or whether it may indicate a more serious underlying disorder. As children start going to nursery school and then primary school, they are exposed to an increasing number of infections, a common feature of which is lymphadenopathy. In the history it is important to gain an impression of how well the child has been in terms of general health, energy level, appetite, weight loss, fevers and frequency of infections. It can be helpful to know how well any siblings have been, and if they have had similar problems. Children with reactive lymphadenopathy are usually well between episodes of swelling of the nodes, and there is no evidence of a progressive illness. Symptoms such as bruising or recurrent nosebleeds, and bone or joint pain with limp, can indicate serious underlying illness such as leukaemia. It is easy to perform initial investigations in the form of a full blood count in primary care, but if there are features suggestive of a general disorder, the child should be referred to hospital for fuller investigations.

The conditions to consider in a child presenting with lymphadenopathy are shown in Box 16.21.

Box 16.21 Differential diagnosis of cervical lymphadenopathy

- Upper respiratory tract infection (notably glandular fever; *see* Chapter 6, page 89)

- Chronic infection (e.g. tuberculosis; *see* Chapter 5, page 78)

- Malignant disease (e.g. leukaemia, Hodgkin's disease)

Acute leukaemia

Acute leukaemia is the commonest form of cancer in children, accounting for approximately one-third of all cases (*see* Figure 16.9), and *acute lymphoblastic leukaemia* (ALL) represents 80–90% of the cases of leukaemia. Most of the others are acute myeloblastic leukaemia (AML), with a small number of very rare forms of leukaemia. The aetiology of acute leukaemia is a topic of extensive investigation, with particular interest in environmental factors such as infection and radiation.

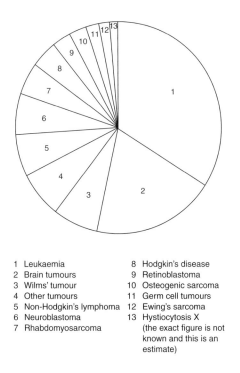

1 Leukaemia
2 Brain tumours
3 Wilms' tumour
4 Other tumours
5 Non-Hodgkin's lymphoma
6 Neuroblastoma
7 Rhabdomyosarcoma
8 Hodgkin's disease
9 Retinoblastoma
10 Osteogenic sarcoma
11 Germ cell tumours
12 Ewing's sarcoma
13 Hystiocytosis X (the exact figure is not known and this is an estimate)

Figure 16.9 Pie chart demonstrating the relative incidence of various childhood cancers.

However, it is known that certain genetic disorders carry an increased risk of developing leukaemia, including Down syndrome and certain immunodeficiency disorders.

Box 16.22 Clinical features of acute lymphoblastic leukaemia (ALL)

- Anaemia

- Increased tendency to infections

- Bleeding/bruising tendency

- Organ infiltration leading to splenomegaly and testicular enlargement

- Uric acid nephropathy may develop with treatment

The clinical features of leukaemia (*see* Box 16.22) are due to bone-marrow failure, with the predictable consequences of anaemia, risk of infection and risk of bleeding (*see* Figure 16.10). Other features that can occur are tissue and organ infiltration, including lymphadenopathy, splenomegaly and testicular enlargement in ALL, and skin rash and gum hyperplasia in monoblastic variants of AML. The diagnosis of leukaemia is established by examination of the bone marrow (*see* Figure 16.11). At the same time a lumbar puncture is performed, as the central nervous system can be involved in the leukaemic process in ALL. Assessment of the bone marrow includes examination of stained films under the microscope, the use of monoclonal antibodies to define cell-surface antigens, and cytogenetic analysis of the chromosomes of the blast cells. By combining all of the information a diagnosis can be made, and certain features may have prognostic significance (*see* Table 16.4).

Discussion with the parents must be undertaken sensitively and at leisure by someone who is skilled in this difficult task. Although the diagnosis of leukaemia is devastating to the parents, there has been a steady improvement in the prognosis over the years, and the majority of children with ALL now have a good prospect of cure.

Ultimately, the prognosis for an individual child will depend on their response to treatment, and the first 4 weeks of induction therapy are of great importance. By the end of the first 4 weeks it is hoped that the child will be in remission, when

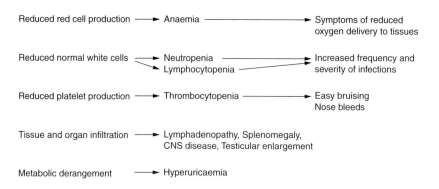

Figure 16.10 Pathogenesis of leukaemia – proliferation of malignant bone-marrow cells with reduction in normal bone-marrow function.

Table 16.4 Prognostic factors in acute lymphoblastic leukaemia (ALL)

	Favourable	Unfavourable
Age	2–10 years	< 2 years and > 10 years
Sex	Female	Male
White-cell count	< 10 × 10⁹/l	> 50 × 10⁹/l
Genetics	Hyperdiploid	Translocation

the blood count is normal and the majority of the bone marrow consists of normal cells with very few or no obvious leukaemic cells. After the child has achieved remission, they move on to CNS-directed therapy, blocks of intensification and then maintenance therapy up to a total of 2 years for girls and 3 years for boys.

The care of a child with leukaemia involves two interrelated parts, namely general supportive care and specific therapy directed at the leukaemic cells. It is important that adequate supportive care is available for the *management* of infection with appropriate antibiotic, antiviral and antifungal therapy, transfusion support with red cells and platelets, and nutritional support if required. Also important is the psychosocial support that is given to the child, their parents and their siblings as they come to terms with the diagnosis.

Modern therapy for acute lymphoblastic leukaemia has improved the prognosis greatly, and in ALL there is a 70% chance of remaining free from disease in the long term with the prospect of cure. As an increasing proportion of children with cancer are surviving, it is becoming apparent that there can be significant late effects of treatment, such as impaired growth and intellectual development after cranial irradiation, cardiac damage due to certain drugs, and impaired fertility. Therefore all long-term survivors require continued follow-up to maintain good health by identifying and treating any late effects that may occur. It should be emphasised that the majority of survivors enjoy good general health.

The management of ALL is summarised in Box 16.23 and Case study 5.

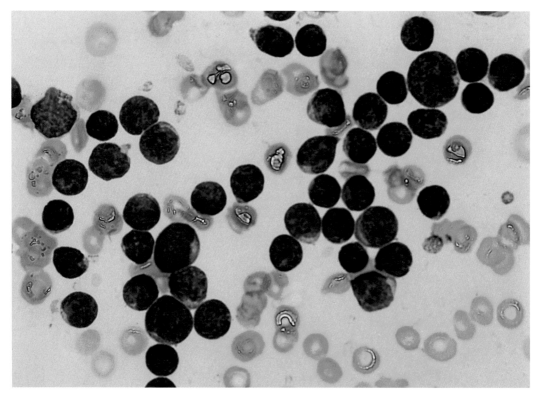

Figure 16.11 Bone-marrow appearance in acute lymphoblastic leukaemia. Note the large number of small uniform blast cells.

Box 16.23 Management of acute lymphoblastic leukaemia (ALL)

General

- Transfusion of red cells
- Transfusion of platelets
- Antibiotics
- Antifungal agents
- Antiviral agents
- Stimulation of neutrophil recovery

Specific

- Chemotherapy
- Radiotherapy
- Bone-marrow transplantation

Psychosocial

- Information to parents and child
- Play therapy
- Early identification and management of behavioural difficulties
- Emotional support

Case study 5

Helen, aged 5 years, had been less well for 3 months, with frequent sore throats and increasing tiredness and pallor. Her parents had noticed swelling in her neck for about a month, and over the previous 2 weeks she had developed a limp. She had previously been well, with normal development and no problems with resistance to infection. There was no family history of note.

On examination, Helen appeared pale and unwell. Her temperature was elevated at 38°C, and she had scattered small bruises of varying ages. Her throat was inflamed, with enlarged tonsils, and there was generalised superficial lymphadenopathy, the largest nodes being about 2 cm in diameter in the neck. Auscultation of the heart revealed a tachycardia with an ejection systolic murmur. In the abdomen the liver was enlarged at 3 cm below the costal margin and the spleen was enlarged at 5 cm.

Helen's blood count showed a haemoglobin concentration of 5.6 g/dl, a white blood cell count of 7.9×10^9/l and a platelet count of 21×10^9/l. Serum biochemistry showed elevation of uric acid and lactic dehydrogenase levels. Examination of the blood film confirmed the anaemia and thrombocytopenia, and demonstrated that the majority of the white cells were small, uniform blast cells suggestive of an acute leukaemia (see Figure 16.11).

Helen was diagnosed as having acute lymphoblastic leukaemia (ALL) of the common type, with an increased number of chromosomes in the blast cells. This combination of factors put her in a favourable prognostic group. After a full explanation had been given to the parents, she was started on chemotherapy according to the current Medical Research Council protocol.

Helen started her chemotherapy with a combination of cytotoxic drugs given orally, intravenously, subcutaneously and by lumbar puncture (the latter being necessary as drugs given by other routes show relatively poor penetration through the blood–brain barrier). By the end of 4 weeks of treatment, Helen was feeling much better and her bone marrow was in remission. She then went on to have blocks of intensification therapy directed at the central nervous system, and continuation therapy for almost 2 years.

Abdominal mass

Abdominal masses in children are rare and frequently asymptomatic. The parents may find them (e.g. at bathtime), or they may be an incidental finding during examination for other reasons.

The possible causes of an abdominal mass are shown in Box 16.24.

Any investigation of a mass in a child's abdomen has to answer four questions. First, what is the structure or organ of origin? Secondly, what is the likely tumour type? Thirdly, is there any other evidence of disease? Finally, is the mass operable?

The most likely organs of origin of a mass in the left side of the abdomen are the kidney, spleen and adrenal gland. The modalities of investigation are chosen to give the best chance of answering the above questions. Blood tests may give a

Box 16.24 Differential diagnosis of abdominal mass

- *Kidney*: hydronephrosis, nephroblastoma, neuroblastoma

- *Liver*: metabolic disease (e.g. Gaucher's disease, secondary malignancy)

- *Spleen*: haemolytic disease (e.g. congenital spherocytosis) or malignancy (e.g. leukaemia)

- *Other*: (e.g. intestinal mass)

clue. For example, the blood count may be consistent with an abnormality related to splenomegaly, while serum biochemistry will give a crude assessment of renal and liver function. However, radiological investigations are the most useful means of assessment of abdominal masses. Plain abdominal films may show calcification of an adrenal mass, suggesting neuroblastoma, while ultrasound may define the structure of origin of the mass. Usually computerised tomography (CT) or magnetic resonance imaging (MRI) scanning is needed to define more accurately the mass, its origin, and its relationship to surrounding structures, so that there can be some assessment of operability or the presence of metastatic disease. *See* Boxes 16.25–16.27 and Case study 6.

Box 16.25   Prognosis of nephroblastoma and neuroblastoma

- Nephroblastoma   5-year survival: 80%

- Neuroblastoma   5-year survival: 30%

Box 16.26   Features of nephroblastoma (Wilms' tumour)

- Around 80% of cases present before 5 years of age

- Presents with large abdominal mass

- Child is usually well

- Associated with hemihypertrophy

- Diagnosis is by ultrasound or computerised tomography

- Treatment is by excision and chemotherapy

Box 16.27   Features of neuroblastoma

- Arises from neural crest tissue in adrenal medulla

- Spontaneous involution is possible

- Occurs mainly in toddlers

- Presents with abdominal mass

- Symptoms of metastasis are common

- Diagnosis is by ultrasound, computerised tomography, raised vanillylmandelic acid (VMA) levels or bone-marrow biopsy

- Treatment is by surgery and chemotherapy; relapse is common

Case study 6

When Daniel was 2 years old, his parents took him to their GP because they thought they could feel a lump in his tummy when they were bathing him. He had previously been a healthy child, achieving all of his milestones at the appropriate time. He had been growing well and his parents had had no concerns about his health until now. There was no past medical history or family history of note.

On examination, Daniel appeared well and not distressed. He was afebrile and there was no bruising or superficial lymphadenopathy. Examination of the cardiovascular and respiratory systems was normal. His abdomen was distended and there was a firm mass to the left of the midline, extending down into the left iliac fossa. The mass was not tender, moved slightly with respiration, and there was no bruit audible over it.

Daniel had a CT scan which confirmed that the mass consisted of an enlarged kidney. There were no enlarged lymph nodes in the abdomen, the liver appeared normal, and there was no evidence of metastatic disease in the lungs. The most likely diagnosis was nephroblastoma (Wilms' tumour). The current management of this tumour is biopsy to confirm the diagnosis, followed by chemotherapy. Daniel had the biopsy performed under general anaesthetic, and a Hickman catheter was inserted for administering chemotherapy. He was given chemotherapy with vincristine and dactinomycin for 4 weeks, and a repeat scan showed the tumour to be smaller. Daniel then underwent surgery to remove the tumour, and this confirmed Stage I disease. After this he completed a further 4 weeks of chemotherapy according to the current international Wilms' tumour protocol. He has an approximately 80–90% chance of remaining free from disease in the long term.

Further reading

- Bolton-Maggs P and Thomas A (2003) Disorders of blood and bone marrow. In: W McIntosh, P Helms and R Smyth (eds) *Textbook of Paediatrics* (6e). Churchill Livingstone, Edinburgh.

- Frewin R, Henson A and Provan D (1997) ABC of clinical haematology: iron-deficiency anaemia. *BMJ.* **314**: 360–3.

- Hann IM and Gibson BES (eds) (1991) *Paediatric Haematology. Bailliere's clinical haematology.* Bailliere Tindall, London.

- Hinchliffe RF and Lilleyman JS (eds) (1987) *Practical Paediatric Haematology.* John Wiley & Sons, Chichester.

- Hoffbrand AV and Pettit JE (2001) *Essential Haematology* (4e). Blackwell Science, Oxford.

- Nathan DG and Look AT (eds) (2003) *Haematology of Infancy and Childhood* (6e). WB Saunders, London.

Self-assessment questions

1 The following conditions may present as iron-deficiency anaemia:
(a) coeliac disease   True/False
(b) Meckel's diverticulum   True/False
(c) leukaemia   True/False
(d) Henoch–Schönlein purpura.   True/False

2 The following features would suggest that bruising is non-accidental:
(a) abnormal coagulation tests   True/False
(b) bruises of several different ages on the body   True/False
(c) bruising mainly on the face and ears   True/False
(d) purpura mainly confined to the legs.   True/False

3 Persistently enlarged cervical lymph nodes require the following management:
(a) biopsy   True/False
(b) full blood count   True/False
(c) a course of antibiotics   True/False
(d) bone-marrow examination.   True/False

4 Haemophilia A has the following features:
(a) it occurs in both sexes   True/False
(b) it often presents with epistaxis   True/False
(c) it is treated by transfusion   True/False
(d) it requires the affected child to stop playing sports.   True/False

17 The newborn

- Measuring birth: definitions
- The prenatal environment
- Birth and adaptation to extrauterine life
- Normal term babies
- Feeding
- Congenital abnormalities
- Small for gestational age
- Multiple pregnancy
- Teenage parents

Measuring birth: definitions

How 'new' is newborn? And what is a neonate, apart from obviously being a newborn baby? The complications of early life are much easier to comprehend when some definitions are understood (see Boxes 17.1 and 17.2). In general, we define babies in terms of the length of their gestation and their birth weight, and the events which may happen to them in terms of the times at which they occur (e.g. the first week, the first month, the first year).

Early infancy is a hazardous time of life, even though in relative terms it became much safer during the twentieth century. So dependent is the welfare of babies on such extraneous factors as whether their fathers are in work, and the economic state of their country, that death rates in early and late infancy are used for international comparisons of socio-economic success and quality of welfare provision, as well as for assessing local factors such as the quality of a maternity service.

Box 17.1 Definitions: weight and gestation

Weight
< 2500 g: low birth weight (LBW)
<1500 g: very low birth weight (VLBW)
< 1000 g: extremely low birth weight (ELBW)

Gestation
≥ 42 weeks: post-term
37–41 weeks: term
< 37 weeks: preterm

Death is a 'hard' outcome – that is, it is relatively easy to ascertain and verify, and is also related to the rate of illness, more formally called 'morbidity'. To describe patterns of mortality in early life, statistics on rates of still birth, perinatal mortality, neonatal mortality and infant mortality (together with further subdivisions) are routinely collected.

The data may be collected over many years and so describe the change of these rates, and their improvement, with time. They may also be used to compare outcomes in different populations, either within or between countries.

Although all of these rates are useful for describing differences between populations, either geographically or over time, they cannot in their crude form be used to measure the relative safety of different hospitals or maternity units. This is because women with high-risk pregnancies are systematically referred from smaller hospitals to centres where fetal medicine services or neonatal intensive care are available. Thus the women delivering in the smaller units tend to be lower risk, and on average have less chance of a perinatal death, whereas their high-risk counterparts are more likely to have an adverse outcome by definition, and these adverse outcomes will tend to occur in the unit to which they are referred.

Measures such as perinatal mortality (*see* Box 17.3) are now less useful for measuring the outcomes of maternity services in general for the following reasons.

- The rates of all perinatal and neonatal deaths are so low that just a few deaths more or less, arising from chance variation alone, tend to give large fluctuations in the rates from year to year in a small population. This can be overcome in part by averaging the rates over a longer period of time, say 3 years.

- Many more very preterm babies are now surviving. It therefore makes sense to aim to avoid fetal loss from mid-gestation onwards, and thus to measure the outcome of pregnancy from 20 weeks. Conversely, some very preterm babies who do not survive do not die until they are several months old. The World Health Organization has therefore recommended that all fetal deaths from 20 weeks, and all postnatal deaths to 364 days inclusive, should be counted and expressed per 1000 births.

- There is an irreducible minimum of 'unavoidable' perinatal death due to lethal congenital malformation, a virtual certainty of death where birth weight is less than 500 g, and a high mortality for babies with a birth weight under 1000 g. Therefore the International Federation of Obstetrics and Gynaecology (FIGO) recommend that the deaths, and mortality rates, should be subdivided as follows: all < 500 g, all < 1000 g, and non-malformed babies ⩾ 1000 g.

The prenatal environment

Life does not start at birth, and the well-being and early life of an infant can only be understood in the context of events that pre-date birth, and may even pre-date pregnancy. Pregnancy may be wanted or unwanted, planned or unplanned, whether or not it occurs within a conventional marriage. The extent to which a family tries to plan pregnancy is a function of the cultural context of that family, and the parents' beliefs about their control over their destiny. Whatever the planning, between 10% and 20% of pregnancies in the UK end in termination.

It has been known for many years that mortality rates among babies of very young (teenage) mothers and older mothers are considerably higher than those for babies of mothers in their twenties. However, young mothers are over-represented among more deprived social groups, while older mothers are frequently those who have delayed childbearing in order to pursue a career or profession.

The estimated date of delivery (EDD) is normally calculated from the first day of the last menstrual period (*see* Figure 17.1), and the EDD is taken as 40 weeks (280 days) later. Routine ultrasound scans are used to confirm the dates of the pregnancy by measurement of the biparietal diameter of the fetal skull, and to screen for major structural malformations such as spina bifida.

The process of forming an attachment to the baby commonly starts with the routine ultrasound scan. Both partners watch the scan and so get their first opportunity to 'see' their baby. Attachment is enhanced with the onset of the perception of fetal movements, is enormously advanced by the birth of the baby, and continues thereafter. The once fashionable concept of 'bonding', whereby the mother and infant were believed to form a permanent attachment at a biologically critical time in the early postnatal period, has not been supported by empirical evidence in humans.

Fetal life is descriptively divided into three trimesters (*see* Figure 17.1). The first trimester is the time of organogenesis, during which the embryo develops from a single fertilised ovum to a complete miniature fetus by completing all of the major stages of organ differentiation and formation. Noxious influences at this stage of gestation may result in fetal loss (miscarriage) or malformation. For example, failure of the embryonic neural tube to close at this stage gives rise to the anatomical malformation known as spina bifida.

After the first trimester, the fetoplacental unit grows and the organs mature, but no new organs are formed. Enormously rapid growth takes place, which is normally accommodated by an expanding uterus and amniotic cavity and sustained by a growing placenta. This process can be disturbed by placental malfunction, leading to intrauterine growth restriction, or by physical constraints on fetal growth, such as an inadequate volume of amniotic fluid. One effect of this may be to mould fetal growth (e.g. to produce the foot and ankle deformity of talipes equinovarus).

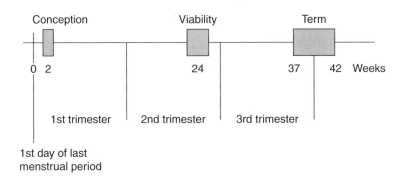

Figure 17.1   The division of human pregnancy into trimesters.

The uterus is generally a benign and protective environment for a fetus, but there are circumstances when this is not so (*see* Box 17.4).

- Alcohol abuse may cause global damage to the fetus, sometimes giving rise to a characteristic syndrome at birth.

- Cigarette smoke is a notorious fetal toxin, reducing birth weight and hampering subsequent neurodevelopment.

- Certain prescribed drugs, such as anticonvulsants (which cannot readily be stopped during pregnancy), may occasionally cause fetal harm, either by increasing the birth prevalence of a malformation (e.g. phenytoin and cleft palate) or by causing a generalised effect (e.g. fetal valproate syndrome).

- Certain prescribed drugs, such as benzodiazepines, may be abused during pregnancy and give rise to a withdrawal state in the baby.

- Abuse of illegal drugs, particularly opiates or cocaine, by the mother can have a devastating effect on the well-being of the neonate. Opiates can cause a severe withdrawal state, and cocaine can give rise to ischaemic brain damage.

- Maternal diseases, such as diabetes, can give rise to malformations in the fetus.

- Apparently minor viral illness in the mother, such as rubella or parvovirus B19 (which causes Fifth disease or 'slapped cheek' in children), may infect the fetus and cause severe damage.

- Maternal protein–calorie malnutrition may reduce birth weight, but most of the variance in birth weight is accounted for by other factors unless maternal malnutrition is severe.

Because many of these noxious influences act on the embryo, they may exert their effects even before a woman knows that she is pregnant. Therefore any public health strategy to minimise the likelihood of fetal harm can only be effective if it is implemented prior to conception. One model for this is the preconception clinic which, if run as a primary care facility, has the opportunity to engage healthy women who may be planning a pregnancy.

Box 17.4   Agents that cause damage *in utero*

- Alcohol abuse
- Cigarette smoking
- Anticonvulsants
- Benzodiazepines
- Cocaine use
- Maternal diabetes
- Rubella, parvovirus

Birth and adaptation to extrauterine life

Most babies are born in a maternity facility rather than at home, and most maternity facilities are in general hospitals. Less than 1% of babies are born outside hospital, but only two-thirds of these are planned ('booked') home deliveries, since it has been UK health service policy for 40 years to encourage hospital birth. The concern about home delivery has been the safety of the mother and the baby, but even though current evidence suggests that planned home delivery is much safer than had previously been thought, there is widespread unwillingness among GPs and community midwives to return to the delivery of a larger proportion of babies at home.

In hospital, it is now routine practice for mothers to be supported throughout labour and delivery by their partner, a relative or a friend, and this commonly extends to elective Caesarean delivery. Such support is not merely emotionally comforting – there are also real benefits in terms of shortening labour, reducing pain and decreasing the likelihood of operative delivery.

Delivery

The vast majority of babies who are born vaginally breathe spontaneously and require no intervention at all.

The mother's own abdomen and chest are ideal sources of warmth. However, it is important to cover the baby with a blanket or towel (a sheet is not enough) to prevent excess heat loss. If the baby requires intervention, drying and wrapping him or her is essential (before active resuscitation) to prevent the addition of thermal stress to the baby's other problems. An overhead radiant heater alone is inadequate to compensate for the evaporative heat loss from a wet baby's skin.

The baby's condition at birth is described in terms of the time to achieve a normal heart rate, time to first breath, and time to regular respiration. The *Apgar score* (devised by Dr Virginia Apgar) is a shorthand way of conveying this information (*see* Table 17.1).

Table 17.1   The Apgar score

Attribute	Score 0	Score 1	Score 2
Heart rate	Absent	< 100 beats/min	> 100 beats/min
Respiratory effort	Absent	Weak, irregular	Strong, regular
Muscle tone	Limp	Some flexion	Weak movement
Reflex response to stimulation of feet	None	Weak movement	Crying
Colour	Blue or pale	Pink body, blue extremities	Pink all over

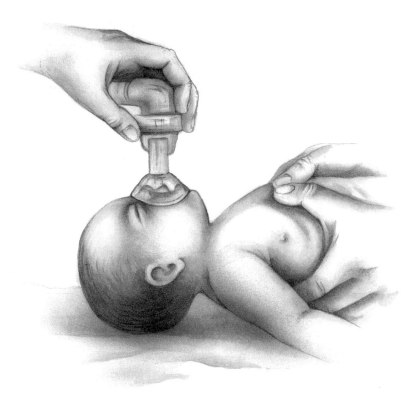

Figure 17.2   Neonatal cardiopulmonary resuscitation, showing the neutral position of the head, mask ventilation, and the two-handed technique for cardiac compressions.

Cardiorespiratory adaptation

There are several stages of adaptation. The baby's first breath initiates a cascade of changes (*see* Figure 17.3), but changes continue to take place over the first 24 hours. Babies are obligatory nose breathers, and only breathe through their mouths when crying.

During the first week, pulmonary arterial pressure continues to fall slowly, and the arterial duct becomes permanently shut by a process of fibrosis. Respiratory control changes over a similar

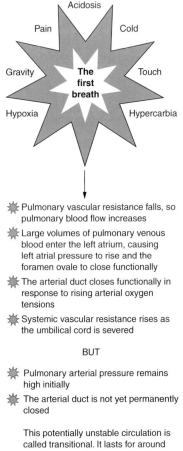

● Pulmonary vascular resistance falls, so pulmonary blood flow increases

● Large volumes of pulmonary venous blood enter the left atrium, causing left atrial pressure to rise and the foramen ovale to close functionally

● The arterial duct closes functionally in response to rising arterial oxygen tensions

● Systemic vascular resistance rises as the umbilical cord is severed

BUT

● Pulmonary arterial pressure remains high initially

● The arterial duct is not yet permanently closed

This potentially unstable circulation is called transitional. It lasts for around 24 hours, by which time pulmonary pressure has fallen considerably and the risk of the baby flipping back into a 'fetal' circulation, with persistent pulmonary hypertension, is much reduced.

Figure 17.3 The mechanism of cardiorespiratory adaptation.

time scale. In particular, the infant's oxygen sensor has been used to the oxygen tension present *in utero*, around 3 kPa. It now has to operate with oxygen tensions in excess of 10 kPa, and cannot immediately do so. It takes about a week to reset.

Adaptation continues long after the first postnatal week. *In utero* the right ventricle of the heart has been dominant. However, after birth the left ventricle assumes the work of pumping against systemic vascular resistance, while the right ventricle has the progressively less arduous task of pumping blood through the low resistance of the lungs. This reversal of dominance from right to left takes many months, as the left ventricle progressively becomes more thick-walled and the right ventricle more thin-walled. The ribs gradually become more calcified and rigid, while the proportions of the thorax and abdomen alter, with relatively greater thoracic growth, and the control of respiration becomes more robust.

Birth asphyxia

This is an unfortunate but widely used term. Babies are mostly robust and designed to withstand hypoxia and circulatory impairment better, and for longer, than at any other time of life. A baby may be born with cyanosis, hypotonia, apnoea, or bradycardia with < 100 beats/minute. However, many will take a first breath, and recover well from this state, simply by being dried and wrapped. If the pH of arterial cord blood is < 7.1, this also suggests that the infant has undergone a significant degree of hypoxic or ischaemic stress.

If the baby needs extensive resuscitation (*see* Box 17.5), including artificial ventilation and cardiac massage, the important feature is the speed of recovery. This is the time to achieve a heart rate of > 100 beats/minute, the time to first gasp and the time to regular breathing movements (whereupon artificial ventilation can usually be stopped). The longer this takes, the more likely it is that the baby will be affected by this perinatal stress.

If a baby has received significant hypoxic or ischaemic injury to the brain or other organs, they might develop some degree of encephalopathy or other organ dysfunction, or they may remain totally asymptomatic. Although they may have appeared to have 'symptomatic asphyxia' at birth, the long-term neurodevelopmental outlook is most closely related to the severity of any subsequent encephalopathy. However, babies who do not establish regular respiration by 20–30 minutes postnatally almost invariably die, or are very severely disabled.

Birth trauma

Serious birth trauma is rare, but occasionally a baby may fracture a clavicle at delivery, or suffer stretching of the nerves of the brachial plexus, resulting in an Erb's palsy. Both of these injuries tend to heal well, although the outlook for a palsy in which avulsion of the nerve roots has occurred is very poor.

Relatively common minor traumas include forceps marks on the face, which may result in localised fat necrosis with the formation of a small subcutaneous lump, and cephalhaematoma, which is a subperiosteal collection of blood over one of the bones of the skull. This can look quite striking, and feels fluctuant on palpation.

Assessing gestation

A dating scan must be performed before 20 weeks to be valid, and where a woman has booked late, concealed her pregnancy or been seriously uncertain about her history, antenatal dating becomes inexact. However, gestation may be estimated by assessing the maturity of a newborn baby. There are several methods for doing this – for example, using neurological features (Dubowitz) or external features (Parkin).

Normal term babies

Around 95% of babies are born between 37 and 42 weeks' gestation ('term'), and most of these are healthy. They need no interventions from any professionals and do not themselves need to be in hospital. They are routinely examined because a reasonably high proportion of them will have a relatively minor problem which, if dealt with appropriately, can have much less impact on the baby's subsequent growth and development. These problems may be so subtle that they are not obvious without an examination to look for them. Examples include the following:

- cataract (*see* Chapter 7, page 99)
- heart murmur (*see* Chapter 21, page 321)
- inguinal hernia (*see* Chapter 18, page 283)
- undescended testes (*see* Chapter 18, page 283)
- hypospadias
- dislocatable hips (*see* Box 17.6 and Chapter 9, page 120)

The head circumference is also measured, not to diagnose hydrocephalus (you would do this with your eyes and fingertips), but to serve as a baseline for future measurements, just as for birth weight.

The timing of the examination is important. If it is done too soon, many babies will have a quiet systolic heart murmur ('flow' murmur) which is of no clinical significance, and the head will still be moulded from the passage through the birth canal, giving a falsely high value for the head circumference. If the examination is done too late, and if a problem is identified, there may not be enough time to sort it out before the mother is due to leave, so that either it must be dealt with as an outpatient, or discharge must be delayed, neither of which is desirable for the parents. The ideal timing for neonatal examination is about 24 hours after birth, although this is unattainable for mothers who wish for rapid (e.g. 6-hour) discharge. There is no evidence that two examinations are of more value than one.

Minor congenital abnormalities are seen infrequently. These include, for example, accessory digits, a two-vessel cord (single umbilical artery), sacral dimple, mongolian blue spot, accessory auricles, single palmar crease, and capillary naevi or haemangiomas. The colour of the baby is a very important guide to general health (*see* Box 17.7).

Box 17.7   Colours of babies

- *Pale pink.* This is normal.

- *Blue.* This is only normal when confined to the hands or feet, and within the first 48 hours postnatally. Central blueness is never normal and requires urgent investigation for cardiac or respiratory disease.

- *Harlequin.* *Red* to the midline on one side and *white* on the other. This unusual and transient phenomenon has never been convincingly explained, but is entirely benign.

- *Very red.* This may occur with polycythaemia, and it is worth checking the baby's haematocrit. Generally the baby has received more than its fair share of blood from the placenta.

- *White.* Anaemia, due to receiving too little blood at birth, occasionally because of a large feto-maternal leak or placental abruption.

- *Grey or mottled.* This is a very sinister colour, often seen with septicaemia, and it requires urgent intervention.

- *Yellow/green.* This is the colour of conjugated jaundice.

- *Yellow/orange.* This is the colour of ordinary 'physiological' jaundice.

Neonatal blood spot screening

Between days 5 and 8 babies have a blood sample from a heel prick taken on to a blood spot card for analysis to detect *phenylketonuria* and *hypothyroidism*. The analytical methods vary, and some will detect other disorders, but the main reason for the tests is as follows (*see* Box 22.7 on pages 335–6):

- The conditions themselves, if not detected early and treated, will lead to permanent learning disability and the real possibility of never leading an independent life.

- With early detection and appropriate treatment, almost all affected children can expect normal neurodevelopment.

- By the time either condition presents clinically (i.e. without screening), substantial brain impairment will have already occurred.

- Both tests are highly specific and very sensitive – that is, they are rarely positive in genuinely normal children, and virtually always positive in genuinely abnormal children.

- Phenylketonuria has a birth prevalence of around 1 in 6000 births, and hypothyroidism has a birth prevalence of around 1 in 3000 births, so neither condition is excessively rare.

- The cost of screening, per case identified, is very much lower than the cost of caring for an undiagnosed or late-diagnosed child.

Blood spot tests for haemoglobinopathies and cystic fibrosis are also to be introduced.

Jaundice

'Physiological' jaundice has its onset on the second or third postnatal day in an otherwise healthy baby. The hyperbilirubinaemia arises because there is an imbalance between the peripheral production of bilirubin from haem, and its disposal by conjugation in the liver. Production is increased because babies are born relatively polycythaemic, and they rapidly break down the excess red blood cells. Disposal is reduced because the hepatic conjugation process is immature and only becomes fully active in the second postnatal week.

Examination is important. A healthy infant with jaundice is common and normal, whereas an ill baby requires immediate investigation (particularly for infection). As a baby can become ill quickly, the fact that they might have been well 12 hours ago is no help. Estimation of the serum bilirubin concentration is usually from a heel-prick sample. The normality of the situation must be explained to the mother. Jaundice can most usefully be considered potentially pathological if it occurs unusually early or is prolonged compared with normal. Additional tests to confirm that jaundice is not associated with underlying disease involve checking the blood group and Coomb's test, and a full blood count. The rationale for these is given below.

Early jaundice is unusual, and physiological jaundice cannot safely be assumed (*see* Box 17.8). After examination, and if one is satisfied with the baby's general good health, investigation is directed towards causes of excess bilirubin production.

> **Box 17.8** Physiology of jaundice
>
> • In babies, unconjugated hyperbilirubinaemia is universal, and clinical jaundice is common.
>
> • Breastfed babies are more often affected.
>
> • Physiological jaundice is benign.
>
> • Only severe, early-onset and prolonged jaundice requires investigation.

> **Box 17.9** Rhesus disease
>
> • The rhesus antigens are D, d, C, c, E and e. Disease most commonly arises from antibodies to D.
>
> • A Rhesus-negative mother can make antibodies to the red cells of a Rhesus-positive fetus as a result of a small feto-maternal leak.
>
> • The maternal IgG anti-D antibodies then cross the placenta, causing destruction of the fetus's own red cells.
>
> • The fetus then becomes anaemic, but excess bilirubin production is dealt with through the placenta until birth.
>
> • After birth, an affected baby may need phototherapy or even exchange transfusion to treat hyperbilirubinaemia. Seriously high bilirubin levels (> 350 mmol/l) can cause bilirubin encephalopathy and sensorineural deafness.
>
> • Rhesus disease has now almost disappeared in the UK as a result of the use of prophylactic anti-D antibodies which are administered to Rhesus-negative women after the delivery of a Rhesus-positive baby, a miscarriage, or a termination of pregnancy. The exogenous antibodies coat any leaked fetal red cells, which are then destroyed in the mother's spleen before they can induce antibody formation.

Haemolytic disease of the newborn used to be caused by rhesus antibodies. Rhesus disease (*see* Box 17.9) is now rare, is unusual in a first pregnancy, and is unlikely if the mother has previously tested negative for rhesus antibody. ABO incompatibility is more common in first than in subsequent pregnancies, but may at best result in a weakly positive direct antibody test, so it can be difficult to diagnose with certainty. Examination of the blood film is performed for the presence of spherocytosis, as this and other abnormalities of red-cell morphology result in short cell lives, but the diagnosis must be confirmed by a red-cell osmotic fragility test. Glucose-6-phosphate dehydrogenase deficiency is an important cause of neonatal jaundice worldwide, and must be considered in families of Mediterranean and Asian origin, but is rare in the UK.

The importance of early jaundice is that when it is caused by haemolysis, mild bilirubin toxicity leads to sensorineural hearing loss, while bilirubin encephalopathy (also called kernicterus) leads either to death or to severe athetoid cerebral palsy. Phototherapy is used to control jaundice non-invasively, and exchange transfusion is used if the jaundice reaches dangerous levels, or if there is severe haemolysis. When haemolysis has been excluded, there is no evidence of any harm being caused to the baby by levels of hyperbilirubinaemia of up to 450 and perhaps 500 micromol/l.

Prolonged jaundice can occur in breastfed babies, but it is always unconjugated, so further testing is not necessary once this fact has been established. Serious causes of prolonged jaundice are rare. Urgent investigation is required, particularly to identify biliary atresia, since the results of surgery to correct this condition are much less good if assessment is delayed for longer than 6 weeks postnatal age (*see* Box 17.10 and Chapter 4).

Box 17.10 Investigation of prolonged jaundice > 2 weeks

- Serum conjugated ('direct') and unconjugated ('indirect') bilirubin

- Urine for bacterial culture, viral culture, bilirubin, reducing sugar (galactose) and amino acids (tyrosine)

- Thyroid function, alpha$_1$-antitrypsin

- Viral serology – rubella, cytomegalovirus, herpes simplex, hepatitis A, B and C

- Abdominal ultrasound for choledochal cyst

Feeding

The neonatal period is not the time to discuss with a new mother the relative merits of breastfeeding or formula – this should have been done antenatally. The role of staff is to support the mother in her chosen method of feeding her baby. Breastfeeding has distinct benefits over artificial (formula) feeding, even in the developed world. The benefits are summarised in Box 17.11.

Worldwide, the lack of availability of clean water makes formula feeding a major cause of death. The relative health benefits of breastfeeding extend far beyond the nutritional and protective effects on the infant, and include the lactational amenorrhoea which ensures wider spacing between consecutive children, and thus more resources for the other children.

Box 17.11 Benefits of breastfeeding

- Protection against infection
- Protection against heart disease in adulthood
- Compensation for insensible fluid loss
- Provision of specialised nutrients
- Cost
- Convenience
- Loss of maternal fat from thighs and hips
- Probable protection against breast cancer

Artificial ('formula') feeds

If a baby is not being breastfed, the only suitable food is highly modified cow's milk (or soya-based milk), often referred to as 'infant-formula' feeds. Unmodified cow's milk, whether skimmed, semi-skimmed or whole, is unsuitable for many reasons, not least the high phosphate load, which can give rise to symptomatic hypocalcaemia if it is fed to very young human babies. Commercial dried milks, evaporated milk and the so-called 'follow-on' formula milks are equally inappropriate for initiating artificial feeding.

Formula feeds must be made up with care to maintain hygiene (*see* Box 17.12). A baby normally takes around 20 minutes to consume the desired amount of formula feed, irrespective of size. If they take longer, certainly over half an hour, there is almost by definition a feeding problem.

There are two kinds of infant formula based on modified cow's milk, namely those in which the protein is predominantly modified from the whey fraction, and those which are predominantly casein (*see* Box 17.13). Each manufacturer markets both types, with different and sometimes confusing brand names. *Whey-based* formulas have a protein composition which approximates to that of 'average' breast milk. *Casein-based* formulas have slightly higher concentrations of protein, carbohydrate and electrolytes.

Box 17.12   Making up a formula feed

- Bottles, teats and utensils must be well cleaned and sterilised.

- Water for the feed should be boiled and then allowed to cool.

- The standard scoop provided with the formula should be used, one scoop to each fluid ounce (30 ml) of water. Granules may be shaken to level them off. Powdered milk should be levelled off with the back of a knife.

- The capped bottle should be shaken well to mix. After putting on the teat, a few drops of milk shaken on to the wrist should feel warm but not hot.

- Feeds can be made up in batches and stored in a refrigerator for up to 24 hours. They can be warmed up in warm water, but should not be heated in a microwave oven because the centre of the feed can become scaldingly hot, while the outside may feel only comfortably warm.

Box 17.13   Curds and whey

- Casein (from Latin *caseus* = cheese) is that fraction of protein in raw milk which is precipitated at pH 4.6 at 20°C.

- Whey is the rest (*c.*20% of protein in cow's milk and *c.*80% of protein in human milk).

- Modified formulas are often described in terms of the whey:casein ratio.

- Infant formulas designed for initiating formula feeding are whey-dominant.

Establishing breastfeeding

Mothers who want to breastfeed are encouraged to put the baby to the breast very soon after birth (*see* Figure 17.4) and maintain skin-to-skin contact as much as possible. Successful breastfeeding is made much easier for a new mother if she is motivated, if she has consistent help, advice and support from midwives, if she has privacy if she wishes, and if her baby is always kept close by her. In addition, the baby should not be offered any fluid other than breast milk, and should be fed on demand. Babies form their own routine with their mother and do not conform to imposed expectations.

Difficulties with breastfeeding most commonly arise from poor positioning of the baby's mouth with respect to the areola of the breast, leading to inadequate milk delivery, prolonged feeds, an unsatisfied child and sore breasts (*see* Figure 17.5). Some mothers find feeding easy, while others need much help and support. Some babies feed very frequently, while others sleep for many hours between feeds. There is no such thing as a 'normal' pattern for breastfeeding.

Breastfeeding is a two-way process, with the baby exerting considerable influence over the mother by stimulating milk production in the act of suckling (the breast–pituitary–prolactin arc) and by provoking let-down (mediated by oxytocin). The content of human milk varies both between different feeds, and within each feed. Most of the water and protein is transferred during the first 5 minutes of the feed in the foremilk, but most of the fat (and hence the energy) is transferred in the last minutes of the feed, in the hind milk. Breastfeeding is a most intimate process that facilitates mother–infant attachment. It is far more than the mere passage of nutrients from a mother to her baby.

Hospitals can do much to promote breastfeeding, while unsatisfactory practices can hinder it. The UNICEF *Ten Steps to Successful Breastfeeding* are designed to encourage good feeding (www. unicef.org/programme/breastfeeding/ and www. babyfriendly.org.uk). *See* Box 22.16, page 341.

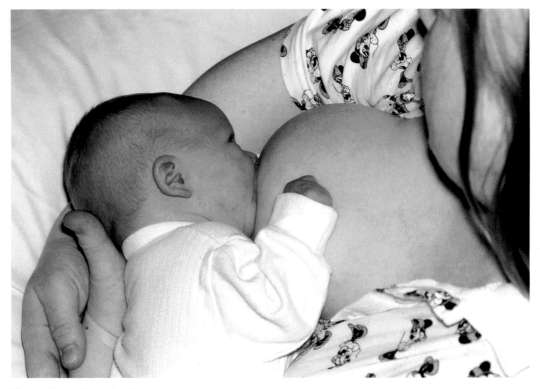

Figure 17.4   Breastfeeding.

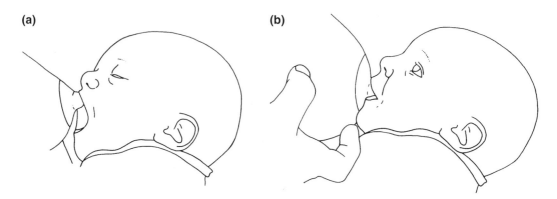

Figure 17.5   Breastfeeding. (a) Correct latching on: wait until the mouth is wide open, then the baby takes the whole areola into the mouth, not just the nipple. (b) Incorrect latching on: the baby sucks on the nipple as if the breast were a bottle.

Bottle-fed babies require, on average, fewer feeds in the day than breastfed babies because the gastric emptying time is greater with formula feeds. Irrespective of the method of feeding, the milk intake increases over the first few days.

There is no fixed amount that any healthy full-term baby should receive on any day. On average, many will be taking in excess of 100 ml/kg/day by day 3. Babies almost always lose weight over the first few days (except those with intrauterine growth restriction, who sometimes do not), and this loss may be up to 10% of their birth weight. The birth weight is usually regained between 1 and 2 weeks after birth, and if feeding is progressing normally the baby will grow at a rate of around 7–10 g/kg/day (or about 200 g/week for an average-sized baby).

Congenital abnormalities

Almost every imaginable congenital abnormality has been described, but the important ones are those which are most often seen, most preventable and most treatable. Congenital abnormalities can usefully be considered to be either of *genetic origin* (pre-dating conception), a *malformation* (originating in the first trimester) or a *deformation* (arising at a later stage of pregnancy). Some, of course, are lethal in early life. Among surviving babies, many have special needs long after discharge from their primary hospital management, and close liaison between hospital staff, the primary care team and the local special needs team must be maintained.

Cleft lip

Behind the cleft lip there may be a cleft palate, but in any case there will be difficulties in feeding the baby. The results of plastic surgery for the defect are extremely impressive, and the parents need to hear this from the surgeon and to see some 'before and after' pictures as soon as possible.

It is always devastating for parents to be confronted by such an appearance at birth. There are three 'golden rules'.

- Keep the baby with the parents unless there is a clear airway problem. Overt rejection at this stage is rare, however much grief and disappointment there may be.

- Explain gently and patiently what the obvious abnormalities are, and don't try to hide anything. While avoiding any attempt to prognosticate, emphasise that expert advice is available and will be sought.

- Do not be afraid to say that you do not have all of the answers immediately.

The community midwife will be a key figure in supporting the family after discharge home (up to 10 days postnatally). Thereafter the health visitor will take on this role together with the GP. Once successful surgery has taken place, the baby will be normal.

Trisomy

This is the single commonest group of chromosomal abnormalities, and of these the most common is trisomy 21 or Down syndrome (*see also* Chapters 10 and 11), followed by trisomy 18 (Edward syndrome) and 13 (Patau syndrome). The last two are virtually always lethal within days or weeks of birth. Trisomy becomes less rare as the age of the mother increases, and mothers over 35 years of age are commonly offered early antenatal screening. Many cases are diagnosed *in utero*, and most of these mothers opt for termination.

Neural-tube defects

These are anencephaly and spina bifida. The defects are due to failure of the neural tube to close in early embryonic life (around 30 days). Anencephaly is always lethal, but spina bifida commonly is not, and has profound repercussions for affected children (*see* Chapter 10). Both may be screened for by measurement of maternal serum alphafetoprotein, detected by antenatal ultrasound, and largely prevented by periconceptional folic acid supplements.

Oesophageal atresia and tracheo-oesophageal fistula

There are a number of variants of this condition, all of which result from maldevelopment of the foregut and lung bud (*see* Figure 17.6).

The inability of the fetus to swallow usually gives rise to polyhydramnios, complicating the pregnancy. In any baby born to a mother with this condition, and without any other explanation for it, it is worth attempting to pass a mucus extractor down into the stomach to prove oesophageal patency (passing a suction catheter or feeding tube is not diagnostic, as it curls up in the oesophageal pouch). Depending on the anatomy of the lesion, it is not always possible to achieve an early primary surgical repair, so the establishment

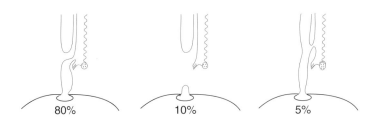

Figure 17.6 The three predominant forms of tracheo-oesophageal fistula.

of a gastrostomy to enable enteral feeding is often the priority.

Other gut atresias: duodenal, anal

Duodenal atresia can be diagnosed antenatally by the 'double-bubble' appearance below the liver on a radiograph or ultrasound, and is associated with Down syndrome, which again may have been diagnosed antenatally by fetal blood sample. Surgical repair is straightforward.

Anal atresia is usually diagnosed shortly after birth by the midwife, who is unable to measure a rectal temperature. In girls there may be a fistula to the vagina, but complete inability to pass meconium means that an urgent defunctioning colostomy is needed, with full corrective surgery when the infant is rather older. The aim is to allow the child to achieve full bowel control whenever possible.

Abdominal wall defects

In *gastroschisis*, the defect is separate from the umbilicus, and loops of fetal bowel float outside the fetal abdomen in the amniotic fluid. There are not usually any other associated abnormalities, and the outlook for the baby is good with early neonatal surgery.

In *exomphalos*, the bowel protrudes in a sac through the umbilicus, and so is not in contact with the amniotic fluid. However, it may be part of an underlying chromosomal defect, part of another syndrome, or have an associated abnormality such as congenital heart disease. The surgical management is relatively straightforward, but the overall outcome is dependent on whatever other anomalies are present.

Explaining the further investigations and counselling the parents requires the distinction between the two conditions to be made.

Diaphragmatic hernia

A malformed diaphragm with a hole in it can allow mobile abdominal contents to herniate up into the chest, more often on the left than the right side because of the site of the liver. The lung on the affected side is compressed and may be hypoplastic. If the mediastinum is pushed across, the other lung will be compressed too. Some of these fetuses are identified *in utero* on ultrasound scanning, but some are missed and may present after birth with cyanosis, either with obvious respiratory distress or with persistent pulmonary hypertension. The treatment is surgical after stabilisation, but the mortality rate is still high (around 40%). Survivors can expect a normal and disability-free life.

Congenital heart disease

A detailed discussion of the many varieties of congenital heart disease and their management is beyond the scope of this chapter (*see* Chapter 21). Those considered here are arranged according to their neonatal presentation. Serious congenital heart disease presents with either cyanosis or cardiac failure (frequently without a murmur), but in the neonate the process is often very rapid.

Isolated heart murmurs are often found to be small ventricular septal defects, most of which will close by themselves over the next few months. The most life-threatening cause of a murmur is critical aortic valvular stenosis, which may well be treatable. Sometimes the murmur of pulmonary stenosis is heard (as in the tetralogy of Fallot, see below), but most often a murmur is functional (no echocardiographic abnormality), or an arterial duct, or peripheral pulmonary branch stenosis which is a normal variant.

Cyanosis

When a baby is found to be dusky and there is no respiratory distress, it is important to measure the oxygen saturation in air by pulse oximetry, and to test the effect of 100% oxygen. A blue baby whose oxygenation does not improve with high inspired oxygen levels and who has no respiratory distress must be considered to have cyanotic congenital heart disease. The most common diagnosis, presenting in the first 24 hours, is transposition of the great arteries.

A baby who becomes rather blue with each feed, and when they are crying, but without any respiratory symptoms, is showing a typical presentation of Fallot's tetralogy (ventricular septal defect, pulmonary stenosis, overriding aorta, and right ventricular hypertrophy). They are generally pink at birth. They may also present with a pulmonary flow murmur.

Cardiac failure

Heart failure of gradual onset is usually secondary to a persistently open arterial duct, or chronic lung disease, in premature babies. It can also complicate septicaemia and result from supraventricular tachycardia. When it complicates structural congenital heart disease, it often presents acutely and without warning as a collapsed baby. Examples include hypoplastic left heart, interrupted aortic arch, and coarctation of the aorta. Such babies have been dependent for their systemic output on the effort of the right ventricle, with systemic blood flow through the arterial duct, and often have a ventricular septal defect which allows the pulmonary venous return to be handled by the right ventricle. The crisis is brought on by closure of the duct. An important and potentially life-saving treatment, following resuscitation, is an intravenous infusion of a prostaglandin to re-open the duct, which allows time for further evaluation and the planning of management.

Small for gestational age

If a baby weighs 2000 g at term, he is on the 1st centile, so he may be pathologically small for his gestational age and may have suffered intrauterine growth restriction (IUGR) (e.g. as a result of maternal hypertension). If measurement of his head circumference reveals that it is not far below the 50th centile, this is called asymmetry of growth. It is quite common, and reflects relative sparing of brain growth in the face of borderline intrauterine nutrition.

Small size causes thermal vulnerability, so small babies need to be kept well wrapped in the delivery room and given an early feed. They are also prone to hypoglycaemia. A reduced level of consciousness is often the only symptom of this (the other important symptom is a seizure). If a baby does not respond quickly to extra feed (or if milk is vomited, which is often a problem with growth-restricted babies), an intravenous glucose infusion is needed as a supplement. Such babies often demonstrate rapid catch-up growth over the next few weeks. *See* Box 17.14.

Box 17.14   Babies with growth restriction

- Are vulnerable to hypothermia
- Need early and frequent feeding
- May develop hypoglycaemia
- Frequently do not lose weight after birth
- Often show rapid postnatal catch-up growth

The near term infant

Those babies who are born between 32 and 36 weeks are preterm, but do not share the 'high-risk' characteristics of babies who are born at less than 32 weeks. Many do not need to be taken for special care. It is now common to have an 'integrated' or 'transitional' care area where babies with needs for extra warmth, tube feeding or intravenous glucose can be looked after beside their mothers. At a gestational age of about 34 weeks babies may start to be able to feed orally, because developmentally they can now coordinate sucking and swallowing. Mothers are often initially afraid to hold or touch preterm babies, but they quickly gain confidence if given appropriate support. *See* Box 17.15.

Serious prematurity (< 32 weeks)

Babies who are born more than 8 weeks early are often described as 'high risk' by virtue of their gestation. Similarly, a pregnancy is described as 'high risk' if there is a potential hazard to the fetus or neonate (or the mother) at any gestation. The term 'high risk' is really a shorthand for 'high risk of death or disability'. There are a number of important reasons for being at 'high risk'. *See* Box 17.16.

Babies are born prematurely either because the obstetrician has identified a situation in which the mother is at risk from continuing the pregnancy (e.g. severe pre-eclampsia), or because the fetus is at higher risk from remaining *in utero* than from being delivered (e.g. severe growth restriction), or because some factor has stimulated preterm labour (e.g. infective chorioamnionitis). Sometimes the factors that cause preterm labour require delivery to be hastened (e.g. antepartum haemorrhage with fetal compromise). Whatever

---

Box 17.15   Near term babies (32–36 weeks)

- They are smaller, need more thermal care, and may not feed effectively in the first days or weeks compared with full-term babies.

- If they develop respiratory distress, it is often due to incomplete clearance of the fetal lung fluid ('wet lung').

- They may develop respiratory distress due to surfactant deficiency, particularly if they are born by elective Caesarean section (without labour).

- They do very well and are not at particularly high risk.

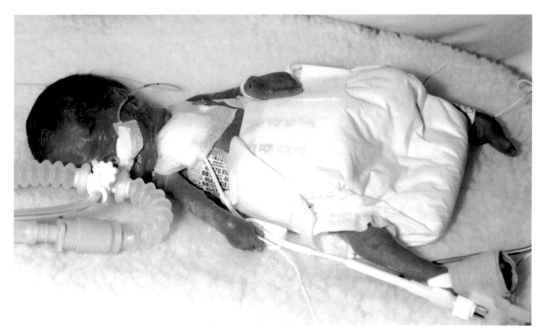

Figure 17.7   Preterm baby being mechanically ventilated.

Box 17.16   Risk factors in pregnancy and at delivery

- Past history of adverse events
- Smoking
- Drug abuse
- Multiple pregnancy
- Maternal diabetes
- Antepartum haemorrhage
- Fetal growth restriction
- Cervical incompetence
- Heavy alcohol consumption
- Pre-eclampsia
- Age over 40 years or under 16 years
- Other maternal disease
- Malpresentation
- Shoulder dystocia

the underlying reason, many premature deliveries are responses to an emergency situation, rather than being planned.

Just over 1% of all live births occur before 32 weeks of gestation, and about 2% of all babies require intensive care. Babies who are born in a hospital without intensive-care facilities must be transferred to one that has them, but the transport of an ill neonate may be hazardous unless it is undertaken by an expert team. If at all possible, a high-risk mother, particularly if she needs delivery before 30–32 weeks' gestation, should be transferred prior to delivery. This also helps to avoid unnecessary separation of mother and baby after delivery.

The first question that parents ask paediatricians when preterm birth appears to be inevitable is 'What are my baby's chances?'. The answer depends more on the gestation than on the birth weight. Other things being equal, by 25 weeks' gestation a live-born baby has a greater than 50% chance of survival, and by 28 weeks this figure is over 85%. The proportion of survivors and the rate of serious disability (compromising the ability to communicate or to lead an independent life) in survivors are shown in Figure 17.8.

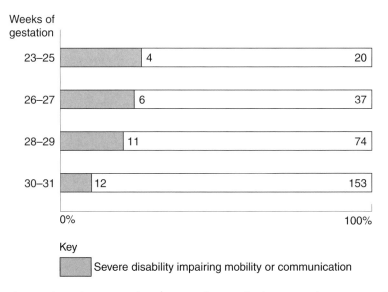

Figure 17.8   The number of survivors, by gestational age at birth, assessed at 2 years of age and their outcome. (From *Report on Perinatal and Late Neonatal Death in the Northern Region*, 1992.)

Mothers can almost always be treated with a short course of corticosteroids, such as betamethasone, prior to delivering a premature baby, provided that the attending obstetricians have some warning of the likelihood of delivery. This helps to mature the fetal lung, and it reduces the severity of the respiratory distress syndrome in the baby (see below). In preterm, high-risk babies the reduction in mortality has been shown to approach 40%.

The next question is 'What will happen to my baby?'. At birth, the paediatric team will be present, and the baby will be resuscitated if necessary. Not all babies, even when born 12 weeks early, require artificial ventilation from birth. All of them need to be transferred to the special care unit, but there is virtually never a situation when a mother (so long as she is not under anaesthetic) is unable to see her baby before transfer to special care. The problems that a baby faces thereafter can best be considered functionally.

Breathing may be a problem due to inadequate production of surfactant molecules within the alveoli of the lung, giving rise to collapse of the small airways. The external signs are listed in Box 17.17. Without added oxygen to breathe, the baby becomes blue and may progress to respiratory failure, which is treated with mechanical ventilation. It is usual to give exogenous surfactant within minutes of birth for very preterm babies.

This disease is termed *respiratory distress syndrome* (RDS) of the newborn, and is also known as hyaline membrane disease (HMD) on account of the histological appearance of the lungs of babies who perish from it. It becomes progressively more likely with increasing prematurity, and is directly related to several secondary problems. The cardiovascular instability caused by RDS may lead to neurological damage (see below), the process of neonatal adaptation is disrupted (which may lead to failure of the arterial duct to shut, which may require medical or surgical treatment), and the lungs themselves may be harmed by mechanical ventilation, leading to prolonged oxygen dependency (bronchopulmonary dysplasia, BPD).

Nutrition is another major issue. The gut of premature babies is immature, and where there has been growth restriction the gut may be markedly hypotrophic. The goal is to establish enteral milk feeding as soon as possible, but this is commonly delayed in the presence of RDS, and a period of intravenous feeding is often needed in very premature babies. The nutritional requirements of premature babies are different from those of full-term babies. Per unit body weight they need more energy and more nitrogen for growth, more calcium and phosphate for bone mineralisation, and more sodium to compensate for the relatively high mandatory renal losses of this electrolyte. The composition of artificial milks for premature babies is designed to reflect these and other requirements. Where breast milk is available from the mother, use of this may enhance future neurodevelopment, but usually it cannot by itself meet the physical growth needs of premature babies.

Neurological damage is the biggest single hazard to the premature baby, and is made more likely by the presence of RDS and its complications. However, it is now known that sometimes the events which give rise to premature delivery can themselves cause hypoxic or ischaemic damage to the fetal brain before birth, so not all of this hazard is postnatal. Evidence for such damage is sought by performing ultrasound scans on the brains of babies who are at high risk of neurological damage, and haemorrhages into the ventricles (intraventricular haemorrhage, IVH) and brain substance are easily seen with this technique. Unfortunately, ultrasound is not good at detecting ischaemic damage to the brain substance, yet this is more important than the presence of IVH. Consequently, the ultrasound appearances are only poorly predictive of subsequent neurodevelopmental outcome, and magnetic resonance imaging is becoming increasingly used.

Infection is much more common in the preterm baby than in any other group of patients except those who are immunosuppressed. Preterm babies are poorly immunocompetent for a number of

---

Box 17.17   Respiratory distress syndrome

- Tachypnoea

- Recession between the ribs

- Bobbing of the head

- Flaring of the nostrils

- Audible grunt or moan with each expiration

reasons, but the most striking is the fact that those born before the third trimester have not received maternal IgG antibodies, which are only transferred to the fetus during the last 3 months of pregnancy. In cases where infection was part of the process giving rise to preterm delivery, the infant may be septicaemic at birth, and congenital bacterial infection has a high mortality rate, particularly when the causative organism is the group B beta-haemolytic streptococcus. *See* Box 17.18.

Box 17.18   Some important neonatal bacterial pathogens

- Group B beta-haemolytic streptococcus (also called *Streptococcus agalactiae*)
- Staphylococci (coagulase negative) (also called *Staphylococcus albus* or *Staphylococcus epidermidis*)
- *Staphylococcus aureus*
- Gram-negative organisms (e.g. *Escherichia coli, Enterobacter, Pseudomonas*)
- *Candida albicans*

Necrotising enterocolitis can be regarded as a special kind of infection. This serious complication of prematurity is also occasionally seen in full-term babies. They develop an acute abdomen, feed intolerance, and a characteristic X-ray appearance of gas in the bowel wall. Breast milk protects against necrotising enterocolitis.

Retinopathy of prematurity is uncommon but serious. It was originally thought to be caused exclusively by an inappropriately high arterial oxygen tension, but it is now known that this is at best only a partial explanation, and that many other factors are important. Low gestational age at birth remains the single most important risk factor. Its detection and management are described in Chapter 7.

The problems faced by the family are considerable, and include the following.

- *Uncertainty.* Will the baby live? Will the baby be damaged? The uncertainties are real and cannot be dismissed. Neurological outcome can only be truly determined in follow-up.

- *Cost.* In the process of supporting each other and being with the baby, jobs are lost, travel expenses mount up, and a high emotional cost is borne by close relatives.

- *Special needs.* A significant number of 'high-risk' babies (*see* Figure 17.8) will have some degree of long-term impairment, and a few of these will be severely disabled. These families then have to cope with a substantial and continuing economic, social and emotional burden.

Multiple pregnancy

The rate of twinning and higher-order multiple pregnancy is increasing with the impact of reproductive medicine. When the total mass of fetus outgrows the capacity of the placentation to support it, the fetuses become growth-retarded. Monozygotic twins may share a placenta, giving rise to the risk of twin-to-twin transfusion. Multiple pregnancies commonly deliver prematurely. Not only is the process of delivery more hazardous than for singletons, but the babies are also subject to the consequences of prematurity as described above. The economic and social consequences of twins and triplets for a family are considerable.

Teenage parents

Young teenagers sometimes become pregnant because of teenage risk-taking behaviour, sometimes out of ignorance, and sometimes because of rape or sexual abuse. Pregnancy is sometimes not noticed, and sometimes deliberately concealed – either way, pregnant children frequently miss out on antenatal care. After delivery at full term, the majority of families look after the baby within the extended family, and placing a child for adoption in these circumstances is now a rare event.

Problems mainly arise when a baby is delivered preterm, since the emotionally immature adolescent girl is then faced with an emotional stress that can be overwhelming. The paediatrician is in effect dealing with two child patients simultaneously, together with a family which may be supportive, but which may be equally likely to be blaming the teenager and wanting to take control of the situation. The putative father may or may not be involved, and may occasionally be blamed for the pregnancy when in fact a male relative is the real father.

Finally, the mother herself is disadvantaged by having her own secondary education interrupted. In some areas, special school-age mothers' facilities have been set up to enable teenage mothers to continue their academic education as well as learning parentcraft skills.

Further reading

- Roberton NRC and Rennie J (eds) (2001) *A Manual of Neonatal Intensive Care* (4e). Arnold, London.
- Speidel B, Fleming PJ, Henderson J *et al.* (eds) (1998) *A Neonatal Vade-Mecum*. Arnold, London.
- Vulliamy DG, Johnston PGB, Flood K and Spinks K (eds) (2002) *The Newborn Child* (9e). Churchill Livingstone, Edinburgh.

Self-assessment questions

1 During fetal life:
(a) malformations, when present, always arise in the second half of pregnancy   True/False
(b) amoxicillin is a well-known teratogen   True/False
(c) dating by ultrasound is most accurate before 20 weeks' gestation   True/False
(d) periconceptional folate supplementation reduces the risk of neural-tube defects   True/False
(e) maternal malnutrition is a common cause of fetal growth restriction in the UK.   True/False

2 Babies born at term:
(a) will have a gestation from the first day of the mother's last menstrual period
   that lies between 36 and 40 weeks   True/False
(b) commonly have quiet heart murmurs in the first 24 hours postnatally   True/False
(c) initially have dominance of the right cardiac ventricle   True/False
(d) need careful thermal care   True/False
(e) cannot breathe through their noses.   True/False

3 The Apgar score relates to:
(a) fetal well-being   True/False
(b) maternal well-being   True/False
(c) cervical dilatation in the first stage of labour   True/False
(d) the condition of a baby at birth   True/False
(e) maternal perineal tears.   True/False

4 Risks in preterm infants include:
(a) hypothermia   True/False
(b) hypoglycaemia   True/False
(c) high rate of congenital abnormality   True/False
(d) intracranial haemorrhage   True/False
(e) liability to a bleeding disorder.   True/False

18 General surgical conditions

- The appropriate surgical environment
- The foreskin: circumcision
- Inguinal hernia and hydrocoele
- Undescended testis
- Scrotal pain
- Acute abdominal pain
- Appendicitis
- Rectal bleeding
- Other abdominal emergencies in children

The appropriate surgical environment

Surgery and anaesthesia in children go hand in hand. Specialist surgery requires specialist anaesthesia, and both should be orientated towards the requirements of children. Paediatric surgery should be carried out in an appropriate environment, with accommodation and facilities for parents, and specialist support services such as nursing, physiotherapy and play therapy. Much minor surgery can be performed on a day-care basis. Such treatment requires careful preparation and high-quality anaesthetic care, and maximising the use of regional anaesthesia gives optimal pain control.

Emergency surgery in children under 5 years of age is taxing both diagnostically and therapeutically. Difficulties include communication, venous access, fluid management and pain relief. These challenges are best met by specialist paediatric surgical units. The significance of bile vomiting in early life and the many manifestations of intussusception in children of any age require familiarity with the conditions as well as confidence in handling young children in order to give high-quality care.

Familiarity with some of the commoner surgical conditions will avoid unnecessary intervention in many of these conditions, which will often resolve with growth. Box 18.1 lists the

10 commonest operations performed in children in order of decreasing frequency.

Box 18.1 The 10 commonest paediatric operations*

- Appendicectomy
- Orchidopexy
- Circumcision
- Herniotomy
- Fracture reduction
- Suture laceration
- Abscess drainage
- Gastrointestinal endoscopy
- Cystoscopy
- Hydrocoele repair

*Excluding ear, nose and throat and ophthalmology.

The foreskin: circumcision

Knowledge of the natural history of the prepuce is essential to avoid unnecessary circumcision. The prepuce is often conical and fused to the glans at birth. Complete retraction of the prepuce may not be achieved until puberty. Forcible retraction of the prepuce is not helpful in assessing the need for surgery, and failure of retraction in itself does not point to a need for operation. Indeed, inappropriate and forcible retraction may cause scarring at the opening of the prepuce. Evaluation should therefore be by gentle forward traction of the prepuce, which will demonstrate the opening of the epithelial lumen of the prepuce in most boys.

Ballooning of the prepuce during voiding represents redundancy of penile skin, and is not in itself an indication for circumcision. Scarring at the tip of the prepuce, with failure to dilate on forward traction, indicates the presence of the rare condition of balanitis xeroderma obliterans, which is a clear indication for surgery. There is also a good case for pre-emptive circumcision to reduce the risk of urinary tract infection in boys with dilatation of the upper urinary tract. Although several religions advocate male circumcision as part of their belief, there is no evidence for the value of routine male circumcision in promoting health.

Box 18.2 lists conditions for which natural resolution can be expected with time and unnecessary operation can be avoided. However, certain other conditions require carefully timed intervention if an optimal outcome is to be obtained (*see* Table 18.1). In particular, children with

---

Box 18.2 Conditions that resolve naturally

- Labial fusion
- Tongue tie
- Hydrocoele in infants
- Umbilical hernia
- Divarication of recti muscles

Table 18.1 Conditions that require prompt elective surgery

Condition	Age at operation
Inguinal hernia	On diagnosis
Undescended testis	Before age 3 years
Supra-umbilical hernia	After age 1 year
Epigastric hernia	After age 1 year
Communicating hydrocoele	After age 3 years

inguinal hernias require prompt operation and should not be left on a waiting-list.

Inguinal hernia and hydrocoele (see Figure 18.1)

Inguinal hernias in infants are important because they can easily become incarcerated and strangulate, and if this happens a baby can become seriously ill very quickly. They may present as an asymptomatic mass that originates in the groin and may extend into the scrotum. They do not transilluminate. If the baby is relaxed and the legs are held up, the hernia can often be gently reduced back into the abdomen, but it will usually reappear when the infant next cries. Hernias are repaired by obliteration of the processus vaginalis with a suture at the inguinal canal (herniotomy), and this is best done as an elective procedure soon after the diagnosis is made.

Hydrocoeles are confined to the scrotum, although they can occasionally be very large. They always transilluminate. They are a common finding in newborn babies, and only rarely need any active treatment.

Undescended testis

The testis, although intra-abdominal for most of fetal life, reaches the groin by week 8 of pregnancy and will enter the scrotum in the following month. About 1 in 14 boys will have an undescended testis at birth, but 90% of these testes will have descended by 3 months of age. Routine neonatal examination should detect most cases of failure of testicular descent, but some children are not diagnosed until much later. Persistent failure of testicular descent beyond 3 years of age has been associated with infertility, torsion of the testis and subsequent malignancy.

Some undescended testes come down during the first 3 months of life, but if the testis has not descended by then, it will need surgery to place it in the scrotum. There are good arguments for screening all boys for undescended testicles either at birth, or at the 6–8 week check. Surgery is usually performed in a day-care setting by the operation of orchidopexy, which is best undertaken in the second postnatal year. The testis is placed in a retaining cavity created in the scrotal wall (the dartos pouch).

Descent can also be complicated by an anomalous final location, most commonly in a superficial inguinal pouch. This is known as an ectopic testis, and the main complication is torsion.

If the testis is impalpable it may be intra-abdominal and it must be found, usually by laparoscopy, so that appropriate surgery can be planned. If no testes can be palpated in an apparent male, it is important to make a careful assessment of the genitalia, involve a paediatric endocrinologist, and determine the sex of the baby (see Chapter 15).

Scrotal pain

When a boy develops acute onset of pain in the scrotum, there are several possible causes (see Box 18.3). Torsion of the testis is the main concern, and prompts surgical exploration of the scrotum in most boys with this symptom. Epididymo-orchitis is usually secondary to either urinary tract infection or mumps.

Box 18.3   The differential diagnosis of acute scrotal pain

- Torsion of the testicular appendages (hydatid of Morgagni)
- Epididymo-orchitis
- Idiopathic scrotal oedema
- Testicular torsion

The diagnosis is helped by ultrasound of the testis with Doppler measurement of testicular blood flow, urine analysis and sometimes isotope imaging. If clinical doubt remains it is safest to explore the scrotum surgically, and it is important to avoid delay. Testicular torsion arises from complete investment of the testis by the tunica vaginalis. Since this anatomical anomaly is common to both testes, the procedure involves untwisting the

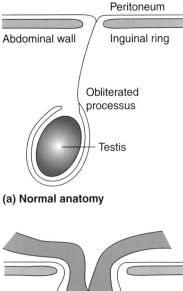

(a) Normal anatomy

Peritoneum

Abdominal wall

Inguinal ring

Obliterated processus

Testis

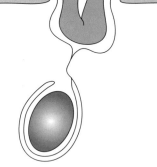

(b) Inguinal hernia

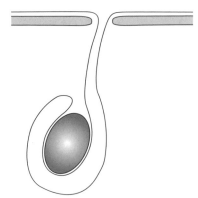

(c) Communicating hydrocoele

Figure 18.1 (a) Normal anatomy of the obliterated processus vaginalis. (b) Anatomy of inguinal hernia. (c) Anatomy of communicating hydrocoele.

affected testis and fixing both testes within the scrotum, using non-absorbable sutures, to prevent recurrence.

Torsion of the hydatid of Morgagni (a structure just above and behind the testis) can be managed conservatively with analgesia, while a diagnosis of epididymo-orchitis implies the need for future imaging of the urinary tract a few weeks after the infection has settled, in order to exclude a structural problem that is predisposing to infection.

Acute abdominal pain

Abdominal pain is a symptom commonly reported by children. It is most often managed at home with or without the aid of a doctor. It may be a symptom of such diverse conditions as intra-abdominal pathology, pneumonia, diabetic keto-acidosis, emotional upset, wind or constipation, and it may also be linked to migraine (abdominal migraine) (*see* Box 18.4). Young children may have great difficulty in localising the pain.

Only 4 in 1000 children will develop abdominal pain that is sufficiently severe to warrant hospital admission in any 1-year period. Of these, two will have an operation for the condition.

Although acute appendicitis is the commonest single condition requiring surgery, more often than not the pain will subside spontaneously without a diagnosis being made. Such children may be said to be suffering from non-specific abdominal pain (NSAP), and they are usually

---

Box 18.4 Conditions that may present with acute abdominal pain

- Constipation
- Urinary tract infection
- Gastroenteritis
- Appendicitis
- Intussusception
- Renal stone
- Pneumonia
- Otitis media
- Diabetes mellitus
- 'Abdominal migraine'

better within 24 hours. In infancy, the differential diagnosis of abdominal pain should include gastro-oesophageal reflux and oesophagitis. The cardinal signs of peritonitis are often difficult to elicit in very young children. (For a discussion of recurrent abdominal pain, *see* Chapter 4.) *See* Box 18.5 for significant clinical features.

Box 18.5   Serious 'abdominal' symptoms and signs

- Unremitting pain for 6 hours
- Bile vomiting
- Dehydration
- Abdominal mass
- Rectal bleeding
- Signs of peritonitis

Appendicitis

Although appendicitis is less common than it was, suspicion of this diagnosis is still the commonest reason for proceeding to surgery in a child with abdominal pain. The diagnosis is most difficult and important in children under 3 years of age, because their less well-developed omentum reduces their ability to confine the spread of inflammation and pus within the abdomen, and their ability to localise their pain is very poorly developed.

The clinical diagnosis is made on the basis of examination and active observation. Sometimes a white-cell count and ultrasound scan of the abdomen (to examine for other possible pathologies) can help. If the child is dehydrated, this requires correction before surgery.

Case study 1

At 10am Colin, aged 8 years, told his teacher that he had a tummy ache, and after he vomited an hour later he was sent home. His mother took him to the GP, who found that he was tender on palpation all over (although Colin said it was worst around his umbilicus) and had him admitted to hospital. By this time his pain had moved to the right lower quadrant, and the admitting house officer found tenderness and guarding in the lower abdomen. The surgical registrar reviewed him and prescribed intravenous fluids because of the vomiting, but being uncertain of the diagnosis decided to review him 2 hours later, according to the unit policy of active observation.

At review the clinical signs had localised to the right iliac fossa, suggesting appendicitis. Appendicectomy was performed together with lavage of the peritoneal cavity using a solution of cephalosporin antibiotic. The anaesthetist gave broad-spectrum intravenous antibiotics to protect against wound infection, and pain relief by injection of bupivacaine into the regional nerves. Postoperatively, Colin received diclofenac suppositories. He was well enough to start drinking fluids the following day, and was discharged home on the third day after his admission.

Rectal bleeding

Rectal bleeding may be associated with diarrhoea, suggesting an infectious cause such as *Campylobacter* or an inflammatory condition such as Crohn's disease or ulcerative colitis. There may be no other symptoms apart from blood in the toilet bowl if the cause is a juvenile polyp. Bleeding may be associated with acute abdominal symptoms in volvulus or intussusception, or be an unexpected finding on the nappy or in the toilet bowl. In infancy, cow's-milk intolerance can cause a haemorrhagic colitis, and in the newborn, necrotising enterocolitis must be considered. A very common cause is an anal fissure, in which case the examination is directed at visualising the fissure if possible, but it is also important to look for evidence of physical or sexual abuse. Initial treatment is with a stool softener. *See* Box 18.6.

Box 18.6   Some common or important causes of lower gastrointestinal bleeding

Neonate
- Necrotising enterocolitis
- Volvulus

Infant
- Anal fissure
- Cow's-milk intolerance
- Intussusception

Child
- Juvenile polyp
- Anal fissure
- Infection: *Campylobacter*, *Shigella*
- Crohn's disease
- Ulcerative colitis

Other abdominal emergencies in children

Intussusception

This typically occurs between 2 months and 2 years of age as a consequence of lymphoid hyperplasia following the introduction of solid foods or recent gut infection. Although lead points (e.g. a Meckel's diverticulum) may precipitate intussusception, hyperplasia of Peyer's patches can cause the ileocaecal region to prolapse through the colonic lumen (ileocolic intussusception) (*see* Figure 18.2 and Box 18.7).

Box 18.7   Intussusception

- A disease of infants and toddlers
- Causes severe intermittent abdominal pain
- The child may pass blood and mucus (a 'redcurrant-jelly' stool)
- There may be a sausage-shaped abdominal mass
- May be reduced under fluoroscopic control with a contrast enema
- Carries an appreciable mortality if the diagnosis is delayed

---

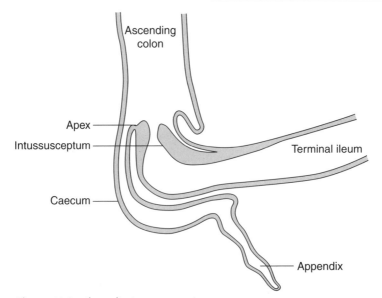

Figure 18.2   Ileocolic intussusception.

Malrotation

This occurs when there is a lack of fixity of the right colon due to disordered return of the hind-gut from the yolk sac into the abdomen during the first trimester of pregnancy. This 'malrotation' of the colon and ileum may allow the midgut to form a volvulus around the superior mesenteric vessels. Bile vomiting is an early presentation of this condition, which can occur in the neonate or later in childhood. If uncorrected, it will progress to ischaemic necrosis of the gut, and death. Diagnosis is made by contrast study of the gut or ultrasound evaluation of the superior mesenteric axis. Surgical correction places the bowel in a state of non-rotation (i.e. with the colon on the left side of the abdomen and the small bowel on the right side). This position is stable and prevents further episodes of volvulus.

Further reading

- Morton NS and Raine PAM (1994) *Paediatric Day Case Surgery*. Oxford University Press, Oxford.

- Nixon A and O'Donnell B (1992) *Essentials of Paediatric Surgery* (4e). Butterworth, Oxford.

Self-assessment questions

1 Bleeding per rectum in a 9-month-old infant:
(a) may be swallowed maternal blood   True/False
(b) with abdominal pain, suggests intussusception   True/False
(c) is diagnostic of necrotising enterocolitis   True/False
(d) with constipation, suggests a possible anal fissure   True/False
(e) is never a serious symptom.   True/False

2 Hernias:
(a) should be repaired without delay in small infants   True/False
(b) if at the umbilicus rarely need surgical repair   True/False
(c) are usually 'indirect'   True/False
(d) always transilluminate   True/False
(e) may disappear, but emerge when the baby cries.   True/False

3 Circumcision:
(a) is desirable in all infants   True/False
(b) can be justified on medical grounds   True/False
(c) is advisable under local anaesthetic   True/False
(d) is indicated if there is ballooning of the prepuce   True/False
(e) will prevent sexually transmitted disease.   True/False

4 Intussusception:
(a) may be reduced without surgical intervention   True/False
(b) is a surgical emergency   True/False
(c) occurs in the first year of life   True/False
(d) may be precipitated by eating bananas   True/False
(e) leads to bloodstained vomiting.   True/False

19 Skin disorders

- Major functions of the skin
- Atopic dermatitis (eczema)
- Psoriasis
- Pigmented skin lesions
- Acne
- Viral warts and molluscum contagiosum
- Nappy rash

First impressions do count. The skin has a social function in addition to its importance as a vital organ of the body. Thus children present because of illness, an uncomfortable symptom such as itching, unhappiness at perceived disfigurement, or because of the reactions of others. Skin conditions are very common in primary care, and the skin may reflect systemic conditions specific to childhood. At one end of the spectrum this may be a non-specific viral rash, less commonly it may be a systemic illness such as Henoch–Schönlein purpura, or rarely, but devastatingly, it may be meningococcal septicaemia.

Patterns of skin disease are changing. There is evidence that atopic dermatitis is becoming even more common. Malignant melanoma, although rare, is increasing in incidence in adults, giving rise to a greater consciousness of the importance of sun protection for children. Campaigns in the media have led to an increase in parental concern about benign pigmented naevi in children.

Major functions of the skin

The dermis is derived from mesoderm, and in the third week of fetal life a single layer of undifferentiated cells precedes the formation of the periderm. The melanocytes migrate from the neural crest. As the true epidermis keratinises beneath it, the periderm is ultimately lost *in utero*, contributing (with sebum) to the vernix caseosa. Keratinisation is progressive, so that by about 32 weeks' gestation the keratin forms a fairly effective barrier to water loss. The skin of the full-term baby is still a delicate structure which is readily susceptible to irritation or mechanical damage. The skin of young children remains particularly susceptible to damage from sunlight, and considerable adult vigilance is required to protect babies and children from sunburn.

As the quality of the skin changes with age, so do the disorders that affect it. For example, the onset of atopic dermatitis, one of the most prevalent skin disorders in childhood, is generally in infancy. With treatment and time most children experience progressively less discomfort. However, it is wise to avoid making predictions, as children rightly resent being told 'they will grow out of it', especially when their experience proves otherwise. Another chronic condition with an unpredictable course is psoriasis. This disorder may suddenly erupt in the early teenage years, and can significantly impair a young person's social development.

The issues of water loss, temperature regulation and infection are especially important for neonates (*see* Chapter 17), and the issue of vitamin D synthesis is of significance for children with heavily pigmented skin. Poor nutrition increases susceptibility to skin infection, and cutaneous infection in older children may be the initial presentation of immune deficiency or a side-effect of immunosuppressive drug therapy. *See* Box 19.1. Some tips for examining the skin are listed in Box 19.2.

Box 19.1 Major functions of the skin

- Protection from:
  - chemicals
  - infections
  - ultraviolet radiation
- Barrier to water loss
- Regulation of temperature
- Sensation
- Synthesis of vitamin D
- Immunological organ

Atopic dermatitis (eczema)

Eczema is the most common disorder of the skin, and much the most troublesome to the child as well as to the parents (*see* Figure 19.1). In an infant

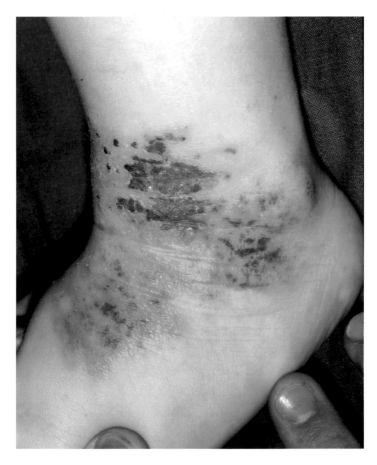

Figure 19.1 Atopic dermatitis. This characteristically affects the flexures in children, causing itchy, inflammatory papules and crusting. In the more chronic lesions there is lichenification.

it leads to generalised distress, sleepless nights and usually huge parental anxiety. Unfortunately, there is no absolute cure. It is important to identify factors that trigger itching. Much relief can be offered through appropriate medication, and newer, more effective treatments are being developed.

Unfortunately, parents are often so concerned about the side-effects of topical steroid preparations that under-treatment is common and flare-ups are inadequately treated (usually by stopping treatment too soon). The continual demands of an itching, fretful child who sleeps poorly and scratches at night are very exhausting for parents.

Diagnosis of eczema is fairly straightforward if there is a family history of atopic conditions (eczema, asthma or hay fever). The differential diagnosis is shown in Box 19.3 and general features in Box 19.4.

Box 19.2   Examining the skin

- Examine all of the skin
- Nappy area in infants
- Flexures
- Hair and scalp
- Nails
- Mucous membranes of the mouth (and tonsils)

Treatment (see Box 19.5)

Emollients (moisturising creams) are the most effective first-line treatment for eczema. They

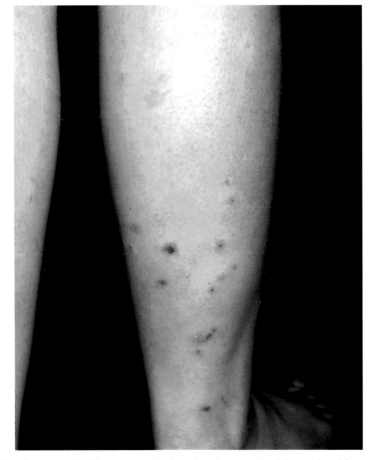

Figure 19.2   Papular urticaria. The characteristic lesion is an urticarial papule with a central punctum. Blisters may be seen, particularly on the legs. Present-day houses appear to be a favourable habitat for cat fleas, which are the usual cause of this condition.

are cheap, readily available and have no side-effects.

For more severe cases of eczema, the mainstay of treatment is a topical steroid ointment or cream (*see* Box 19.7). The golden rule is 'the least amount of the weakest preparation which gives relief'. The amount used must be charted and a schedule of reducing to weak topical steroids or emollients given. Combination products (e.g. antibiotic with corticosteroid) can stain clothes and carry a greater risk of inducing allergic contact dermatitis, so they are better avoided. The way in which a preparation is used is as important as what is used.

Children with atopic dermatitis are often colonised by *Staphylococcus aureus*, and the inappropriate use of antibiotics, either topically or systemically, can allow the emergence of resistant strains.

If there is an inadequate response to appropriate strengths of topical steroids, or if these agents are not tolerated, there is a clear need for non-steroidal topical immunosuppressives. Tacrolimus is available for moderate to severe disease, and pimecrolimus can be used for mild to moderate disease.

It is important to offer assessment for every exacerbation, as occasionally herpes simplex may be responsible. In this situation steroid cream is contraindicated, and systemic therapy with acyclovir is required.

Systemic antihistamines given 1 hour before bedtime are effective in reducing night-time scratching, mainly through their sedative effect. It is important to specify sucrose-free syrups to reduce the risk of dental caries.

Box 19.4 Atopic dermatitis

An itchy skin condition (or parental report of scratching or rubbing by the child) plus at least three of the following:

- a history of flexural involvement (elbows, knees, fronts of ankles or around the neck, or cheeks in children under 4 years)

- a personal history of asthma or hay fever (or history of atopic disease in a first-degree relative in children under 4 years)

- a history of generally dry skin in the last year

- visible flexural dermatitis (or dermatitis involving the cheeks/forehead or outer limbs in children under 4 years)

- onset under the age of 2 years.

Box 19.5   Management of atopic dermatitis

- Identify avoidable/treatable factors:
  - overbathing
  - pets
  - food
  - allergy to any medication
  - infection by bacteria, virus or fungus
  - infestation by scabies or lice.

- Explain the natural history.

- Consider prescribing:
  - a soap substitute
  - an emollient (moisturising cream)
  - topical corticosteroid
  - oral antihistamine, especially at night
  - oral antibiotic, if secondary infection.

- Offer a review appointment.

Box 19.6   Treatment of scabies

- Record everyone who is in close personal contact with the child.

- Ascertain how these people are to be informed of their need for treatment.

- Explain that treatment has to be synchronised within a family group.

- Advise on appropriate products and the method of use (e.g. if permethrin cream is used, there is a maximum dose that depends on the child's age).

- Arrange any required practical help from community nurses.

- Include a warning that repeated unnecessary treatments cause irritation.

Box 19.7   Topical corticosteroids

- Prescribe the lowest dose of the weakest preparation that works.

- Sometimes needs a short course of stronger topical steroid to get control.

- Ointment may work better than cream, but children like it less.

- Should be lightly spread, not rubbed in vigorously.

- Should be applied once or twice daily – there is no advantage in more frequent use.

- Should be continued for 4 or 5 days after the surface of the skin has healed, to deal with the deeper inflammation.

Case study 1

For some weeks Alexander, aged 2 years, has been very itchy. His mother tells the GP that he wakes every night scratching, and his sheets are bloodstained. The 1% hydrocortisone cream which was initially prescribed has been helpful, but his mother is reluctant to continue using it daily since she read in a magazine that steroid creams have side-effects. His mother is exhausted.

Alexander has had dry, itchy skin since he was 3 months old. Initially there was scaling of his scalp, which the health visitor described as 'cradle cap'.

His two elder brothers also had atopic dermatitis in infancy, but have not had troublesome skin since they were 5 years old. One brother has asthma.

A swab for bacteriological culture is taken. Acute flares, including pustule formation, may be caused by group A haemolytic streptococci, so Alexander is given erythromycin pending the results of culture. He is also prescribed a topical antibiotic for the crusted lesions. On examination he is fretful but cooperative. At any opportunity he scratches his wrists, and when undressed he scratches his legs. His skin is generally dry and there are painful fissures on his right thumb. There are pustules on his knees and legs. At his elbows and wrists, popliteal fossae and ankles there is dermatitis (*see* Figure 19.1). At his ankles there are weeping, crusted areas. There are no scabies burrows on his hands, wrists, feet or genitalia (*see* Figure 19.3). The lymphatic glands in both groins are enlarged.

Three weeks later Alexander's mother brings him back for review. She reports that he appeared to be scratching more on two occasions after eating a particular brand of potato crisps. She is advised to exclude these from his diet, and this helps to reduce the symptoms.

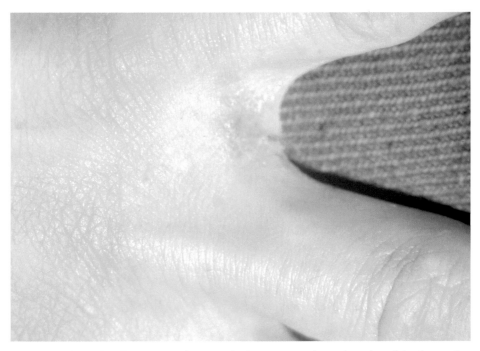

Figure 19.3 Scabies. The characteristic lesion is the burrow. In infants, the soles of the feet or the groin are commonly affected. In older children with a persisting infestation, the generalised truncal rash may be difficult to distinguish from atopic dermatitis.

Psoriasis

Psoriasis is an inflammatory condition charac-terised by scaling plaques, often on the elbows and knees. There is often a family history of the condition.

It may present with nappy rash, or in the older child with a scaly lesion. Nappy rashes may occur as a result of irritation or from infection by *Candida*. Children with a genetic predisposition to psoriasis can present with a sudden severe nappy rash, often with a more generalised rash (*see* Figure 19.4 and Box 19.8).

In older children it is not uncommon for guttate psoriasis to develop after tonsillitis due to strepto-coccal infection. It is relevant to take a throat

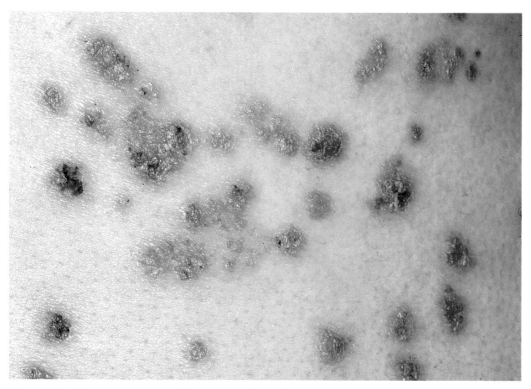

Figure 19.4   Guttate psoriasis tends to erupt. The erythematous scaling lesions are widely distributed over the trunk, but may also affect the scalp.

Box 19.8   Guttate psoriasis

- Often follows streptococcal sore throat

- Presents acutely in the guttate form and resolves within a few weeks

- Treatment is required if the itch is severe

- An emollient cream can minimise the scaling

- Shampoos containing prepared coal tar can help

- Avoid further trauma to the already irritated skin

swab, since if group A haemolytic streptococci are isolated, penicillin should be prescribed. If episodes of tonsillitis are frequent, referral for consideration of tonsillectomy is appropriate.

The response to scratching is called the *Koebner phenomenon*. This term is used in several conditions for the isomorphic response. For example, after trauma the Koebner phenomenon can develop in the damaged areas, and it may also occur in surgical scars if the psoriasis is in an active phase.

Both the patient and his or her parents require an explanation of the natural history of psoriasis. They need to know that childhood psoriasis often presents acutely in the guttate form, and that it usually resolves. Treatment is required if the itch is severe, and an emollient cream can minimise the scaling. Shampoos containing prepared coal

---

Case study 2

Elaine, aged 11 years, is distraught. Over the past 16 days, itchy red spots have appeared on her body, arms and now her neck. She is frightened that they will extend to her face. In addition, her scalp is scaly and she has dandruff. Three weeks previously she had had a severe sore throat. She has been rubbing in a variety of handcreams and body lotions. Her mother is anxious because she remembers an uncle who had severe psoriasis and was very disabled by arthritis. Looking at Elaine's medical records, her GP notes state that she had a very florid nappy rash as a baby.

Elaine has enlarged tonsils and associated lymphadenopathy. On her scalp there are hard, scaly areas, but there is no loss of hair. Scattered diffusely over the trunk there are oval lesions that are red and superficially scaling. Where she has scratched, tiny circular lesions are developing. The diagnosis is guttate psoriasis (*see* Figure 19.4). Treatment is discussed, and coal-tar shampoo is recommended.

The practice nurse has a video of the treatments available for psoriasis. She also has a leaflet illustrating how to get the most benefit from the prepared tar shampoo prescribed for Elaine.

---

tar can be beneficial. It is important to apply the therapies gently in order to avoid further trauma to the already irritated skin.

Pigmented skin lesions

Moles

Moles are the usual name given to acquired pigmented lesions. In general these are benign.

Moles may suddenly develop during adolescence, and existing lesions may alter, either by increasing in thickness or by darkening in colour. At this age, some compound naevi also involute, giving the characteristic halo naevus. In addition, it is important to be aware of the type known as Spitz naevus, which has a spindle-cell cellular pattern (*see* Figure 19.5).

Box 19.9   Pigmented skin lesions

- *Freckle*: tiny areas of increased pigmentation after sun exposure.

- *Naevus* (plural *naevi*): an imprecise term applied to a variety of hamartomas in the skin.

- *Café au lait lesion*: irregular area of even pigmentation which is not raised; if numerous, they may suggest neurofibromatosis.

- *Compound naevus*: the most frequently seen lesion; the centre tends to be darker and more raised.

- *Spitz naevus*: spindle-cell tumour which histologically resembles melanoma.

Although rare, malignant melanoma may occur in childhood. There is no formula which may be applied at this age to aid the decision as to whether to excise a pigmented lesion, and it remains a difficult area of clinical judgement. Several factors may influence the decision to remove pigmented lesions (*see* Boxes 19.9 and 19.10).

Sun protection is important. It has been argued that the introduction of sun blocks which reduce the erythema from short-wavelength ultraviolet rays (UVB: 295–320 nm) result in longer overall

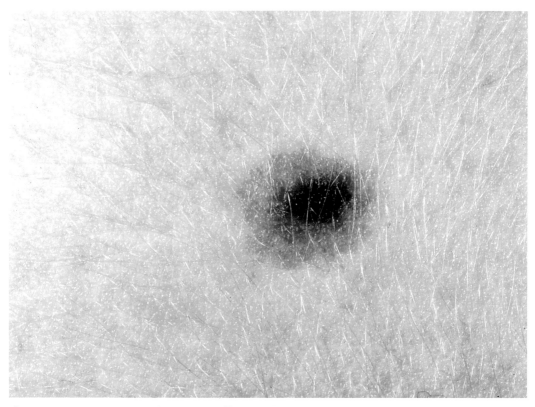

Figure 19.5 Spitz naevus. Characteristically a single red or red-brown nodule suddenly develops on sun-exposed skin. After a period of rapid growth it stabilises and persists. Excision is recommended.

Box 19.10 Factors that influence the need to remove pigmented lesions

- First-degree relative treated for melanoma

- Multiple atypical lesions

- Spitz naevus (*see* Figure 19.5)

---

sun exposure. Thus sunscreens now generally also contain protection from longer-wavelength ultraviolet rays (UVA: 320–400 nm). Dermatologists recognise that sunburn in childhood is a risk factor for the subsequent development of multiple naevi and malignant melanoma. It is wise to avoid exposure to the sun between 11am and 3pm. Clothing and an appropriate hat may also be useful barriers to ultraviolet radiation. Thus wearing a cotton T-shirt makes sense, especially for activities such as water sports,

when there is additional reflection of ultraviolet rays from the water.

A compound naevus is the type of naevus most frequently seen. The centre tends to be darker and more raised (*see* Figure 19.6).

Another naevus is the halo naevus (Sutton's naevus), which has a halo of non-pigmented skin (*see* Figure 19.7).

A further cause of pigmentation is sunshine which whilst generally very enjoyable, can have adverse effects on the skin (*see* Box 19.11).

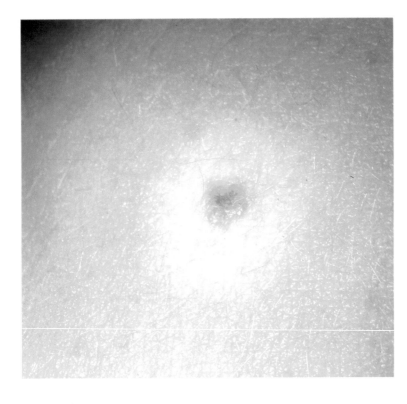

Figure 19.6   Compound naevus. Adolescents develop such lesions, which often have an irregular border and a darker raised centre.

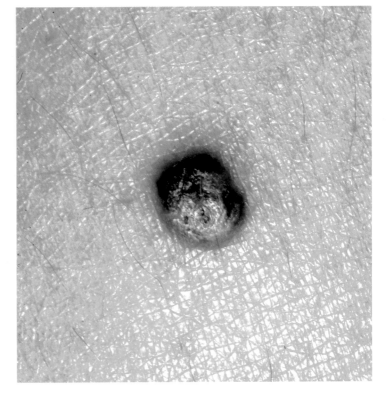

Figure 19.7   Halo naevus (also known as Sutton's naevus) is a pigmented lesion which is spontaneously regressing and has a rim of depigmentation.

> **Box 19.11** Sunburn
>
> • Risk factor for malignant melanoma
>
> • Avoid sun exposure between 11am and 3pm
>
> • Clothing and a hat are useful barriers
>
> • Additional ultraviolet rays are reflected from water

Acne

Acne affects the face and trunk of most teenagers. It is characterised by comedones and pustules. In severe cases it progresses to cysts and scarring.

Teenagers with acne are usually very self-conscious and may be embarrassed to ask for help (*see* Figure 19.8). It is worth suggesting a preparation that contains benzoyl peroxide, taking care to explain that it is likely to cause some dryness of the skin and that it will not bring about instant resolution of the problem. This is another situation where an explanatory leaflet, which the young person can read in their own time, may be a useful means of providing information. A thoughtfully written publication may help a teenager to realise that a number of treatment approaches are available. There are additional topical preparations available, such as tretinoin, systemic antibiotics and, for severe cases, oral isotretinoin (*see* Box 19.12).

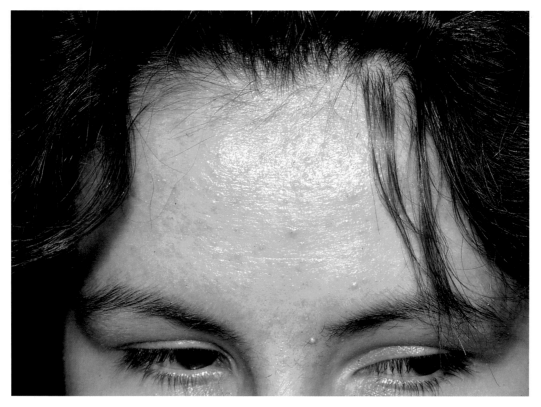

Figure 19.8 Acne. This is the epitome of teenage years. The characteristic lesion is the comedone, but the more obvious lesions are pustules and cysts. Treatment aims to lessen the severity and to limit the extent of long-term scarring.

> **Box 19.12** Acne
>
> • Is a cause of undivulged teenage unhappiness
>
> • May be helped by topical benzoyl peroxide
>
> • May need systemic tetracycline or erythromycin
>
> • In severe cases, may require oral isotretinoin

Viral warts and molluscum contagiosum

Warts are lumpy swellings that usually occur on the hands in young children, and which are caused by a virus infection. They are unsightly, but are otherwise symptomless and of nuisance value only. They normally resolve spontaneously with time (*see* Box 19.13).

The viruses that cause warts and verrucas are papilloma viruses, of which many types are now recognised (*see* Figure 19.9).

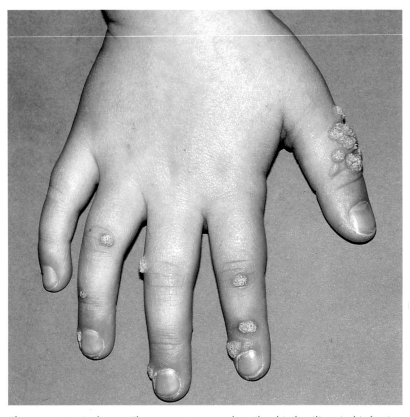

Figure 19.9 Viral wart. The correct term to describe this familiar viral infection is 'verruca vulgaris' on the hand, and 'verruca plantaris' on the foot. However, the term 'wart' is acceptable as a description of these benign virus-induced tumours. The pain from a verruca on the sole of the foot may be lessened by using a ringed dressing to reduce pressure. Whichever treatment is adopted, persistence is required.

Box 19.13 Viral warts

- Are common

- Are caused by papilloma virus

- Usually resolve spontaneously after a few months

- May be treated with topical keratolytics

- Plantar warts (verrucas) are often painful and need treatment

- Respond to cryotherapy (with topical anaesthetic cream)

Molluscum contagiosum is also a cutaneous viral infection (*see* Figure 19.10 and Box 19.14). It has been usual not to treat either warts or molluscum with cryotherapy (liquid nitrogen) because this treatment is painful. Unfortunately, molluscum contagiosum may become very

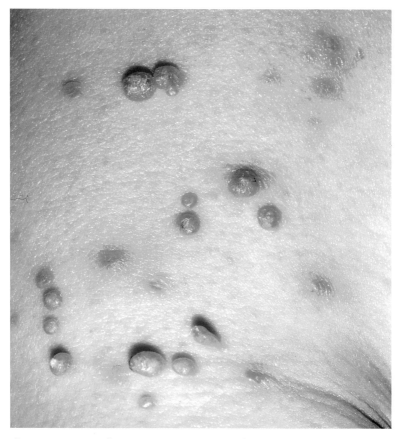

Figure 19.10 Molluscum contagiosum. Early lesions are skin-coloured papules. More chronic lesions have an umbilicated appearance or become very inflamed. In some children, pustular areas develop. The cause is a pox virus, and if left untreated the lesions will resolve, but the condition may persist for months.

widespread, and the lesions do not always resolve without scarring. The introduction of effective local anaesthetic cream means that children are often able to tolerate cryotherapy if this cream has first been applied under occlusion for 1 hour. However, young children who are untroubled by their warts need not be treated, and older children may respond to topical podophyllin. Molluscum contagiosum is generally more troublesome in children who have atopic dermatitis. It is important to employ emollients and to avoid the use of topical corticosteroids at the affected sites.

Box 19.14 Molluscum contagiosum

- Is caused by a pox virus
- Is often associated with dermatitis
- May spread widely
- Usually resolves with no treatment, but may persist for a few years
- Responds to cryotherapy (with topical anaesthetic cream)

Nappy rash

Nappy rash is common in infancy. It is very troubling to parents, who are both concerned about the distress of the baby and also feel that it is their own fault.

It is certainly true that close contact with decomposing urine will cause a rash (ammoniacal dermatitis), but nappy rash can also be caused by the yeast *Candida*, and by seborrhoeic dermatitis, which is a skin disorder associated with cradle cap (heaped-up yellow scales on the scalp), as well as by napkin psoriasis. *See* Box 19.15.

Ammoniacal dermatitis tends to spare the flexus, whereas yeast infection covers them and has noticeable satellite lesions. Seborrhoeic dermatitis is diagnosed by the presence of cradle

---

Box 19.15 Causes of nappy rash

- Ammoniacal dermatitis
- *Candida* (thrush)
- Seborrhoeic dermatitis
- Napkin psoriasis

---

cap, and the rash tends to be in all the flexures (neck, axillae and also behind the ears). Napkin psoriasis resembles true psoriasis, with well-defined, slightly raised scaly plaques in the napkin area, which may spread up the trunk. The flexures are usually involved.

Resistant cases are best treated by exposure and with a topical corticosteroid, mixed with an antibacterial and antifungal agent if appropriate. *See* Box 19.16.

Box 19.16 Treatment of nappy rash

- *Ammoniacal dermatitis*: exposure, good hygiene, protective cream, topical corticosteroids.
- *Candida*: nystatin orally and topically, exposure.
- *Seborrhoeic dermatitis*: scalp – clean with olive oil; bottom – exposure, topical steroid, possibly with antifungal agent.
- *Napkin psoriasis*: weak topical steroid.

Further reading

- Harper JI, Oranje A and Prose N (eds) (2000) *Textbook of Paediatric Dermatology* (2e). Blackwell Science, Oxford.
- Verbov JL (2002) *Handbook of Paediatric Dermatology*. Martin Dunitz, London.

Case study 3

Jane, aged 3 months, is brought by her mother to the practice baby clinic for weighing and immunisation. Anne, the health visitor, notices that she has a bad nappy rash which extends over the whole area of the buttocks and down the legs. There are also some red satellite lesions extending on to the abdomen. The mother is quite upset about it, saying that she has tried several creams but it is getting worse. She has also noticed that Jane has some white spots in her mouth and is not feeding so well. The health visitor examines Jane carefully and notices that the rash covers the skin creases at the hips and there are satellite lesions on the abdomen. It appears very red, with sharply demarcated edges. She also has small white spots on her tongue and on the gums which look like 'thrush'.

These are all signs of *Candida* infection, so the health visitor treats Jane with oral and topical nystatin, an antifungal agent, and advises the parents to expose the baby's bottom after changing the nappy. A week later the rash has nearly disappeared.

Self-assessment questions

1 Eczema:
(a) can affect a child of any age from infancy onwards   True/False
(b) may be superinfected by herpes virus   True/False
(c) is best treated with powerful steroids   True/False
(d) tends to improve with time.   True/False

2 Nappy rash:
(a) is indicative of poor hygiene   True/False
(b) is distressing for the infant   True/False
(c) responds well to treatment   True/False
(d) may be infective in origin.   True/False

3 Scabies:
(a) only occurs in poor families   True/False
(b) is associated with intense itching   True/False
(c) is most obvious around the wrists and ankles   True/False
(d) requires systemic treatment.   True/False

4 Warts:
(a) are caused by a virus   True/False
(b) are readily transferred from one part of the body to another   True/False
(c) require surgical ablation   True/False
(d) often remit spontaneously.   True/False

20 Renal disease

- Urinary tract infection
- Haematuria and glomerulonephritis
- Proteinuria and nephrotic syndrome
- Acute renal failure
- Haemolytic–uraemic syndrome
- Chronic renal failure

Disease of the urinary tract in children is common, important, and may have far-reaching effects into later life. Reflux uropathy remains a depressingly frequent reason for end-stage renal failure in adults. Congenital abnormalities of the renal tract are relatively common, and some may be detected on routine antenatal ultrasound. Unfortunately, the ability to detect congenital disease outstrips current knowledge of how best to manage it postnatally.

Urinary tract infection is the commonest renal tract disease in childhood.

Surveys of school-age children have suggested that 3–5% of girls and 1–3% of boys will have at least one urinary tract infection (UTI) in childhood. Despite being so common, UTI generates more uncertainty and controversy than almost any other area in general paediatrics.

UTI is also non-specific in its presentation, so young children with symptoms such as fever or abdominal pain commonly have their urine investigated for infection. Such infections need treatment in their own right, and infection prompts investigations to elucidate an underlying congenital cause.

Renal disease outside the urinary tract may present with an obvious symptom such as haematuria, but is frequently silent, and may only be identified during investigation of a presenting symptom, such as failure to thrive. Renal disease may occur alone or it may be a more variable part of a multisystem syndrome. In childhood, the two commonest ways in which renal disease may be identified are through the detection of haematuria and/or proteinuria. *See* Box 20.1.

Box 20.1 Renal disease: presenting patterns

- Haematuria
- Proteinuria
- Systemic hypertension
- Acute renal failure
- Effects of chronic renal failure
  - failure to thrive, short stature
  - malaise and tiredness
  - anaemia
  - renal osteodystrophy
- Effects of tubular dysfunction
  - acidosis
  - amino-aciduria
  - hypokalaemia
  - hypophosphataemia
  - normoglycaemic glycosuria

Urinary tract infection

Presentation

Urinary tract infection may present with specific symptoms or as non-specific fever, or it may be asymptomatic (*see* Table 20.1). It should always be suspected in an unwell child, including an infant.

The incidence of UTI in pre-school children remains unknown, but it is in this group that infections complicated by vesico-ureteric reflux may cause progressive renal scarring. If such damage is sufficiently severe, it can in turn lead to progressive glomerulosclerosis of the remaining kidney substance with gradual loss of function, despite precautions to prevent further scarring due to infection.

After many years, chronic pyelonephritis may lead to hypertension or chronic renal failure. The proportion of children who will eventually go on to develop these serious complications is unknown. However, the experience of adult renal dialysis/transplant programmes suggests that childhood reflux nephropathy is still the commonest cause of end-stage renal failure in adults under the age of 50 years. Paediatricians aim to prevent these late sequelae by early diagnosis and treatment of childhood UTI. Table 20.2 shows the sex ratio and percentage admitted in different age groups.

Diagnosis

The key to diagnosis of UTI is finding infection in the urine. However, collecting a urine specimen

Table 20.1 Features of urinary tract infection in childhood

Age < 12 months	Age > 12 months
Asymptomatic	Abdominal pain
Failure to thrive (growth faltering)	Back pain
Febrile convulsion (> 6 months)	Change in urinary frequency
Fever	Febrile convulsion
Septicaemia	Unexplained fever
Irritability	Visible haematuria
Persistent neonatal jaundice	Pain on micturition
Poor feeding	Rigors
Vomiting	

Table 20.2 Characteristics of urinary tract infection

Age (months)	Female:male ratio	Percentage admitted to hospital	Total
0–6	0:5	69%	45
7–12	0:9	68%	31
13–18	1:7	57%	28
19–24	5:3	56%	25
> 24	3:1	7%	574

Unpublished data from the Royal Aberdeen Children's Hospital.

from a child is not particularly easy. Some methods of doing this are listed in Box 20.2.

> **Box 20.2**   Collecting urine from a child
>
> *From a baby*
> - Sit with a sterile bottle while the baby has the nappy off, and try to collect a specimen when they urinate (easy in boys!).
> - Use a urine collection pad in the nappy.
>
> *From a potty-trained toddler*
> - Wash the potty with ordinary washing-up liquid. It will then be clean enough to use to collect a urine sample.
>
> *From an older child*
> - Collect the sample in a sterile bottle when the child urinates.
>
> *Suprapubic aspiration*
> - The bladder is aspirated with a needle in an ill infant.

Once the specimen has been collected it must be examined for infection. The simplest method is microscopy for bacteriuria and white cells, which is a reliable screening test. Treatment should not be started until either a urine specimen has been examined under the microscope or a specimen has been sent for culture.

Urine cultures are potentially problematic. If there is a delay between urine collection and its arrival with the GP, any growth is impossible to interpret. Ideally, the urine would be collected and transferred at $< 5°C$ directly to the laboratory, but even then the loss of pus cells can be rapid. A number of strategies for urine collection and transfer have therefore evolved. Urine culture can be obtained by means of dipslides, which are rectangular culture plates that are wetted in the urine flow and then sent for incubation at the local laboratory. An alternative is to use sterile containers with boric acid, a reversible bacteriostatic which is sufficiently effective to allow postal transfer, or direct immediate microscopy of the urine. If the child is unwell, it is reasonable to start an antibiotic pending the result of urine culture.

Treatment

The treatment of choice in UTI is an oral broad spectrum antibiotic (e.g. amoxicillin).

The length of antibiotic courses for UTI has been the subject of some controversy, but both single high-dose treatments and short (5-day) courses are associated with a small proportion of relapses.

The *management of vesico-ureteric reflux* (*see* Box 20.3) is either medical with prophylactic antibiotics, or an attempt to correct the reflux surgically. Studies to date have not shown a clear difference between medical and surgical strategies. Children with evidence of renal scarring require long-term follow-up, measurement of blood pressure, urinary surveillance for new episodes of infection, and repeat imaging of the kidneys and urinary tract.

> **Box 20.3**   Managing vesico-ureteric reflux
>
> - Antibiotic prophylaxis
> - Regular urine cultures
> - Repeat renal imaging
> - Regularly check blood pressure
> - Consider surgery
> - Long-term follow-up

Further investigation

The optimal investigation of UTIs in childhood is a hotly debated area, which reflects the limitations of the methods currently available. The main aims of investigation are as follows:

1. to determine the presence or absence of renal scarring; depending on the child's age and the presence or absence of scarring, exclude vesico-ureteric reflux
2. to exclude an obstructive lesion
3. to screen for the rarer underlying problems, such as renal calculi or evidence of autosomal-dominant polycystic kidney disease.

(*See* Box 20.4.)

It is currently believed that initial renal scarring in association with vesico-ureteric reflux occurs in pre-school children (under 5 years). However,

> **Box 20.4** Possible lesions in children with urinary tract infection
>
> • Renal scarring
> • Vesico-ureteric reflux
> • Obstructive uropathy
> • Renal calculi
> • Renal polycystic disease
> • Any congenital abnormality of the urinary tract

when scarring has already occurred, and if vesico-ureteric reflux continues, further scarring may occur up to the age of 10 years. Thus, in children under 5 years of age it is necessary to know both whether there is scarring and whether there is reflux, while in older children the critical feature is the presence or absence of scarring.

Scarring is best demonstrated by the dimercapto-succinic acid (DMSA) isotope scan. Its ability to show up abnormal renal scan patterns during or immediately after infections has led to the suggestion that it may be possible to avoid imaging for reflux in children over 12 months of age who have a normal DMSA scan. However, in children

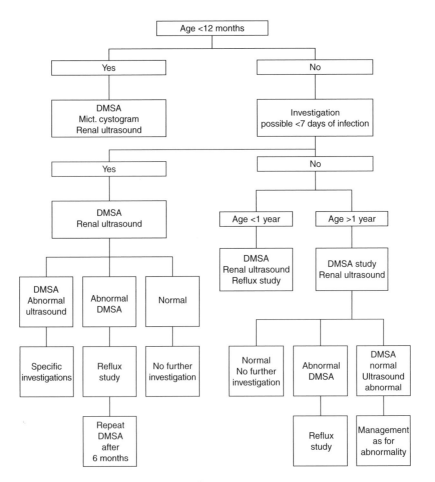

Figure 20.1 Algorithm for the investigation of urinary tract infection.

under 12 months reflux must be sought. This is the basis of the algorithm for renal investigation of UTI shown in Figure 20.1. Traditionally, the micturating cysto-urethrogram (MCUG) has been used to demonstrate vesico-ureteric reflux, but children with bladder control can be imaged successfully using an indirect micturating isotope scan. A 5-point scale is used to describe reflux. This ranges from 1 for reflux into the ureter only to 5 for gross dilatation with reflux up to the calyces and loss of the normal papillary impression.

All children with proven UTI require investigation.

Case study 1

Laura is a 3-year-old girl whose parents contact their GP after she has been generally unwell for a few days with intermittent abdominal pain and lethargy. Having been dry at night for about 8 months, she has also started to wet the bed again. Her parents have become concerned because during the night she has been feverish and having shivering episodes. She is seen later that morning by a doctor, and no focus of infection is found. Her parents are asked to collect a sample of urine for analysis and culture.

One part of the sample is sent to the local laboratory for culture and microscopy, and the remainder is checked by a reagent strip and shows moderate blood and protein but no glucose. Laura remains feverish and is started on an antibiotic pending the culture results.

Microscopy shows numerous pus cells, red blood cells and organisms.

The urine culture is reported as *E. coli* > 100 000 colonies/ml. The organism is sensitive to the antibiotic that has been prescribed, and within 48 hours Laura is afebrile and much improved. Her parents are asked to continue giving the antibiotic for 10 days.

Laura is reviewed after completing her course of antibiotics, and a repeat urine culture is sterile. After 3 months she has a second UTI very similar to the first, and then a third UTI a few months later. The GP arranges a renal ultrasound scan and DMSA scan (*see* algorithm in Figure 20.1 for investigation) at the local X-ray department. Ultrasound is reported as normal.

The DMSA scan shows that Laura has scarring in the upper pole of the left kidney, which contributes 25% of the total functioning renal mass. MCUG shows grade III vesico-ureteric reflux on the left side.

Laura has recurrent UTI. This problem is most common in girls, and can occur despite an anatomically normal renal tract and no vesico-ureteric reflux. The mechanism is not fully understood, but the most likely explanation is a dysfunctional voiding pattern.

Haematuria and glomerulonephritis

Haematuria is relatively common in childhood, and is most often associated with urinary tract infection (*see* Box 20.5). Causes are listed in Box 20.6. It is important always to consider the possibility of acute glomerulonephritis, which is an autoimmune disorder that usually follows an infection. The history and examination are summarised in Boxes 20.7 and 20.8, and Figure 20.2.

Post-streptococcal glomerulonephritis (*see* Box 20.9) follows infection with group A

Box 20.5   Haematuria

- Haematuria is the presence on microscopy of more than 5 red blood cells per high-power field.

- Normal urine contains a small number of erythrocytes.

- Urine that is positive for blood on reagent strips may contain haemoglobin but no red cells.

Box 20.6 Some causes of haematuria

• Exercise

• Benign familial haematuria

• Fever-associated

• Trauma

• Coagulation disorders

• Infection – any urinary tract infection, TB

• Glomerulonephritis
 – post-streptococcal
 – crescentic
 – membrano-proliferative
 – IgA nephropathy

• Henoch–Schönlein purpura

• Haemolytic–uraemic syndrome

• Hypercalciuria (some with calculi)

• Autosomal-dominant polycystic kidney disease

• Tumours – Wilms' tumour, rhabdomyo-sarcoma of bladder

• Factitious (Münchausen's syndrome by proxy)

Box 20.7 The history in haematuria

• Preceding episodes of haematuria
 – dysuria, loin pain
 – skin rashes
 – joint pains

• Family history of haematuria, renal failure, kidney stones or urological surgery

---

alpha-haemolytic streptococci, which is most commonly pharyngeal but can be associated with impetigo. The condition is characterised by hypertension, haematuria, and sometimes by acute renal failure. Investigations are listed in Box 20.10.

Measurement of blood pressure is of central importance in any child presenting with a possibility of renal disease (including UTI). It is essential to ensure that a large enough cuff (covering at least two-thirds of the upper arm) has been used, as smaller sizes give falsely high readings. It is also wise to ensure that several readings are taken before diagnosing hypertension, as an elevated blood pressure may be related to the stress of being in hospital rather than to renal disease itself.

Box 20.8 Examination in haematuria/renal disease

1 Oedema: peripheral and periorbital

2 Blood pressure

3 Skin: rashes

4 Heart: enlargement, mitral murmur

5 Abdomen: palpable kidneys or bladder

6 Vulvo-vaginitis or a local injury

The long-term prognosis should be good, with end-stage renal failure occurring in less than 1% of cases. Treatment is summarised in Box 20.11. Rarely, a child may present with a nephritic/nephrotic picture. This is a combination of nephritis as above combined with massive proteinuria, resulting in the nephrotic syndrome (see below). This combination may occur in a number of other acute glomerulonephritic conditions, such as Henoch–Schönlein nephritis, and is associated with more glomerular damage and a higher risk of developing end-stage renal failure.

Box 20.9 Glomerulonephritis

• Usually presents with haematuria

• Urine contains casts, protein, and red cells of glomerular origin

• Common causes are post-streptococcal and IgA nephropathy

• May be complicated by hypertension

• Post-infective causes have a good prognosis

Box 20.10   Investigations for glomerulonephritis

- Urine culture
- Plasma urea, creatinine, electrolytes, albumin, immunoglobulins
- Urine culture
- Urinary protein:creatinine ratio (early morning)
- Timed protein excretion
- C3 and C4 components of complement
- Renal ultrasound
- Coagulation screen
- Antistreptolysin O level (ASO)
- Auto-antibodies
- Renal biopsy

Box 20.11   Treatment of acute glomerulonephritis

- Fluid balance to avoid overload
- Penicillin
- Low-salt, low-protein diet
- Monitor renal function
- Treatment of hypertension
- Diuretics if necessary

Case study 2

Allan is a previously healthy 7-year-old boy whose mother brings him to see his GP with a sore throat. The doctor finds inflamed tonsils with some tender enlarged anterior cervical lymph nodes. She says that antibiotics are not required and that Allan should be given paracetamol for his fever and discomfort. A few days later he feels better and returns to school. Twelve days after first noticing the sore throat, his parents observe that his face is looking rather puffy around the eyes, and they take him back to his GP. The presumptive diagnosis is hay fever, and he is given an antihistamine. The following day the facial swelling is worse. He is taken back to the doctor, who requests a sample of urine. The urine looks 'smoky' and on testing shows blood +++ and protein +++. Allan is referred to hospital for further assessment.

Examination in hospital shows that he has some ankle oedema as well as facial swelling. His blood pressure is 125/85 mmHg. There is no rash and no cardiac murmur. Examination is otherwise normal. Urine microscopy shows red cell casts. A presumptive diagnosis is made of acute post-streptococcal glomerulonephritis.

Investigations show Allan's urea concentration to be 11.4 mmol/l (normal range < 6.5 mmol/l) and his creatinine level is 85 micromol/l (normal range for age up to c.70 micromol/l). The plasma albumin concentration is 35 g/l (normal range 36–48 g/l). A throat swab grows normal upper respiratory flora only. Allan's antistreptolysin O (ASO) level is elevated at 320 IU/ml (normal range < 160 IU/ml). Complement studies show a C3 of 23 mg/dl (normal range 88–200 mg/dl) and a C4 of 32 mg/dl (normal range 12–40 mg/dl) (see Box 20.10 and Figure 20.3).

Allan's blood pressure rises to 130/105 mmHg.

His hypertension is confirmed, and he is treated with fluid restriction, a low-salt diet and nifedipine (see Box 20.11). Five days after admission his urine output suddenly increases and his blood pressure returns to normal. His blood biochemistry also returns to normal. His urinalysis still shows blood +++, but now with protein +.

Six weeks after his admission the urine still shows blood ++++, but there is only a trace of protein. His blood pressure and C3 are now both normal.

Six months after his admission the urine shows blood ++ but is negative for protein. At 10 months the urinalysis is negative for both blood and protein, and remains so 2 years later.

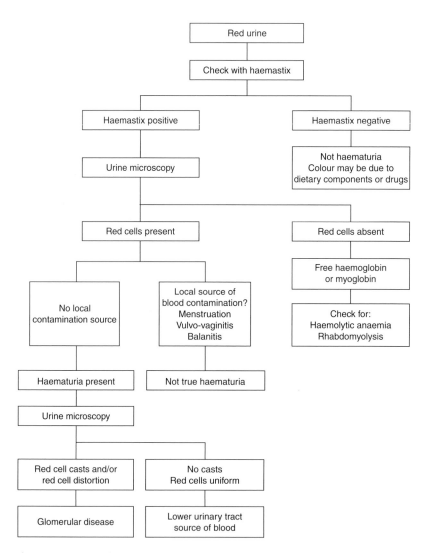

Figure 20.2   Initial assessment of red urine for possible haematuria.

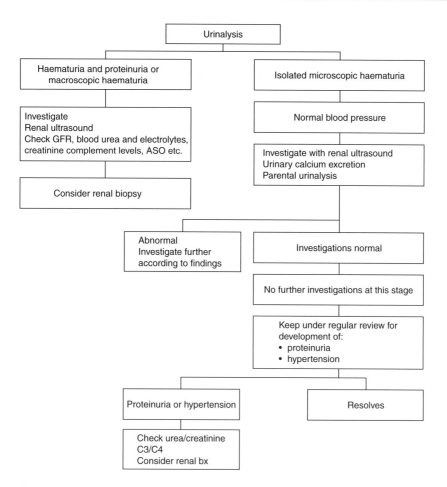

Figure 20.3   Further assessment of microscopic haematuria.

Proteinuria and nephrotic syndrome

Intermittent proteinuria is a fairly common and benign finding (*see* Box 20.12). Persistent proteinuria is less common, and is more likely to be associated with a significant underlying condition. Massive proteinuria with symptoms is always pathological.

Nephrotic syndrome (*see* Box 20.13 and Figure 20.4) is defined as massive proteinuria causing hypoalbuminaemia with consequent oedema. Hyperlipidaemia (low-density-lipoprotein fraction) is the fourth and least well understood component of the syndrome. In over 75% of

---

Box 20.12   Benign causes of proteinuria

• Orthostatic (postural)

• Fever

• Exercise

---

children under the age of 5 years this is due to light 'negative' or 'minimal-change' glomerulonephritis (MCG), where the glomerular appearances on both light and electron microscopy are normal apart from the non-specific features found in any condition with massive proteinuria.

Box 20.13 Nephrotic syndrome

- Massive proteinuria
- Hypoalbuminaemia
- Oedema
- Hyperlipidaemia

Children with nephrotic syndrome are intrinsically vulnerable to infection, particularly from *Streptococcus pneumoniae*, during the active phase when their immune system is compromised. It is therefore usual to prescribe prophylactic penicillin. It is important to monitor the blood pressure, as hypotension may be a consequence of the fluid leak from the vascular compartment.

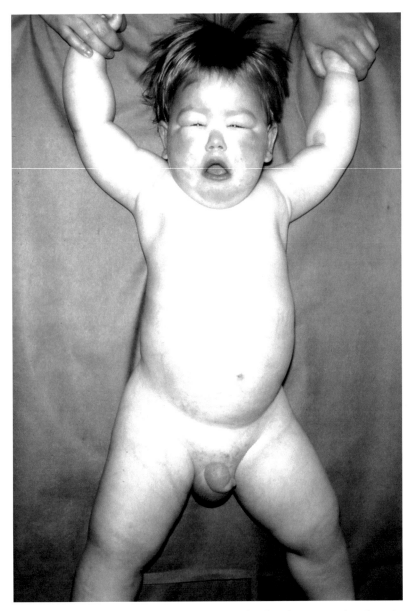

Figure 20.4 Nephrotic syndrome. Note the marked generalised oedema. Facial oedema is usually more marked in the mornings. Ascites and hydrocoeles can also develop.

Nephrotic syndrome is normally very responsive to treatment with steroids. Some children relapse frequently, and in time may become either steroid dependent (relapsing when steroids are reduced below a certain dose) or resistant to steroids. In these children, a single course of cyclophosphamide can restore steroid sensitivity or allow a reduction in steroid dose. The cyclophosphamide cannot be repeated because of its cumulative toxicity. Cyclosporin can also be used to maintain remission, but is again nephrotoxic.

The risk of end-stage renal failure in MCG is very low ($< 1\%$), so the long-term prognosis is very good. Even those who are frequent relapsers or steroid resistant eventually go into remission, although this may take many years and the condition can persist into early adult life.

Screening for proteinuria is most easily carried out using a urine reagent strip. This is accurate for albumin but will miss the lower-molecular-weight proteins that are found in some renal diseases, such as tubular disorders.

A simple test for orthostatic proteinuria is to collect two urine samples, one in the early morning and a second sample later in the day, and to check the protein:creatinine ratio in both samples. In addition, the family can be asked to check two urine samples in a similar way with dipsticks and to record the results.

Where investigations show persistent proteinuria there are many possible causes. It is always important to remember that glomerular and other diseases may have an orthostatic component, so it is important that the early-morning protein level is normal and not just lower than the later sample. The different stages in the investigation of proteinuria are shown in Table 20.3.

Table 20.3   Investigation of proteinuria

Primary
- Urine culture
- Urinalysis for blood and glucose
- Urine microscopy
- Early-morning and late-in-the-day urine for protein:creatinine ratio

Secondary
- For history of renal disease, abnormal physical findings, abnormal primary investigations
- Plasma urea, creatinine, electrolytes, phosphate, calcium, alkaline phosphatase and plasma proteins
- Urine biochemistry
- Glomerular filtration rate (GFR)
- Timed urinary protein excretion
- ASO level
- Complement C3 and C4
- Renal imaging

Tertiary
- For heavy proteinuria, reduced GFR, persistently reduced C3 or possible familial nephritis
- Renal biopsy

Case study 3

Anne is a previously healthy 3-year-old girl who is taken to her GP with a 2-day history of increasing facial swelling. On examination, her doctor notes that she has ankle oedema and ascites. A sample of urine shows protein ++++, but with no blood.

Anne is sent to hospital for further assessment. Her blood pressure is found to be 80/55 mmHg. Her urea concentration is 6.1 mmol/l, creatinine is 58 μmol/l and albumin is 17 g/l (normal range 36–50 g/l). Complement C3 and C4 are normal, as is a renal ultrasound scan. Her overnight urine protein excretion rate is 48 mg/m^2/hour (normal range < 4 mg/m^2/hour), with a protein:creatinine ratio of 1500 mg/mmol (normal range < 20 mg/mmol).

The diagnosis is nephrotic syndrome, and there are no atypical features such as hypertension, haematuria or renal failure.

When the initial investigations have been completed, Anne is started on prednisolone (2 mg/kg ideal weight/day) and penicillin. She becomes progressively more oedematous, but her blood pressure remains normal and her urine continues to show protein only. After 13 days the proteinuria falls to + and then the following day there is only a trace. The oedema clears and her albumin level is found to have returned to normal. There is a high risk of relapse (c.80%) which needs to be identified early and treated. Parents can be asked to check the urine on alternate days with a protein dipstick. If the latter shows ++ or more, the urine should then be checked daily, and if the proteinuria remains at or above that level, steroids should be started again at the recommended dose. Early treatment in steroid-sensitive nephrotic syndrome often helps to limit the severity of relapses.

Over the next 5 years Anne has three relapses, which are treated at home without problems. She has subsequently gone into a longer-term remission of 3 years.

Anne's response to steroids was good, but if no improvement had been seen by 28 days of treatment, she would have been considered steroid resistant. Diagnoses other than MCG would then be considered, particularly focal segmental glomerulosclerosis and mesangial proliferative glomerulonephritis. The possibility of these diagnoses is increased if features such as haematuria, hypertension or renal failure are present. These diagnoses can only be made on a renal biopsy.

Acute renal failure

This rare and life-threatening event may be a side-effect of acute nephritis or of haemolytic–uraemic syndrome. It may also be related to intrinsic renal disease or post-renal causes such as urethral obstruction or calculi. Oliguria is the key feature, with excretion of less than 300 ml/m^2/day. Circulation and fluid balance must be monitored very closely, and peritoneal dialysis may be required.

Haemolytic–uraemic syndrome

This disturbing condition is the commonest cause of acute renal failure in children. It follows an enteric infection (usually *E. coli*) and presents with thrombocytopenia and haemolysis. Management is by dialysis and the prognosis is usually good (*see* Box 20.14).

Box 20.14   Haemolytic–uraemic syndrome (HUS)

- Acute renal failure
- Haemolytic anaemia
- Thrombocytopenia
- Commonest renal cause of acute renal failure
- May be secondary to gastrointestinal infection
- Diarrhoea-associated haemolytic–uraemic syndrome has a good prognosis

---

Chronic renal failure

Fortunately this condition is rare in childhood. The commonest cause is a structural malformation, followed by glomerulonephritis and hereditary nephropathies. Presenting features include poor growth, anaemia, anorexia and bone deformities, with hypertension developing later. Peritoneal dialysis is preferred to haemodialysis, and the eventual aim should be renal transplantation.

Hypertension in children is most commonly of renal origin. Other causes are listed in Box 20.15.

Box 20.15   Causes of hypertension

- Coarctation of the aorta
- Catecholamine excess (phaeochromo-cytoma, neuroblastoma)
- Endocrine causes
- Renal disease
- Essential hypertension

Further reading

- Barrat TM, Avner ED and Harmon WE (1999) *Pediatric Nephrology* (4e). Williams and Wilkins, Baltimore, MD.
- Webb NJA and Postlethwaite RJ (eds) (2003) *Clinical Paediatric Nephrology*. Oxford University Press, Oxford.

Self-assessment questions

1 Urinary tract infection:

(a) is unlikely before the age of 1 year   True/False

(b) a first UTI in a boy or girl should be investigated   True/False

(c) urine microscopy is the best method of diagnosis   True/False

(d) should not be treated before a urine specimen has been collected.   True/False

2 Haematuria:

(a) is normally associated with pain on micturition   True/False

(b) is best tested for by urinalysis   True/False

(c) is an adverse feature if seen in nephrotic syndrome   True/False

(d) is an indication for renal biopsy.   True/False

3 Nephrotic syndrome:

(a) is an indication for renal biopsy   True/False

(b) has a good prognosis   True/False

(c) normally responds well to steroids   True/False

(d) normally occurs only once.   True/False

4 Hypertension:

(a) does not occur in infancy   True/False

(b) is common in nephrotic syndrome   True/False

(c) is common in acute nephritis   True/False

(d) is life-threatening in children.   True/False

21 Heart disease

- Aetiology
- Clinical assessment
- Murmurs
- Cyanosis
- Cardiac failure
- Pyrexia and congenital heart disease
- Congenital heart disease in the neonate

Almost all heart disease in children is congenital in origin, with a birth prevalence of 8 in 1000 live births. Heart defects account for over 30% of all congenital anomalies. The mortality rate for children with congenital heart lesions has fallen over the last two decades, mainly due to earlier recognition of symptoms, the skill of cardiac surgeons, and the significant improvement in cardiopulmonary bypass techniques. There are eight common structural congenital heart defects (accounting for over 80% of the total) (see Box 21.1), and rhythm disturbances such as heart block and supraventricular tachycardia can also present as congenital lesions.

Acquired heart disease (see Box 21.2) is uncommon, and the incidence of rheumatic fever in children fell from 12 in 100 000 in the 1960s to 0.2 in 100 000 in the late 1980s. However, myocarditis, infective endocarditis and Kawasaki disease (mucocutaneous lymph node syndrome) are still rare causes of death and disability in children. The heart can also be involved in a number of systemic diseases, such as Marfan's syndrome, muscular dystrophy and the connective tissue disorders.

Children with actual or suspected heart disease require specialist evaluation, and resources and

---

Box 21.1 The eight commonest congenital heart defects

- Ventricular septal defect
- Patent arterial duct
- Atrial septal defect
- Tetralogy of Fallot (cyanotic)
- Pulmonary stenosis
- Coarctation of the aorta
- Aortic stenosis
- Transposition of the great arteries (cyanotic)

Box 21.2 Acquired heart disease

- Rheumatic fever
- Myocarditis (viral)
- Infective endocarditis (bacterial)
- Kawasaki disease (mucocutaneous lymph node syndrome)

expertise are concentrated in tertiary centres in the UK. However, GPs and paediatricians in general hospitals will see most children with their initial presentation of cardiac disease, and have to decide when it is appropriate to seek the services of the specialists.

As with other surgical conditions of the newborn, many congenital cardiac anomalies are now diagnosed antenatally on routine ultrasound, enabling management plans to be formulated before the delivery of the baby.

Aetiology

Both genetic and environmental factors (*see* Box 21.3) have been implicated as a cause of congenital heart disease (CHD). Multifactoral inheritance is the most likely genetic base for most CHD, with the abnormal genes only expressing themselves in the presence of external environmental stimuli. Over a third of children with chromosomal problems will have CHD, and just under 10% of all children with CHD will have a chromosomal anomaly. A number of children with a q11 deletion on chromosome 22 have abnormalities of the aortic arch and ventricular septum. Other organs are also involved, and the association is known as *Catch 22* (*see* Box 21.4). A number of syndromes and chromosomal abnormalities

(such as trisomy of chromosomes 21, 18 and 13) have associated cardiovascular anomalies (*see* Box 21.5).

As well as 'Why did it happen?', one of the commonest questions asked by parents is 'Will it happen again?'. If normal parents have had a child with a congenital heart defect, the risk of the next child being affected is increased threefold. If one of the parents has a heart defect, the risk of them having an affected child is increased fourfold. Subsequent pregnancies can be monitored using fetal echocardiography or, in the case of chromosomal problems, amniocentesis or chorion villus biopsy.

Box 21.4 'Catch 22'

- Cardiac defects
- Abnormal facies
- Thymic hypoplasia
- Cleft palate
- Hypocalcaemia
- Chromosome 22 q11 deletion

Box 21.3 Environmental factors and congenital heart disease

- Maternal infection
  - *Toxoplasma*, rubella, cytomegalovirus
- Maternal disease
  - Diabetes mellitus (TGA, transient cardiomyopathy)
  - Systemic lupus erythematosus (complete heart block)
- Drugs
  - Alcohol: TGA
  - Warfarin: ventricular septal defect
  - Phenytoin: pulmonary/aortic stenosis
  - Amphetamines: atrial and ventricular septal defects

TGA, transposition of the great arteries.

Box 21.5 Syndromes with associated heart disease

- *Down syndrome (trisomy 21)*: atrioventricular septal defect.
- *Turner's syndrome*: coarctation of the aorta.
- *Noonan's syndrome*: pulmonary stenosis.
- *William's syndrome* (D): aortic stenosis.
- *Marfan's syndrome* (D): dilatation and aneurysm of the aorta.
- *Holt–Oram syndrome* (D): atrial and ventricular septal defects.
- *Ellis–van Crefeld syndrome* (R): atrial septal defect.
- *Friedreich's ataxia* (R): cardiomyopathy.

R, autosomal recessive; D, autosomal dominant.

Clinical assessment

The majority of children with heart disease present in one of three ways:

- detection of a heart murmur
- cyanosis
- signs of heart failure.

Other presenting symptoms, especially in older children, include syncope and dizziness, chest pain, poor exercise tolerance and palpitations.

Electrocardiography (ECG) and a chest X-ray should be carried out on all children with suspected heart disease. The ECG provides information on chamber size, evidence of hypertrophy and conduction disturbances. There are several features of cardiovascular disease on a chest X-ray, and important non-cardiac diagnoses may be made (*see* Box 21.6). Echocardiography confirms most anatomical abnormalities of the heart, and can provide functional and haemodynamic information. Magnetic resonance imaging (MRI) is also a useful non-invasive investigation of cardiac and great-vessel anatomy, but most young children need to have this investigation performed under light general anaesthesia. Cardiac catheterisation and angiography provide more detailed functional and anatomical information, especially in complex cardiac cases.

Normal heart sounds are described in Box 21.7. Abnormal heart sounds include ejection clicks, found in aortic and pulmonary stenosis and occasionally in abnormalities of the mitral valve. A loud second heart sound is heard in the presence of pulmonary hypertension. The time between the closure of the aortic and pulmonary valves is increased during inspiration, and the second heart sound is said to be *split*. In cases of atrial septal defect, an excess of blood in the right

> **Box 21.6** Cardiac disease and the chest X-ray
>
> - Increased cardiac size and cardiothoracic ratio
> - Altered cardiac contour: absence or dilatation of pulmonary artery
> - Lung fields: plethora, oligaemia, oedema
> - Rib notching (coarctation of aorta)

> **Box 21.7** Normal heart sounds
>
> - *First*: closure of the mitral and tricuspid valves.
> - *Second*: closure of the aortic and pulmonary valves.
> - *Third*: rapid ventricular filling in diastole.
> - *Fourth*: increased flow into left ventricle caused by atrial contraction.

ventricle delays pulmonary valve closure and the splitting does not vary with respiration. This is termed *fixed splitting*.

Murmurs

Heart murmurs are classified as innocent or organic, and can be heard in either systole or diastole, or both (continuous murmurs) (*see* Table 21.1). The intensity of the murmur is usually graded from 1 to 6, and all murmurs that are graded 4 to 6 or greater are associated with a palpable thrill. Murmurs may be located to one site on the praecordium, but some may radiate throughout the praecordium, to the head and neck, and through to the back. In cases of suspected aortic coarctation, listen over the scapula for the continuous murmur of collateral blood vessels. The murmur of a patent arterial duct can also be heard over the left scapula.

Table 21.1 Heart murmurs

Murmur	Defect
Ejection systolic	Aortic stenosis Pulmonary stenosis Coarctation of the aorta
Pansystolic	Ventricular septal defect Mitral incompetence Tricuspid incompetence
Early diastolic	Aortic incompetence Pulmonary incompetence
Mid-diastolic	Mitral stenosis Tricuspid stenosis
Continuous	Patent ductus arteriosus Venous hum Systemic collaterals

Over 50% of children will be heard to have a murmur at some stage. An innocent murmur is usually detected at a routine clinical examination or when a child presents with an intercurrent febrile illness (*see* Box 21.8). These murmurs, caused by turbulence in a normal heart or great vessels, are also accentuated by exercise. The murmurs can present at any time in childhood, but to be considered innocent they have to satisfy a number of criteria (*see* Box 21.9). Most innocent murmurs are diagnosed and dealt with by GPs. Children are referred for further investigation if there is any doubt about the diagnosis or if the parents request a second opinion. Once the diagnosis of an innocent murmur has been made, the parents and the child should be reassured, and no follow-up is necessary.

Murmurs are also frequently heard in the neonatal period and may be due to a closing ductus arteriosus, mild tricuspid regurgitation or flow through the branch pulmonary arteries (*see* Chapter 17). These murmurs usually disappear within the first few weeks of life.

Some types of CHD may be asymptomatic, and the murmur may be detected on routine examination of the neonate or young child. The differential diagnosis includes small ventricular septal defect, atrial septal defect, coarctation of the aorta and mild pulmonary or aortic stenosis. These murmurs are usually louder than innocent murmurs, and may radiate through to the back.

The murmur of a ventricular septal defect has a maximum intensity at the lower left sternal border. Over 60% of small intramuscular ventricular septal defects will close spontaneously. The aortic stenosis murmur may radiate to the neck, and the pulmonary stenosis murmur is best heard at the upper left sternal border. In coarctation of the aorta there may be a collateral circulation over the scapula, and there will be weakness and delay of the femoral pulses. The classic finding in an atrial septal defect is *fixed splitting* of the second heart sound.

Box 21.8   Common innocent murmurs

- *Vibratory murmur (Still's murmur)*: 'buzzing' in quality, mid systolic in timing, varies with position, age group 3–7 years, best heard between the apex and lower left sternal border.

- *Pulmonary flow (ejection murmur)*: soft and 'blowing' in quality, early systolic ejection murmur in timing, age group 8–14 years, best heard at upper left sternal border.

- *Venous hum*: caused by blood cascading into great veins, continuous murmur, age group 3–6 years, best heard above and below clavicles, can be diminished by Valsalva manoeuvre or turning neck.

Box 21.9   Characteristics of an innocent murmur

- Asymptomatic
- Systolic (except venous hum)
- Accentuated by fever and exercise
- Varies with position
- Does not radiate

- No accompanying cyanosis
- Normal pulses
- Normal heart sounds
- No associated thrills
- Normal ECG and chest X-ray

Case study 1

Jack, aged 5 years, is the second child of unrelated parents. He was born at term by spontaneous vaginal delivery, and received all of his immunisations. He had developed normally.

He became ill with a cough and a fever, followed by loss of appetite and vomiting, so his mother took him to the GP. A diagnosis of viral gastroenteritis was made, but clinical examination revealed a soft mid-systolic heart murmur localised at the apex.

On examination, Jack showed no signs of respiratory distress (intercostal and subcostal indrawing), and there was no tracheal tug. He was pink, and there was no finger clubbing. His apex beat was not displaced. There was no evidence of a forceful right or left ventricle and no palpable precordial or suprasternal thrill. His brachial pulse rate was 80 beats/minute, with unremarkable volume, character and regularity. His femoral pulses were of good volume, with no delay between the upper and lower limb pulses (and therefore no clinical evidence of aortic coarctation). He was not visibly anaemic, nor did he have hepatomegaly or peripheral oedema. His blood pressure in the right arm was 90/45 mmHg, making both aortic stenosis and coarctation of the aorta unlikely, since both may cause hypertension.

Jack made a good recovery from his gastroenteritis, but on subsequent review 2 weeks later, the systolic murmur was still present. He was referred for a second opinion because of parental anxiety, but an ECG and chest X-ray were normal, and echocardiography revealed a structurally normal heart. This was therefore confirmed to be an innocent murmur.

Cyanosis

Transposition of the great arteries (TGA)

This is the commonest cyanotic heart defect presenting in the first postnatal days. Cyanosis occurs when there is a right-to-left shunt of blood, allowing oxygenated and deoxygenated blood to mix together (e.g. in a common atrium or single ventricle), or when the infant has TGA (*see* Box 21.10).

In TGA, the aorta arises from the right ventricle and the pulmonary artery arises from the left ventricle. This arrangement creates two parallel circulations. If the ductus arteriosus is open or if there is an accompanying ventricular septal defect, the two circulations can mix and some oxygenated blood reaches the aorta. If mixing does not occur, the infant will become very ill with acidosis and heart failure soon after birth. Emergency management consists of the infusion of prostaglandins E_1 or E_2 to open the duct and allow time for the baby to be transported to the intensive-care unit. This may be followed by the *Rashkind's procedure*, in which an artificial atrial septal defect is created, allowing mixing of oxygenated and deoxygenated blood. A definitive repair involves transposing the aorta on to the pulmonary root and the pulmonary artery on to the aortic root in the first or second week of life (the *switch* operation).

Box 21.10   Transposition of the great arteries (TGA)

- Commonest type of cyanotic congenital heart disease

- Associated with maternal diabetes mellitus

- Presents with neonatal cyanosis when the arterial duct shuts

- Immediate treatment is by prostaglandin infusion to open the duct

- Definitive corrective treatment is a 'switch' procedure

Tetralogy of Fallot

Intermittent episodes of cyanosis during the first year of life are the usual presentation of tetralogy of Fallot, which is the most common cyanotic congenital heart defect. It may present at birth with cyanosis or be picked up on routine clinical examination if a murmur has been heard. Cyanotic episodes may occur early in the morning, with activity or with intercurrent illness. During the cyanotic episodes the child may be breathless, irritable and crying.

The two main components of Fallot's tetralogy are the right ventricular outflow tract obstruction and the ventricular septal defect (*see* Box 21.11). As the obstruction increases, the right ventricular pressure rises, becomes suprasystemic and blood flows from right to left across the ventricular septal defect, causing cyanosis. When flow to the lungs improves, the right ventricular pressure falls and the infant becomes pink once more.

Box 21.11 Tetralogy of Fallot

- Ventricular septal defect
- Pulmonary or infundibular stenosis
- Overriding aorta
- Right ventricular hypertrophy

Other signs include a right ventricular 'tap' and systolic thrill with an associated loud ejection systolic murmur at the upper left sternal border. There will be right axis deviation and right ventricular hypertrophy on the ECG. Chest X-ray shows oligaemic lung fields, a 'concave' pulmonary artery bay and a right-sided aortic arch ('boot-shaped' heart) (*see* Figure 21.1). The diagnosis of tetralogy of Fallot is confirmed by echocardiography.

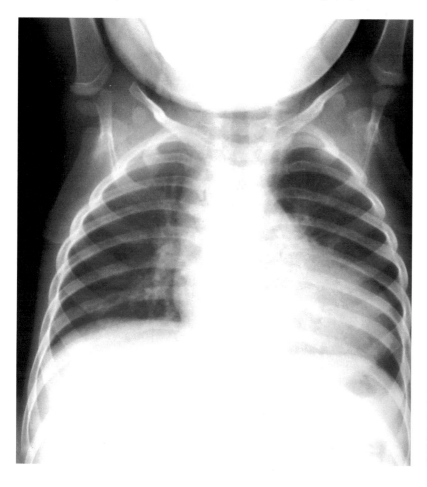

Figure 21.1 Chest X-ray showing a typical boot-shaped heart and poor pulmonary vascular pattern seen in tetralogy of Fallot.

Infants and children with tetralogy of Fallot characteristically have 'spells' or hypoxic episodes due to insufficient blood flow to the lungs. During these spells, the heart murmurs may be reduced or inaudible. Squatting delays venous return, increases systemic vascular resistance and improves blood flow to the lungs (*see* Figure 21.2). Because the cyanotic episodes are caused by infundibular spasms, the spasm can be relieved by squatting, placing young infants in the knee–elbow position, or treating with propranolol. The definitive treatment is surgical. Complications are listed in Box 21.12.

> **Box 21.12**   Complications of tetralogy of Fallot
>
> - Cyanotic episodes ('spells')
> - Polycythaemia/anaemia
> - Exercise limitation
> - Bleeding tendency
> - Cerebral thrombosis
> - Cerebral abscess
> - Bacterial endocarditis
> - Cerebral anoxia/death

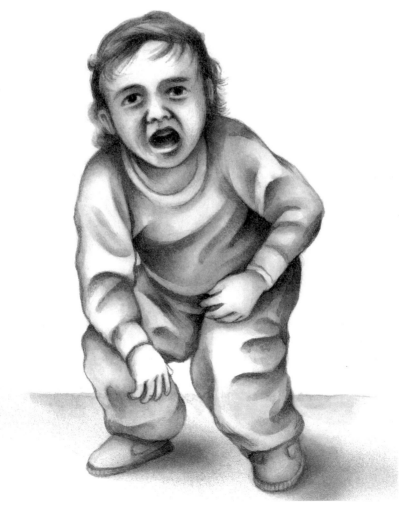

Figure 21.2   A 1-year-old child, breathless and squatting during a cyanotic episode. Squatting improves blood flow to the lungs.

Cardiac failure

The classic symptoms of heart failure in childhood are dyspnoea and tachypnoea with poor weight gain. Sweating is a cardinal sign in the first few months of life. The liver increases in size and becomes firm. Chest X-ray shows cardiomegaly and increased pulmonary vascular markings (*see* Box 21.13).

The commonest cause of heart failure in early infancy is a large left-to-right shunt through either a ventricular septal defect, a patent ductus arteriosus or an atrioventricular septal defect (*see* Boxes 21.14 and 21.15). Although these defects are present at birth, they do not become symptomatic until the pulmonary vascular resistance falls, thus creating a pressure difference between the left and right side of the heart. The additional blood flow to the right heart may cause hypertrophy and

Box 21.13 Signs and symptoms of heart failure
• Restlessness
• Excessive weight gain (acutely)
• Poor weight gain (chronically)
• Tachypnoea
• Tachycardia
• Sweating
• Gallop rhythm
• Cyanosis
• Hepatomegaly
• Oedema

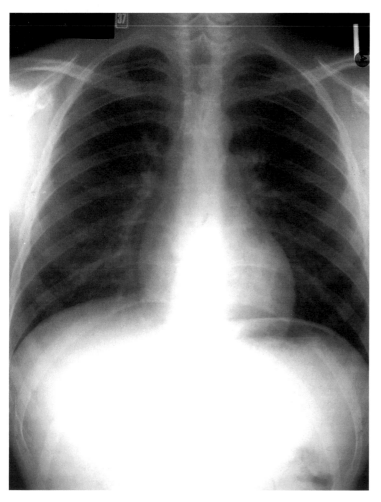

Figure 21.3 Chest X-ray showing a normal heart.

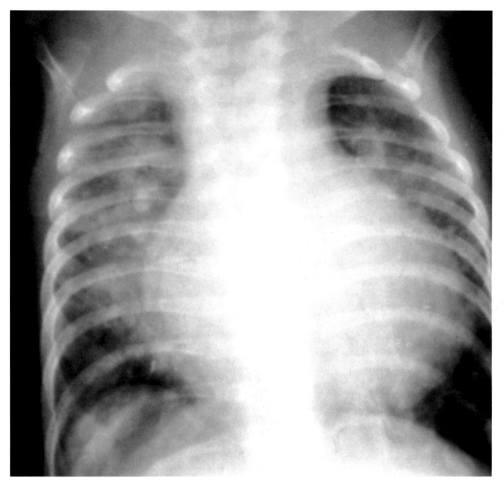

Figure 21.4   Chest X-ray showing an enlarged heart with pulmonary plethora.

dilatation of the right ventricle. The extra blood flows through the lungs, leading to pulmonary plethora (*see* Figure 21.4 contrasted with normal in Figure 21.3). Failure of the right ventricle leads to oedema, weight gain and hepatomegaly. The extra blood flow eventually compromises the left ventricle, which leads to pulmonary venous congestion and the symptoms of tachypnoea, dyspnoea, feeding difficulties and poor weight gain.

Around 30% of atrioventricular septal defects occur in children with Down syndrome, and all children with that syndrome need an echocardiogram to exclude this and other forms of congenital heart disease. In atrioventricular septal defect (AVSD), a mid-diastolic murmur may be heard (due to a relative narrowing of the mitral/tricuspid valve) and the ECG shows a 'superior' axis (i.e.

the QRS axis between –10° and –150°). (For other causes of heart failure in the first weeks and months, *see* Boxes 21.14 and 21.15.)

Box 21.14   Causes of heart failure in the neonate

- Coarctation of the aorta
- Hypoplastic left heart syndrome
- Critical aortic valve stenosis
- Myocardial ischaemia (secondary to birth asphyxia)
- Supraventricular tachycardia
- Severe cardiomyopathy/myocarditis

> **Box 21.15**   Causes of heart failure in infancy
>
> • Ventricular septal defect
>
> • Patent ductus arteriosus
>
> • Large ostium primum atrial septal defect
>
> • Atrioventricular septal defect
>
> • Anaemia
>
> • Supraventricular tachycardia
>
> • Arteriovenous fistula

The mainstay of treatment for acute cardiac failure is a combination of inotropic drugs (digoxin, dobutamine) to support cardiac contraction, diuretics to decrease preload, and vasodilators to decrease the afterload on the left ventricle. If medical management is not successful, blood flow to the lungs can be decreased by placing a band around the pulmonary artery, or the defect can be closed or corrected surgically.

If the excess pulmonary blood flow is not decreased, the pulmonary arterioles react by contracting. This increases the pulmonary vascular resistance which, if unabated, can cause irreversible pulmonary hypertension. As the pulmonary pressure increases to a value greater than that in the left ventricle, deoxygenated blood flows across the ventricular septal defect (a right-to-left shunt), causing permanent cyanosis. This is called Eisenmenger's syndrome, and the only hope of cure is a heart transplant.

Pyrexia and congenital heart disease

Children with congenital heart disease are at great risk of infective endocarditis (sometimes called subacute bacterial endocarditis) (*see* Box 21.16). Turbulent blood flow across the heart defect leads to platelet adhesion to the endocardium. Organisms in the bloodstream are caught within the platelet clot, and subsequently multiply and create vegetations. Pieces of these vegetations may slough and create septic emboli. Management consists of a 6-week course of the appropriate intravenous antibiotic(s).

The disease can be prevented by scrupulous dental hygiene and prophylactic antibiotics prior to and after dental or surgical procedures. It is imperative that children and their parents are educated about the prevention of infective endocarditis.

> **Box 21.16**   Infective endocarditis
>
> *Symptoms*
> • Fever
> • Malaise/lethargy
> • Loss of appetite
> • Pallor/anaemia
>
> *Signs*
> • Loud or new heart murmur
> • Splenomegaly
> • Splinter haemorrhages
> • Skin/conjunctival petechiae

Congenital heart disease in the neonate

In the first week of life, infants with congenital heart disease may present with signs of cardiac failure, cyanosis, or a mixture of the two (*see* Chapter 17). Most of these defects do not manifest themselves *in utero* because of the fetal circulation, but become apparent as the neonatal circulation is established (*see* Box 21.17), and particularly as the pulmonary arterial pressure falls.

Presentation of congenital heart disease in the first few weeks of life is commonly related to the

> **Box 21.17**   Circulation changes at birth
>
> • Pulmonary vascular resistance falls
>
> • Pulmonary blood flow increases
>
> • Systemic vascular resistance rises
>
> • Arterial duct closes
>
> • Foramen ovale closes
>
> • Ductus venosus closes

closure of the ductus arteriosus. When systemic blood flow is dependent on the arterial duct, the infant presents with heart failure. A common cause of duct-dependent systemic blood flow is critical coarctation of the aorta. If the coarctation is very narrow, blood can only reach the descending aorta from the pulmonary artery via the ductus arteriosus. When the ductus closes, the lower half of the body becomes poorly perfused, and acidosis and heart failure ensue.

When pulmonary blood flow is dependent on the arterial duct, the infant presents with cyanosis (*see* Box 21.18). In lesions such as atresia of the pulmonary or tricuspid valves, blood flow to the lungs is dependent on an open duct, since blood can only reach the pulmonary artery via the duct from the descending aorta. When the ductus closes, severe cyanosis ensues. The immediate treatment for any lesion whose presentation is precipitated by duct closure is the infusion of prostaglandin to keep the duct open while definitive diagnosis and management plans are made.

Box 21.18   Causes of cyanosis in the first postnatal week

- Transposition of the great arteries
- Pulmonary atresia
- Severe tetralogy of Fallot
- Tricuspid atresia
- Ebstein's anomaly of the tricuspid valve
- Total anomalous pulmonary venous drainage

Case study 2

Hannah was born at 36 weeks' gestation by emergency Caesarean section for breech presentation. She spent 1 week in special care because of feeding problems. She was breastfed for the first 4 months of life. At her 8-month assessment her mother commented that Hannah had developed blue lips and face while crawling and moving in her baby walker. She was still feeding well and thriving. On clinical examination she was pink, but had a harsh, pansystolic murmur best heard at the lower left sternal border radiating through to the back. There was an associated precordial thrill. In view of the history and clinical findings (which were not suggestive of an innocent murmur), she was referred for a cardiac opinion.

On clinical examination she was pink with normal pulses, but there was a systolic thrill with an associated loud ejection systolic murmur at the upper left sternal border. The ECG showed right-axis deviation and right ventricular hypertrophy, and the chest X-ray revealed oligaemic lung fields and a right-sided aortic arch. The diagnosis of tetralogy of Fallot was confirmed on echocardiography.

Hannah started to walk unaided at 10 months of age. By the age of 1 year, her mother noted that she had a tendency to squat after she had been walking. She was again cyanosed and slightly breathless. On one occasion she developed deep cyanosis, lost consciousness for a few seconds, and became extremely pale. In view of these symptoms she was started on propranolol, which improved her considerably until the time came for definitive surgery.

Further reading

- Moss AJ *et al.* (2000) *Moss and Adams Heart Disease in Infants, Children and Adolescents.* Lippincott, Williams & Wilkins, Baltimore, MD.

- Anderson RH *et al.* (1998) *Paediatric Cardiology.* Churchill Livingstone, Edinburgh.

- Jordan SC and Scott O (1989) *Heart Disease in Paediatrics* (3e). Butterworth Heinemann, Sevenoaks.

Self-assessment questions

1 Squatting is a phenomenon:
(a) of pulmonary atresia — True/False
(b) of Fallot's tetralogy — True/False
(c) of respiratory embarrassment — True/False
(d) related to circulatory adjustment — True/False
(e) seen in infants who are not yet walking. — True/False

2 Factors that increase the risk of congenital heart disease include:
(a) Down syndrome — True/False
(b) group B streptococcal infection — True/False
(c) cytomegalovirus infection — True/False
(d) a family history of asthma — True/False
(e) maternal insulin-dependent diabetes. — True/False

3 Femoral pulses:
(a) should be felt as part of any examination of a child — True/False
(b) may be difficult to palpate in normal children — True/False
(c) are absent in cases of ventricular septal defect — True/False
(d) are absent if there is a patent arterial duct — True/False
(e) can only be assessed by using a Doppler probe. — True/False

4 Cyanotic congenital heart disease:
(a) is unlikely to be apparent at birth — True/False
(b) is immediately life-threatening — True/False
(c) may be mimicked by a metabolic disease — True/False
(d) may develop after a ventricular septal defect — True/False
(e) is associated with Down syndrome. — True/False

22 Prevention of illness and promotion of good health

- Prevention of illness
- Health promotion
- Health education
- Parent empowerment
- Community-based programmes
- Public policy and child health
- Health promotion programmes
- Health services for children
- Adolescent health services

In paediatrics, prevention is even more important than in other areas of medicine because of the impact that illness has on children's social life and achievement. Chronic illness has a major effect on educational attainment, and disability can entirely constrain a child's life chances. Prevention is also of proven effectiveness, and the means are well established. Yet still prevention in child health does not have the high profile in the UK which is conferred on it in other countries in Europe, in particular in Scandinavia. Prevention is best integrated with a curative approach, although the most effective preventive measures of all are outside the responsibility of the health sector (e.g. improvement in housing quality).

The term *prevention* is used when the aim is to reduce the prevalence or severity of particular illnesses or conditions. The term *health promotion* is used when the aim is to promote good health and well-being. Thus the former is narrower in scope and perhaps more easy to measure in terms of outcome, whereas the latter is broad in scope and ultimately more likely to achieve a healthier society of children. Prevention falls clearly within the paediatric remit, whereas health promotion is a multisectoral activity (i.e. different sectors, such as education and roads departments, work together) and will usually be led by public health professionals or by politicians (*see* Box 22.1).

Box 22.1   Working together

- *Multidisciplinary*: several disciplines within healthcare working together (e.g paediatrics, general practice, nursing and speech therapy).

- *Multi-agency*: several different agencies working together (e.g. health, social services, education and voluntary organisations working together to provide services in a locality).

- *Multisectoral*: different sectors within the local authority working together at a high level (e.g. health, housing and recreation working together on a local environmental improvement).

This chapter covers both prevention and health promotion, and will provide examples demonstrating evidence of effectiveness and opportunities for incorporation into everyday work.

Prevention of illness

Prevention can be classified as primary, secondary or tertiary.

- *Primary prevention*: reduction in the number of new cases of a disease, disorder or condition (e.g. immunisation, accident prevention).

- *Secondary prevention*: reduction in the prevalence of a disease by shortening its duration or decreasing its impact through early detection and prompt intervention (e.g. screening).

- *Tertiary prevention*: reduction in impairment and disability, and minimisation of suffering (e.g. team management of cerebral palsy).

Primary prevention

This is the most effective and desirable form of prevention, but unfortunately there are few examples of it in real life. The best and perhaps only good example is *immunisation* to prevent infectious disease. Other examples are listed in Box 22.2.

Box 22.2   Primary prevention

- Immunisation

- Prevention of suddent infant death syndrome through *Back to Sleep* campaign

- Prevention of smoking through banning tobacco advertising

- Prevention of pedestrian accidents through traffic calming

- Prevention of head injury in child cyclists through use of cycle helmets

- Prevention of fire deaths through smoke alarms

- Prevention of ingestion of medicines through issue of child-proof containers

- Antenatal prevention by genetic counselling and provision of folic acid supplements to the mother

---

Note that immunisation is the best example of primary prevention which is organised within the health system and where paediatricians play a key role. Thus it is vital that all doctors have a thorough understanding of how it works and the main schedules.

There follows a detailed discussion of immunisation as an example of primary prevention.

Rationale for immunisation in the UK

Immunisation is the central tool for the prevention of infectious disease. It has been shown to be effective in the control of the diseases listed in Box 22.3, and Figures 2.1 and 2.2 (*see* Chapter 2) illustrate the benefit for measles and for *Haemophilus influenzae*, respectively. Although other factors are important for infectious disease control, specifically good hygiene, clean water and effective sewage, once these are present then immunisation has been critical in further reducing incidence and leading towards eradication, which should now be the goal in the UK and Europe.

Box 22.3   Immunisable diseases in the UK

• Pertussis

• Diphtheria

• Tetanus

• Polio

• Measles

• Mumps

• Rubella

• *Haemophilus influenzae*

• Meningococcus type C

• Tuberculosis (TB)

• Hepatitis B (not part of routine programme)

Problems and controversies of immunisation

There have been two public issues in relation to immunisation in the last two decades which illustrate how important the issue of public confidence is, and also how significant the role of the press is.

Pertussis

In the 1970s, reports began to emerge of 'brain damage' following the whooping cough immunisation. It has always been known that side-effects of this immunisation are relatively common, including prolonged crying, high temperature, occasionally convulsions and also local effects of redness and swelling at the site of injection. These were not considered to cause lasting damage, whereas whooping cough itself is a very nasty illness. However, public confidence suffered and

a support group of parents started to report cases of children who developed encephalopathy with convulsions after the injection, and there was a subsequent drop in vaccine uptake. This in turn led to a resurgence of pertussis between 1975 and 1985 (*see* Figure 22.1).

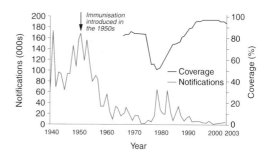

Figure 22.1   Pertussis notifications and vaccine coverage for children by their second birthday in England and Wales, 1940–2003. *Source*: Health Protection Agency; Department of Health.

It was not until a nationwide study of children with encephalopathy was published in 1981 that it was established that there was no increased incidence after vaccine and the association in time was coincidental rather than causal. It was concluded that the risk of a normal child developing a serious central nervous system illness due to pertussis immunisation was 1 in 110 000 immunisations, and the risk of suffering permanent brain damage was 1 in 310 000.

Over this period many articles in the tabloid press warned against the dangers of whooping cough vaccine, yet the scientific basis for the concerns was slight. However, this crisis did highlight the need for the public to be given more detailed and accurate information about the side-effects of vaccines, something that had not really happened until that time.

Measles

A similar situation developed during the 1990s in relation to measles vaccine. This was at a time when public confidence in Government announcements on the safety of food had been blunted following the BSE epidemic. A study was published in *The Lancet* in 1998 which proposed a link between measles immunisation and both

Crohn's disease and autism. The scientific evidence for this link has now been disproved. However, as with pertussis, this report was taken up by the press and a support group was set up by parents who thought that their child's autism had been caused by immunisation. There is a temporal association, as autism is often identified around the beginning of the second year of life, which is when the MMR vaccine is administered. Autism is a very serious disorder that puzzles parents and leads to lifelong disability, and its cause is not known.

Some parents were also concerned about the ability of the body to mount a response to three vaccines given at one time.

The purported links between measles immunisation and autism were widely taken up by the press and led to very widespread anxiety among parents, with a not surprisingly adverse impact on the vaccine coverage (see Table 22.1).

Table 22.1 Proportion of 2-year-olds receiving the MMR vaccine in the UK

Dates	Percentage vaccine coverage
April–June 1995	92.5%
April–June 1998	89.7%
April–June 2001	84.2%
April–June 2002	81.0%

There was also a demand from parents' groups for the Department of Health to provide single-agent vaccines for measles, mumps and rubella, rather than the combined vaccine, so that parents who wished to do so could choose to omit measles. The Department of Health was adamant that this should not be done, as it would impair uptake and would be less effective as well as more painful for the child. However, private clinics sprang up which offered the monovalent vaccines, and some of these practised unethically.

Meanwhile, further studies were being conducted which failed to substantiate the early paper, and showed no link between autism and measles vaccination. Health professionals and their organisations are united in the view that MMR is effective and not the serious risk to health that the media portrayed it to be.

So what were the lessons of this unfortunate story? First, the Government and health professionals should be as open and honest about side-effects as possible, otherwise they will be accused of a cover-up. Secondly, parents' lobbying groups can be very effective in pursuing interests which are sometimes misguided, and we have to listen to and work with them. Thirdly, the tabloid media in the UK in general pays little attention to science and will take up issues largely on the basis of whether they will increase sales.

Immunisation schedule in the UK

The current UK immunisation schedule is shown in Box 22.4.

Box 22.4 Immunisation schedule

2 months	DPT + HIB + Men C (combined), oral polio
3 months	DBT + HIB + Men C (combined), oral polio
4 months	DBT + HIB + Men C (combined), oral polio
13 months	MMR 1
3 years	MMR 2, DPT, oral polio
11 years	BCG for children testing Heaf negative
16 years	DT, oral polio

DPT, diphtheria, pertussis, tetanus; DT, diphtheria, tetanus; MMR, measles, mumps, rubella; HIB, *Haemophilus influenzae* type b; Men C, meningococcus C.

Contraindications to immunisation are shown in Box 22.5.

Box 22.5 Contraindications to immunisation: genuine and mythical

Genuine	Mythical
Severe reaction	Epilepsy
Egg anaphylaxis	Febrile convulsion
(measles)	Mild reaction to egg
	Temperature
	Teething
	Eczema

Secondary prevention

This is the type of prevention practised most often in the health service, but only a small number of conditions are amenable to this approach. The main types of secondary prevention are shown in Box 22.6.

Secondary prevention is potentially a very effective type of prevention, and as applied to phenylketonuria has virtually ended the severe handicap which resulted from this debilitating condition.

Box 22.6 Secondary prevention

- Screening for phenylketonuria, hypothyroidism, cystic fibrosis, sensorineural hearing loss, etc. (see under description of child health promotion programme)

- Early detection of growth failure, short stature, developmental delay, parenting problems

---

However, for an effective screening programme to be established, certain criteria have to be fulfilled (*see* Box 22.7) and this can be difficult to achieve. In addition, setting up a screening programme is fraught with difficulty. A high coverage of the population for the test must be achieved and maintained, and there must be an efficient system for dealing with those who are test positive. Parents undergo a period of severe anxiety when told that their child may have a severe condition, and therefore this period should be kept as short as possible.

The pathway of screening for phenylketonuria is shown in Box 22.8, and the schedule for screening for childhood conditions in the UK is shown in Box 22.9.

Box 22.7 Criteria for a successful screening programme

1 The condition should be an important public health problem as judged by the potential for heath gain achievable by early diagnosis.

2 There should be an accepted treatment *or other beneficial intervention* for patients with recognised *or occult* disease.

3 Facilities for diagnosis and treatment should be available and shown to be working effectively for classic cases of the condition in question.

4 There should be a latent or early symptomatic stage, and the extent to which this can be recognised by parents and professionals should be known.

5 There should be a suitable test or examination. It should be simple, valid for the condition in question, reasonably priced, repeatable in different trials or circumstances, sensitive and specific. The test should be acceptable to the *majority* of the population.

6 The natural history of the condition *and of conditions which may mimic it* should be understood.

7 There should be an agreed definition of what is meant by a case of the target disorder, and also an agreement as to (i) which other conditions are likely to be detected by the screening programme and (ii) whether their detection will be an advantage or a disadvantage.

8 Treatment in the early, latent or presymptomatic phase should favourably influence the prognosis, *or improve the outcome for the family as a whole.*

9 The cost of screening should be economically balanced in relation to expenditure on the care and treatment of individuals with the disorder and to medical care as a whole.

10 Case finding may need to be a continuous process and not a 'once and for all' project, but *there should be explicit justification for repeated screening procedures or stages.*

Source: adapted from Wilson and Jungner, by Elliman D and Hall D (2003) *Health for All Children* (4e). Oxford University Press, Oxford.

Box 22.8 Screening for phenylketonuria

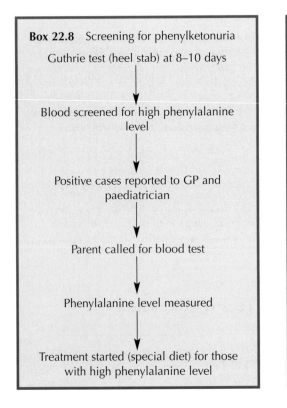

Guthrie test (heel stab) at 8–10 days

↓

Blood screened for high phenylalanine level

↓

Positive cases reported to GP and paediatrician

↓

Parent called for blood test

↓

Phenylalanine level measured

↓

Treatment started (special diet) for those with high phenylalanine level

---

Box 22.9 Screening schedule in UK child health promotion programme

- *Birth*: physical examination for cataract, congenital heart disease, congenital dislocation of the hips and undescended testes; test for sensorineural hearing loss under development.

- *10 days*: Guthrie test for hypothyroidism, phenylketonuria, cystic fibrosis.

- *6 weeks*: physical examination for cataract, congenital heart disease, congenital dislocation of the hips and undescended testes.

- *7–9 months*: distraction test for hearing (now being phased out in favour of neonatal screening).

- *4 years*: orthoptic test for visual defects.

- *4–5 years (school entry)*: height measurement for short stature.

Source: Elliman D and Hall D (2003) *Health for All Children* (4e). Oxford University Press, Oxford.

Child health surveillance has been used to cover the oversight of the physical, social and emotional health and development of all children. *Health for All Children* suggests that child health surveillance should be regarded as synonymous with secondary prevention.

Tertiary prevention

This term is applied to chronic and disabling conditions which, if inadequately treated, will lead to increasing handicap. A good example is cerebral palsy. If neglected, this condition could result in a child who is immobile with a very limited independent life. If treated by physiotherapists, surgeons and paediatricians, the same child could achieve independent mobility and pursue a full-time education, perhaps in a mainstream school. The ingredients of tertiary prevention are a multidisciplinary team of therapists and physicians, and support from social services and education with full partnership with the parents, together with effective coordination between the various arms of the service.

Box 22.10 lists examples of conditions for which tertiary prevention is necessary.

Box 22.10   Tertiary prevention

- *Cerebral palsy*: mobility and education.
- *Spina bifida*: mobility and education.
- *Muscular dystrophy*: mobility.
- *Diabetes mellitus*: prevention of blindness and ischaemic damage.
- *Down syndrome*: prevention of side-effects of heart disease, thyroid disease, education.

Box 22.11   Faculty of Public Health Medicine: 10 areas of public health practice

- Surveillance and assessment of the population's health and well-being
- Protecting and promoting health and well-being
- Developing quality within an evaluative culture which puts research evidence into practice and manages risk
- Managing, analysing and interpreting information, knowledge and statistics
- Prioritising and providing professional advice in health and healthcare
- Policy and strategy development and implementation
- Developing communities, advocating for health and reducing inequalities
- Strategic leadership for health and well-being across all sectors
- Education, research and development
- Managing self, people and resources and practising ethically

---

Health promotion

Health promotion is any planned measure which improves physical or mental health or prevents disease, disability and premature death. Child health promotion can encompass interventions in curative medicine, education, the environment or public policy.

Public health can be defined as 'the science of preventing disease, prolonging life and promoting health through the organised efforts of society'. The *fields of public health practice* are listed in Box 22.11.

Child public health has been defined as the organised efforts of society to promote child and young people's health, to prevent disease and to foster equity for children and young people within a framework of sustainable development.

Health education

Health education is any activity that promotes health through learning. Thus it is aimed at areas where there is a deficiency of knowledge or information. Health education is a very important component of health promotion, but will only succeed in changing health-related behaviour in parents or children (i) if knowledge is lacking in the first place and is wanted by the person concerned, and (ii) if the individual has the capacity to change their behaviour. Thus, for example, information on the prevention of home accidents is desirable and may be appreciated, but if the parent cannot afford to buy stairgates or fireguards, change is unlikely to occur.

Parent empowerment

This means improving the ability of parents to take decisions for themselves. Many parents, particularly from disadvantaged backgrounds, do not feel in control when talking with professionals and others in positions of influence. They also do not sense that they can change their own lives, but rather they feel that they are the victims of events and of those around them. For paediatricians, parent empowerment means helping the parent of their patient to be in charge of the child's management. This requires knowledge and support which should be reduced as the parent becomes more confident.

Community-based programmes

An important theme within health promotion is working with communities to bring about change in the factors that affect health. Such programmes involve health professionals and social workers joining with community groups and following local priorities for improvement. A current Government initiative entitled 'SureStart' works to these principles in order to improve the health and education of children up to 4 years of age.

The aims of the national programme are described below (*see also* Box 22.12).

Box 22.12 'SureStart'

SureStart is a Government-funded scheme that aims to target poor inner-city areas and provide additional services for children under 4 years of age and their parents. The aim is to overcome the effects of early deprivation on child health and development, by providing enhanced health, educational and social services in an integrated way. This could include additional health visiting, early reading support for children, nurseries and parents' groups. Priorities are set by local residents, who play an important part in the service development.

The targets for one local scheme are as follows.

1 *Improving social and emotional development*
   - 100% of families with young children to have been contacted by local programmes within the first 2 months of birth
   - Early identification and appropriate support of parents with postnatal depression
   - A reduction in the number of children aged 0–3 years re-registered on the Child Protection Register

2 *Improving health*
   - Smoking: a reduction in the percentage of children in the SureStart area whose parents smoke during the child's first 2 years of life
   - Parenting support and information to be available for all parents in SureStart areas
   - All local programmes to give guidance on breastfeeding hygiene and safety, with particular emphasis on the increasing uptake at birth, 6 weeks and 4 months
   - A reduction in the number of children aged 0–3 years admitted to hospital as an emergency with gastroenteritis, a respiratory infection or severe injury.

Aims and objectives of SureStart

SureStart aims to achieve better outcomes for children, parents and communities by:

- increasing the availability of childcare for all children

- improving health, education and emotional development for young children

- supporting parents in their role and in developing their employment aspirations.

This will be achieved by:

- helping services to develop in disadvantaged areas, while providing financial help to enable parents to afford quality childcare

- rolling out the principles that drive the SureStart approach to all services for children and parents.

Principles of SureStart

SureStart supports families from pregnancy right through until children are 14 years of age, including those with special educational needs, and for those with disabilities up to age 16 years. The guiding principles, drawing on best practice in early education, childcare and SureStart local programmes, are described below.

Working with parents and children

Every family should have access to a range of services that will deliver better outcomes for both children and parents, meeting their needs and stretching their aspirations.

Services for everyone

The same service is not appropriate for everyone. Families have distinctly different needs, both between different families, in different locations and over time in the same family. Services should recognise and respond to these varying needs.

Flexible at point of delivery

All services should be designed to encourage access. For example, issues such as opening hours, location, transport issues and care for other children in the family need to be considered. Wherever possible we must enable families to get the health and family support services that they need through a single point of contact.

Starting very early

Services for young children and parents should start at the first antenatal visit.

This means not only advice on health in pregnancy, but also preparation for parenthood, decisions about returning to work (or indeed starting to work) after the birth, and advice on childcare options and support services available.

Respectful and transparent

Services should be customer driven, whether or not the service is free.

Community driven and professionally coordinated

All professionals with an interest in children and families should be sharing expertise and listening to local people about service priorities. This should be done through consultation and by day-to-day listening to parents.

Outcome driven

All services for children and parents need to have as their core purpose better outcomes for children. The Government needs to acknowledge this by reducing bureaucracy and simplifying funding to ensure a 'joined-up' approach with partners.

Public policy and child health

Improving child health has a lot to do with politics. Box 22.13 illustrates some of the problems relating to children's health which require Government policy before they can be relieved. A change in policy can only come about by political lobbying or advocacy.

Box 22.13 Child health problems that require a political action

Problem	Political action
Alcohol and drug misuse	Greater control over under-age sales
Obesity	Control of advertising of convenience foods
Child abuse	Banning of corporal punishment
Pedestrian and bicycle accidents	Traffic calming and cycle lanes
Dental caries	Fluoridation of water
Smoking	Control of sales and banning of smoking in public places

---

Health promotion programmes

The following brief examples illustrate how programmes in three key areas might operate.

Injury prevention through the use of cycle helmets

Cycle helmets are known to prevent head injuries in cyclists but are not widely used in the UK, particularly by children, who are the main users of bicycles. This is partly because of cost and partly related to image. Most teenagers consider that helmets are not 'cool' to wear. Also there is little support for helmet wearing from cycle organisations, which consider that they target the victim (the cyclist) rather than the culprit (the motorist).

However, this point of view is not helpful to a teenage victim who is brain damaged after a serious injury on a bike. It would seem sensible to try to increase helmet use while also improving facilities for cyclists and slowing down traffic speeds.

Box 22.14 lists some possible ways of increasing helmet usage by children.

Box 22.14 Possible ways of increasing helmet usage by children

- Legislation to make it compulsory
- Providing low-cost helmets through schools
- Giving media publicity to local youth leaders or celebrities who wear helmets
- Ensuring that all children in cycle clubs wear a helmet
- Providing publicity for helmets on head-injury wards
- Cycle safety classes in primary schools with information on helmet use
- Local newspaper to run a campaign on helmets, with a competition for a slogan

The promotion of breastfeeding

Breastfeeding is known to improve health by reducing both intestinal and respiratory infections, and may well have several other health benefits to both child and mother. Yet the percentage of mothers who start breastfeeding in the UK languishes at around 70%, with a very high social class divide and a rapid fall-off after 6 weeks, when the maximum benefit accrues. What can be done to improve this unfortunate situation? There are many factors outside the health service which need to be addressed (e.g. maternity leave which recognises the advantages of breastfeeding), and few interventions of proven effectiveness. Some of these are listed in Box 22.15.

Box 22.15 Interventions to promote breastfeeding that have been demonstrated to work

- Placing the infant on the breast shortly after birth

- Good advice and support with regard to 'latching on'

- No separation of the infant from the mother in the first week (baby rooms in with mother)

- No use of supplementary milk or water in the first few weeks

- Peer support after discharge from hospital

Box 22.16 UNICEF Baby Friendly hospital criteria: 10 steps

1 Have a written policy that is routinely communicated to all healthcare staff.

2 Train all healthcare staff in the skills necessary to implement the policy.

3 Inform all pregnant women about the benefits and management of breast-feeding.

4 Help mothers to initiate breastfeeding within half an hour of birth.

5 Show mothers how to breastfeed and how to maintain lactation even if they are separated from their infants.

6 Give newborn infants no food or drink other than breast milk, unless medically indicated.

7 Practise rooming-in, allowing mothers and infants to remain together 24 hours a day.

8 Encourage breastfeeding on demand.

9 Give no artificial teats or pacifiers to breastfeeding infants.

10 Foster the establishment of breastfeeding support groups, and refer mothers to them on discharge from hospital.

UNICEF has developed the Baby Friendly award, which will denote hospitals and community facilities which ensure that staff follow the above standards. The 10 steps to successful breastfeeding to be followed by a hospital before it is designated Baby Friendly are listed in Box 22.16.

Thus the first steps to be taken to improve uptake should be to introduce baby-friendly criteria both in hospital and in the community, and to establish peer support for breastfeeding mothers after discharge from hospital.

The promotion of good parenting to prevent behavioural problems

Behavioural problems are extremely common in children at present, and lead to poor child mental health, family stress and reduced individual achievement. Such problems are known to stem from the ways in which parents manage their infants at an early age.

Parents state that they need more support and information both on infant development and on how to respond to infant and child behaviour. It is known that parent training is effective in enabling parents to improve their management. Yet such training is not universally available. There is an evidence base for the development of such training based on the work of Webster-Stratton.

Box 22.17 lists ways in which good parenting can be promoted in order to reduce the prevalence of behaviour problems.

Box 22.17 Ways to promote good parenting

- Group parenting programme

- Information and support from health visitors

- Age-paced parenting newsletter (information sent out every month to new parents)

- Support given to parents through child-care and nursery (e.g. SureStart)

- Poverty reduction programmes

- Adequately funded parental leave

Health services for children

This section covers the organisation of health services for children in the UK. Only a brief summary will be given, as the services are prone to frequent reorganisation.

Primary care

Primary care is the first level of care for child and family health. It is provided by general practitioners working as part of a *primary care team*, whose membership is shown in Box 22.18.

> **Box 22.18**   Primary care team members
>
> - GPs
> - Practice nurse
> - Health visitor (mainly pre-school children)
> - School nurse (school-aged children)
> - Practice nurse (nursing duties in the surgery including immunisation)
> - Nurse practitioner (nurse who is trained to make a diagnosis and give treatment without a doctor present)
> - District nurse (undertakes nursing duties in the home, mainly with chronically ill adults and the elderly)
> - Midwife
> - Receptionist
> - Secretaries
> - Practice manager (manages practice staff)
>
> Note: many practices will also have a counsellor and a visiting psychologist and dietitian.

Secondary care

Secondary healthcare consists of the specialist services to which the primary care team refers patients. These services are usually hospital based, but increasingly specialist services are provided in the community. Secondary child health services are listed in Box 22.19.

> **Box 22.19**   Secondary child health services
>
> - Consultant paediatrician
> - Paediatric surgeon
> - Speech therapist
> - Physiotherapist
> - Occupational therapist
> - Child psychiatrist
> - Child psychologist
> - Play therapist
> - Specialist children's nurse (e.g. diabetic nurse)

Other children's services: education and social services

The local authority provides a number of services for children that work closely with the health services. These services mainly come under social services and education, and are summarised in Boxes 22.20 and 22.21.

> **Box 22.20**   Social services work with children
>
> - Child protection (for children at risk of abuse)
> - Children being looked after (children in care)
> - Children in need
> - Children's homes
> - Adoption and fostering
> - Youth offender teams
> - Children with a disability

Box 22.21   Special education services for children

- Special schools

- Special units in mainstream schools

- Local education authority support services (e.g. visually disabled, hearing impaired)

- Educational psychology service (for assessment of children with learning difficulties)

- Educational welfare service (for school non-attenders)

- School support:
  - Special educational needs coordinator
  - Teaching assistant
  - Behaviour support teacher
  - Guidance teacher

Social services are the lead agency for child protection, and are responsible for the initial assessment, organising child protection case conferences, maintaining a Child Protection Register, setting up a management plan and monitoring the care of children on the Child Protection Register. They have important preventive functions with families, too, but in view of the high media profile of child protection work, the latter tends to dominate their staff time, sometimes to the disadvantage of children in need. Social workers have a close working relationship with child health services, especially with paediatricians and health visitors, in relation to families in need and children on the Child Protection Register.

Adolescent health services

Adolescent or teenage health has been largely ignored in the UK in the past, but is now being considered an important area for health investment. It is known that adolescents have distinctive health needs, which include mental health, sexual health, sports injuries, chronic illness and disability. At present adolescents do not readily access services themselves, and in hospitals there are rarely separate facilities for teenagers either as inpatients or as outpatients. A more adolescent-friendly service would enable more effective treatment, and would also help young people to take responsibility for their own health. (*See* Chapter 23 for further discussion of this period of transition.)

Further reading

- Blair M, Stewart-Brown S, Waterston T and Crowther R (2003) *Child Public Health*. Oxford University Press, Oxford.

- Department of Health (1996) *Immunisation Against Infectious Disease – 'The Green Book'*. DoH, London. Updated information is now available via the DoH website, www.dh.gov.uk.

- Elliman D and Hall D (2003) *Health for All Children* (4e). Oxford University Press, Oxford.

- Polnay L (ed.) (2002) *Community Paediatrics*. Churchill Livingstone, Edinburgh.

Useful website

- UNICEF Baby Friendly; www.babyfriendly. org.uk

Self-assessment questions

1   Which of the following are immunisable diseases?
(a) measles   True/False
(b) RSV bronchiolitis   True/False
(c) polio   True/False
(d) rotavirus infection   True/False
(e) *Haemophilus influenzae.*   True/False

2   Which of the following meet the criteria for an effective screening test?
(a) Guthrie test for phenylketonuria   True/False
(b) Denver developmental screening   True/False
(c) measurement of weight at school entry   True/False
(d) Ortolani test on hips at 6 weeks.   True/False

3   SureStart:
(a) is an injury prevention programme   True/False
(b) is aimed at all children in the UK   True/False
(c) brings together health, social services and education   True/False
(d) includes early reading programmes.   True/False

4   The primary care team:
(a) is for primary-school children   True/False
(b) may include a psychologist   True/False
(c) may include a paediatrician   True/False
(d) covers patients only in a defined geographical area.   True/False

23 Looking forward to adult life

- Definitions
- Legal aspects
- Hazards of adolescence
- Sexual health
- Transition to 'adult' care

Definitions

Transition from childhood to adult life (adolescence) has a broad range of definitions. In North America it has developed as a medical specialty in its own right within an age band spanning 15–25 years. It encompasses a period of life when physical, psychological and sociological maturity and independence are intermingled. The North American definition is one of convenience, as it recognises the transition from paediatricians who care for families and children to the physicians and surgeons who care for adults. Physical maturation becomes established in girls at around the age of 12 years, with the onset of menarche or first menstrual period at approximately 13 years of age, although this has a wide variation (from 9 to 18 years). There is no such clear-cut identifier in boys, but peak height velocity, which is associated with sexual maturation, occurs at around the age of 12 years in girls and approximately 2 years later in boys. This gender difference has important implications, as girls not only mature physically in advance of boys but they also tend to achieve adult attributes ahead of them. This is reflected by the fact that young women tend to leave the family home and establish their independence several years ahead of their male counterparts.

Legal aspects

Ratification of the *UN Convention on the Rights of the Child* by the UK Government in 1991 has been reflected in national legislation and has significant consequences for parents, young people and their carers. The Children Act (England and Wales 1989, Scotland 1995) enshrines some of the rights of young people and responsibility of their carers. This legislation supports previous legislation on the age of majority. Although 18 years is commonly regarded as the age of achieving full adult rights and responsibilities,

345

children of any age who are able to understand what is being proposed for them, whether it be medical or surgical treatment or custody arrangements, must be involved in the decision-making process. With regard to the age at which a child must be included in these important decisions there is not a lower age limit, but certainly by the age of 12 years children and young people need to be involved in consent for any medical or surgical interventions that are proposed for them. Confidentiality must also be maintained unless there are overriding reasons why this should not be so. Young people have the right to have confidential information about them withheld from their parents/guardians if they so desire. This has been tested in the English courts for contraceptive advice in young people under 16 years of age.

Hazards of adolescence (see Boxes 23.1 and 23.2)

Growing up involves the adolescent in a variety of learning experiences, experimentation, and 'testing the boundaries' of rules and accepted social practices. A desire to take part in 'risk taking' is normal during the transition to adulthood.

Box 23.1   Adolescence

- Age range 12–25 years
- Physical and psychological maturation occurs earlier in girls
- A period of physical change and emotional turbulence

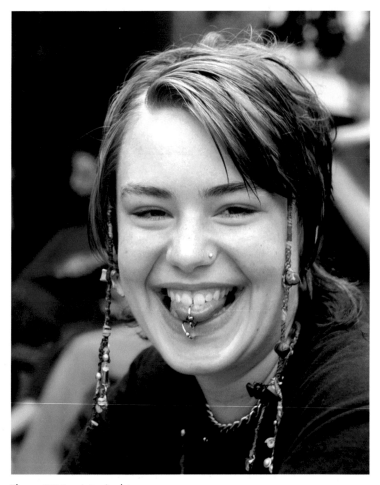

Figure 23.1   A typical teenager.

> **Box 23.2**   Characteristics of adolescence
>
> - Changing physiology
> - Establishing independence
> - Experimentation and risk taking
> - Setting of lifetime patterns (e.g. smoking, sexual behaviour)
> - Developing self-esteem and value system

Some of the commonest reasons for admission to hospital at this age are attributable to behavioural factors rather than to any disease process. In male adolescents, the most common reason for hospital admission is head injuries and open wounds. The incidence of deliberate self-poisoning increases with age. One-third of all legal abortions are in females under the age of 20 years, and young people between 16 and 24 years of age account for almost 60% of driver fatalities, although they represent only 20% of licensed drivers.

In addition to these demands on health services by young people, the development of various lifestyles can have important implications for emerging adult patterns of living across the lifespan, as the evidence about smoking, drinking, diet and physical inactivity reveals. Young people with a chronic health problem such as asthma or diabetes may be particularly 'at risk' in adolescence by taking on embryonic forms of certain aspects of lifestyle, such as smoking (*see* Figure 23.2) or drug use in association with their peers or in order to imitate an admired adult role model or protest against parental values. Attempting to prevent the development of unhealthy lifestyles in adolescence may be the best way of reducing a number of health risks in adulthood, particularly for those with a chronic illness.

A number of models of adolescent behaviour have been proposed, including the 'focal' theory of Coleman (1990), which suggests that concerns about gender role peaks at around the age of 13 years, concerns about acceptance or rejection by peers become more important at around 15 years of age, while issues relating to the gaining independence from parents climb steadily to peak beyond 16 years and then tail off towards the early to mid twenties (*see* Figure 23.3). The fact that adolescents do not usually cope with all of these crises at the same time but meet them

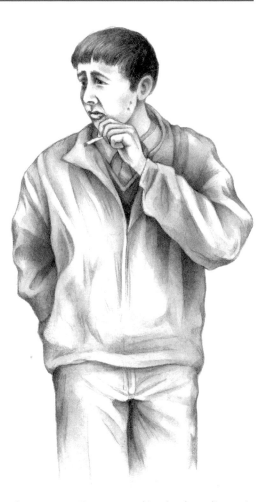

Figure 23.2   Teenage smoking leads to disease in later life.

sequentially may provide some resolution of the paradoxes of the huge amount of disruption and crisis implicit in adolescence, yet the relatively successful adaptation to adulthood and maturity in the majority of cases.

In young people with the additional burden of chronic illness, attention needs to be given to their and their parents'/guardians' coping skills. A recurrent theme is the need to establish independence while helping parents to come to terms with the 'loss' of their dependent sick child, for whom they have hitherto taken full responsibility. Compliance with treatment is also a major concern, as failure to maintain a regular therapy can have serious immediate and long-term consequences for the health of the affected individual.

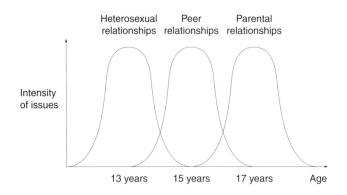

Figure 23.3 Coleman's focal theory.

General underlying principles in the Convention on the Rights of the Child

Box 23.3 Themes from the UN
Convention on the Rights of the Child

- Best interests of the child to be considered, particularly in family disputes
- Right to survival and development
- Respect and support for parents/carers
- Seek the child's view
- Maintain privacy and confidentiality
- Provide access to relevant information
- Protect from violence
- A right to education
- Rights of disabled
- Rights of minorities, protection from discrimination

The Committee on the Rights of the Child, the international body established to monitor governments'

progress in implementing the Convention, has identified five underlying principles that must be considered in the implementation of all other rights (*see also* Box 23.3).

- *Article 2*. All of the rights in the Convention apply to all children without discrimination on any grounds.

- *Article 3*. In all actions that affect children, their best interests must be a primary consideration.

- *Article 6*. All children have the right to life and optimal survival and development.

- *Article 12*. All children who are capable of expressing a view have the right to express that view freely and to have it taken seriously in accordance with their age and maturity.

- *Article 24*. All children have the right to the best possible health and access to healthcare.

For adolescents with a chronic illness there are a number of barriers that restrict their access to services. These are outlined in Box 23.4.

In addition, parents are less likely to be aware of their health needs at this age, and are therefore less likely to be in a position to encourage them to seek help. Good practice in privacy and confidentiality is described in Box 23.6.

Box 23.4   Barriers to access to services by adolescents with a chronic illness

- Health services are often not designed to accommodate the needs of teenagers.

- Adolescents are often reluctant to talk to doctors because they fear that their parents will be contacted. They want privacy but are not offered confidential advice and treatment.

- They are often embarrassed and uncomfortable talking with adults about personal issues.

- They may fear criticism or moral censure if they are seeking help with sexual or reproductive health issues.

Sexual health

There is no doubt that this area of human activity is a major challenge for young people and their parents and carers. The World Health Organization has defined sexual health as 'the integration of somatic, intellectual, emotional and social aspects of sexual being in ways that are positively enriching and that enhance personality, communication and love'. In making the transition to full adult maturity, many pitfalls await the adolescent. Social pressures on young people are enormous, with messages from the media portraying sex as glamorous and abstinence and contraception as dull and boring. Partner pressure may present the adolescent with challenges that he or she is unable to deal with. Recent surveys from Exeter in England have revealed that approximately 50% of all young people are sexually experienced by the age of 17 years, with 40% having engaged in sexual intercourse before the legal age of 16 years. Young people are not only at risk from their own experimentation and risk taking, but also they are at risk of exploitation. This further highlights their need for the principles of accessibility and confidentiality that are enshrined in the UN Convention. Sexual abusers can take advantage of young people's insecurity and need for acceptance (see Chapter 14, page 217).

Transition to 'adult' care

The pattern of transitional care outlined in the case study on page 351 is commonly adopted for children in their early teens, and is the first step towards full independence and regular follow-up in an adult-oriented service. Transfer to the adult service would traditionally take place somewhere between 16 and 18 years of age. Parents often find it difficult to separate from their children, particularly when they have hitherto been largely responsible for their medical management (see Figure 23.4). Unless responsibility for day-to-day management is transferred to young people, there is a danger that the medical management itself may become part of the natural testing of boundaries and the need to establish independence. In a life-threatening illness, such as cystic fibrosis, this compliance with therapy can quite literally mean the difference between early death and extended survival in relatively good health. Parents are aware of this fact, but with many young people their behaviour is not often linked to long-term consequences, and the young person him- or herself therefore has a rather different view. Peer pressure and the need to be accepted as 'one of the crowd' are other influences that are particularly strong in girls and young women. Having to take up to 10–12 pancreatic enzyme capsules with meals draws attention to oneself, and constant coughing and sputum production (a feature of the disease) are the kind of reasons often cited by young people for poor compliance or adherence to regular therapy. Establishing trust between healthcare professionals and young people and transferring responsibility for disease management and a healthy lifestyle to young people themselves are prerequisites for long-term future health, not only in the presence of chronic illness but also in those without health problems (see Boxes 23.5 and 23.6).

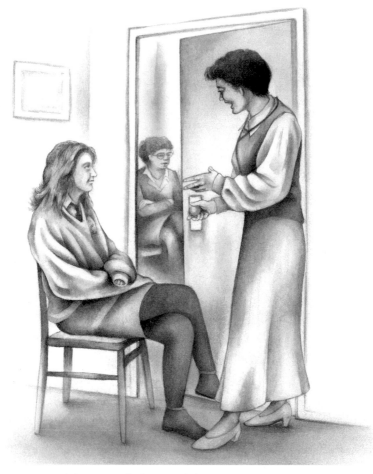

Figure 23.4 Adolescent with doctor, while parent looks on.

Box 23.5 Health service needs of adolescents

- Collaborative, not directive
- Confidentiality
- Managed transfer to adult services

Box 23.6 Confidentiality and privacy

We (medical practitioners) will:

- see you on your own, in private, if that is what you want
- always keep what you want to tell us confidential (unless there is a very good reason why we should not). If we do have to tell someone else, we will tell you who and why
- give you all the support you need if we are going to tell someone else
- make sure all our staff know about these rules on confidentiality.

Source: Child Health Rights (1995).

Case study 1

Anita, aged 13 years, was first diagnosed with cystic fibrosis after she presented with rectal pro-lapse and failure to thrive at 11 months of age. She has a brother John who is 2 years older than her, and her parents made the decision not to have any more children after the diagnosis was estab-lished. Anita has maintained normal growth and development on her pancreatic supplements, and has had three hospital admissions with respiratory exacerbations, one at age 7 years, one at age 11 years, and one 6 months ago. She acquired chronic *Pseudomonas* carriage in her sputum between the first and second admission. She has moderately severe disease with an FEV_1 of 70% predicted and no chest deformity. She is a regular sputum producer. She is a tall slim girl, with height on the 75th centile and weight on the 25th centile. She is well established in puberty, breast stage 3, but she has not started to menstruate yet. Her parents have both been very involved in her treatment, with most of the twice daily physiotherapy by postural drainage and percussion being performed by her mother. Both parents are active members of the local Cystic Fibrosis Group.

Anna's parents have a keen interest in recent genetic advances, and are anxiously awaiting the introduction of gene therapy or gene replacement. They hope that these advances may extend Anita's life well beyond her expected survival. In the mean time their objective is to keep her as well as possible with currently available treatments, for which they have hitherto been largely responsible. All responsible parents invest huge amounts of time and emotional energy in child-rearing, but these efforts are redoubled by the presence of chronic disease and illness. For most families living in industrialised countries the threat of chronic illness and risk of premature death is not an issue, making the burden of serious chronic illness even harder to bear and accept. Most parents experience feelings of loss at the passing of childhood and the changes in their children as they make the transition to adult life. A common challenge is to achieve a balance between accept-ance of the illness by the child and their parents and, at the other extreme, denial of the severity of the disease and resultant harm by failing to comply with the best possible medical treatments.

At Anita's next clinic visit both parents come with her, as is their usual practice. Anita appears uncharacteristically remote and does not take part in the interview. Her mother appears to show some irritation with Anita's persistent rudeness. Dr Jones suggests to Anita and her parents that perhaps Anita is reaching an age when she should be seen for at least part of the visit on her own. Anita's mother seems somewhat hurt and perplexed at this suggestion, but she agrees to it. Anita becomes more forthcoming and communicative when she is seen for 5 minutes on her own, and it is agreed that in future she will come into the consulting room at the beginning of the interview, and then invite her parents into the room to discuss the current situation and plans for the future. Anita is also taught how to perform chest physiotherapy herself using a forced expiration tech-nique, reserving the traditional postural drainage and percussion (which requires another person to perform the treatment) for significant respiratory exacerbations.

Further reading

- British Association of Community Child Health (1995) *Child Health Rights. A practitioner's guide.* British Association of Community Child Health, Royal College of Paediatrics and Child Health, London.

- Brook CGD (ed.) (1993) *The Practice of Medi-cine in Adolescence.* Edward Arnold, London.

- Coleman JC and Hendry LB (1990) *The Nature of Adolescence.* Routledge, London.

- McFarlane A (ed.) (1996) *Adolescent Medi-cine.* Royal College of Physicians, London.

- McFarlane A and McPherson A (1996) *The New Diary of a Teenage Health Freak.* Oxford University Press, Oxford.

- Royal College of Paediatrics and Child Health (2003) *Bridging the Gaps. Health care for ado-lescents.* Royal College of Paediatrics and Child Health, London.

Useful website

- www.teenagehealthfreak.org

Self-assessment questions

1 During adolescence:
(a) self-poisoning increases with age   True/False
(b) boys develop social skills more rapidly than girls   True/False
(c) experimentation and risk taking behaviours are common   True/False
(d) concerns about gender role peaks at around 18 years   True/False
(e) compliance with medical treatment becomes more reliable.   True/False

2 With regard to medical procedures:
(a) young people under 16 years require parental consent   True/False
(b) parents and legal guardians must be consulted   True/False
(c) completion of puberty is required before consent is regarded as legal   True/False
(d) consent without parental consultation is only legal for minor procedures   True/False
(e) competence in giving consent is not age dependent.   True/False

3 With regard to rights and responsibilities:
(a) young people have a right to confidentiality in all areas of sexual behaviour   True/False
(b) healthcare professionals can override young peoples' requests for
    confidentiality   True/False
(c) these have been defined in a UN Convention   True/False
(d) parental rights are paramount until the young person achieves 18 years   True/False
(e) if healthcare professionals disclose confidential information about young
    people they must explain why.   True/False

Answers to the self-assessment questions

Chapter 2

1
- (a) True
- (b) True
- (c) True
- (d) True

2
- (a) True
- (b) True
- (c) False
- (d) False

3
- (a) True
- (b) True
- (c) True
- (d) False

4
- (a) True
- (b) True
- (c) False
- (d) True

Chapter 3

1
- (a) False
- (b) False
- (c) True
- (d) True
- (e) True

2
- (a) True
- (b) False
- (c) True
- (d) True
- (e) False

3
- (a) True
- (b) False
- (c) False
- (d) True
- (e) True

4
- (a) False
- (b) True
- (c) True
- (d) True
- (e) False

Chapter 4

1
- (a) True
- (b) False
- (c) True
- (d) False
- (e) False

2
- (a) True
- (b) False
- (c) True
- (d) True
- (e) True

3
- (a) False
- (b) True
- (c) True
- (d) False
- (e) False

4
- (a) True
- (b) False
- (c) False
- (d) True
- (e) True

Chapter 5

1	2	3	4	5
(a) True	(a) True	(a) True	(a) True	(a) True
(b) False	(b) False	(b) False	(b) True	(b) False
(c) False	(c) True	(c) True	(c) False	(c) False
(d) True	(d) False	(d) False	(d) False	(d) True
(e) False	(e) True	(e) False	(e) True	(e) False

Chapter 6

1	2	3	4
(a) False	(a) False	(a) True	(a) True
(b) False	(b) True	(b) True	(b) False
(c) True	(c) True	(c) True	(c) False
(d) True	(d) True	(d) True	(d) True

Chapter 7

1	2	3	4
(a) True	(a) False	(a) False	(a) False
(b) False	(b) True	(b) False	(b) False
(c) False	(c) True	(c) True	(c) True
(d) True	(d) False	(d) True	(d) True
(e) True	(e) False	(e) True	(e) True

Chapter 8

1	2	3	4
(a) False	(a) False	(a) True	(a) True
(b) True	(b) False	(b) True	(b) False
(c) False	(c) True	(c) False	(c) True
(d) False	(d) False	(d) False	(d) False
(e) False	(e) True	(e) False	(e) True

Chapter 9

1	2	3	4
(a) False	(a) True	(a) True	(a) True
(b) True	(b) True	(b) True	(b) True
(c) False	(c) False	(c) False	(c) False
(d) True	(d) False	(d) False	(d) False

Chapter 10

1
- (a) False
- (b) False
- (c) True
- (d) True

2
- (a) False
- (b) True
- (c) False
- (d) False

3
- (a) True
- (b) False
- (c) False
- (d) True

4
- (a) False
- (b) True
- (c) False
- (d) True

Chapter 11

1
- (a) True
- (b) True
- (c) True
- (d) False

2
- (a) True
- (b) True
- (c) False
- (d) True

3
- (a) False
- (b) True
- (c) True
- (d) True

4
- (a) False
- (b) False
- (c) False
- (d) True

Chapter 12

1
- (a) True
- (b) True
- (c) True
- (d) False

2
- (a) False
- (b) False
- (c) True
- (d) True

3
- (a) True
- (b) False
- (c) True
- (d) True

4
- (a) False
- (b) True
- (c) True
- (d) False

Chapter 13

1
- (a) False
- (b) False
- (c) True
- (d) True

2
- (a) True
- (b) False
- (c) True
- (d) False

3
- (a) False
- (b) False
- (c) True
- (d) False

4
- (a) False
- (b) True
- (c) True
- (d) True

Chapter 14

1
- (a) False
- (b) True
- (c) True
- (d) True

2
- (a) True
- (b) True
- (c) True
- (d) True

3
- (a) True
- (b) True
- (c) True
- (d) True

4
- (a) False
- (b) True
- (c) False
- (d) True

Chapter 15

1	2	3	4
(a) False	(a) True	(a) True	(a) True
(b) True	(b) True	(b) True	(b) False
(c) False	(c) False	(c) True	(c) True
(d) True	(d) True	(d) False	(d) True
(e) True	(e) True	(e) False	(e) False

Chapter 16

1	2	3	4
(a) True	(a) False	(a) False	(a) False
(b) True	(b) True	(b) True	(b) False
(c) False	(c) True	(c) True	(c) False
(d) False	(d) False	(d) False	(d) False

Chapter 17

1	2	3	4
(a) False	(a) False	(a) False	(a) True
(b) False	(b) True	(b) False	(b) True
(c) True	(c) True	(c) False	(c) False
(d) True	(d) True	(d) True	(d) True
(e) False	(e) False	(e) False	(e) False

Chapter 18

1	2	3	4
(a) False	(a) True	(a) False	(a) True
(b) True	(b) True	(b) False	(b) True
(c) False	(c) True	(c) False	(c) True
(d) True	(d) False	(d) True	(d) False
(e) False	(e) True	(e) False	(e) False

Chapter 19

1	2	3	4
(a) True	(a) False	(a) False	(a) True
(b) True	(b) True	(b) True	(b) True
(c) False	(c) True	(c) True	(c) False
(d) True	(d) True	(d) False	(d) True

Chapter 20

1
(a) False
(b) True
(c) True
(d) True

2
(a) False
(b) True
(c) True
(d) False

3
(a) False
(b) True
(c) True
(d) False

4
(a) False
(b) False
(c) True
(d) True

Chapter 21

1
(a) False
(b) True
(c) False
(d) True
(e) False

2
(a) True
(b) False
(c) True
(d) False
(e) True

3
(a) True
(b) True
(c) False
(d) False
(e) False

4
(a) True
(b) False
(c) True
(d) True
(e) True

Chapter 22

1
(a) True
(b) False
(c) True
(d) False
(e) True

2
(a) True
(b) False
(c) False
(d) True

3
(a) False
(b) False
(c) True
(d) True

4
(a) False
(b) True
(c) False
(d) False

Chapter 23

1
(a) True
(b) False
(c) True
(d) False
(e) False

2
(a) False
(b) False
(c) False
(d) False
(e) True

3
(a) False
(b) True
(c) True
(d) False
(e) True

Index